Human Well-Being Research and Policy Making

Series Editors

Richard J. Estes, School of Social Policy & Practice, University of Pennsylvania, Philadelphia, PA, USA

M. Joseph Sirgy (iD), Department of Marketing, Virginia Polytechnic Institute & State University, Blacksburg, VA, USA

This series includes policy-focused books on the role of the public and private sectors in advancing quality of life and well-being. It creates a dialogue between well-being scholars and public policy makers. Well-being theory, research and practice are essentially interdisciplinary in nature and embrace contributions from all disciplines within the social sciences. With the exception of leading economists, the policy relevant contributions of social scientists are widely scattered and lack the coherence and integration needed to more effectively inform the actions of policy makers. Contributions in the series focus on one more of the following four aspects of well-being and public policy:

- Discussions of the public policy and well-being focused on particular nations and worldwide regions
- Discussions of the public policy and well-being in specialized sectors of policy making such as health, education, work, social welfare, housing, transportation, use of leisure time
- Discussions of public policy and well-being associated with particular population groups such as women, children and youth, the aged, persons with disabilities and vulnerable populations
- Special topics in well-being and public policy such as technology and well-being, terrorism and well-being, infrastructure and well-being.

This series was initiated, in part, through funds provided by the Halloran Philanthropies of West Conshohocken, Pennsylvania, USA. The commitment of the Halloran Philanthropies is to "inspire, innovate and accelerate sustainable social interventions that promote human well-being." The series editors and Springer acknowledge Harry Halloran, Tony Carr and Audrey Selian for their contributions in helping to make the series a reality.

More information about this series at http://www.springer.com/series/15692

el-Sayed el-Aswad

Countering Islamophobia in North America

A Quality-of-Life Approach

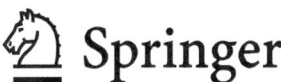 Springer

el-Sayed el-Aswad
Bloomfield Hills
Michigan, MI, USA

ISSN 2522-5367 ISSN 2522-5375 (electronic)
Human Well-Being Research and Policy Making
ISBN 978-3-030-84672-5 ISBN 978-3-030-84673-2 (eBook)
https://doi.org/10.1007/978-3-030-84673-2

This Springer imprint is published by the registered company Springer Nature Switzerland AG.
The registered company address is: Gewerbestrasse 11, 6330 Cham, Switzerland

This book is dedicated to all those who have suffered from Islamophobia and all forms of discrimination, Muslims and non-Muslims.

When we turn a blind eye to discrimination against our Muslim neighbors, we cannot claim to remain true to our American values, and if we tolerate discrimination against those of another faith, we undermine our own cherished religious freedom.

President Jimmy Carter, Countering the Islamophobia Industry *(2018, 4).*

Preface

Lack of accurate information and knowledge about Islam and Muslims in North America and elsewhere poses problems hindering policymakers from designing and implementing effective policies countering Islamophobia regionally and globally. Islamophobia means unfounded hostility toward Islam as well as irrational fear of Muslims. The monograph is directed to a broad audience of academics, practitioners, and policymakers interested in the topic of Islamophobia and counter-Islamophobia. This study demonstrates how Islamophobia, hatred, discrimination, race, and racism intersect in North America. Terms such as Islamophobia, xenophobia, anti-Muslim racism, anti-Muslim sentiment, anti-Muslim hatred, anti-Muslim discrimination, and anti-Muslim prejudice are interchangeably used in this monograph as well as in public and private zones. Islamophobia shows a clear connection between the fear, distrust, hostility, and hate exhibited toward Muslims and Islam.

Islamophobia has been a pressing issue for academics, policymakers, and advocates of public and private sectors. The right of freedom of expression has been used as a justification for attacking Muslims in North America and other countries. The institutionalized apprehension or distrust of Muslims is both a drive and an outcome of Islamophobia. The phenomenon of Islamophobia derives from a complex set of ideological, racial, religious, social, economic, political, media, and other drivers. Islamophobia results in a negative impact on the well-being of Muslims living in North America (Fig. 1.1) Islamophobia prevents Muslims from contributing to social, economic, and political development of their North American communities. The trouble with the ideology of the anti-Muslim prejudice and fear of Muslims or Islamophobia is that the fight against politically oriented Muslim extremists is viewed as a "fight against Islam as a whole" (el-Aswad, el-S. 2013, p. 42).

This monograph focuses on the peoples of the USA and Canada who share all-encompassing social histories represented in their experience as former European colonies; the magnitude of their economies and natural resources; the large scope of their human capitals; and the diversity of their social, cultural, religious, political, racial, and ethnic construction. The inhabitants of both countries travel easily across borders into one another's country (Estes et al., 2017). However, Muslims have been accused of not being able to assimilate into the mainstream life of North America.

This study provides a holistic understanding of Islamophobia, hate rhetoric, and racism in challenging socio-political climates in North America, particularly the USA and Canada, in which Muslims have experienced discrimination based on their religion, race, ethnicity, customs, language, names, and attire. This book introduces the reader to a quality-of-life perspective that identifies the drivers of Islamophobia from which counter-Islamophobic programs can be constructed. Special focus will be placed on the economic, political, cultural, religious, and media outcomes and drivers of Islamophobia. Additionally, this study addresses issues of minority versus majority as well as of aggressive policies and actions of the extreme right wing and other racist groups against Muslim minorities in North America. The Islamophobic discourse that employs a center/periphery binary focusing on *difference* and subordinate status of minorities has resulted in narratives of inequality, conflict, delegation, and resistance leading to illness and negative impact on Muslims' well-being.

This study examines the role media, the white supremacist movement, anti-immigrant policy, and right-wing or alt-right ideology play in the negative depiction of Islam and Muslims in North America. Muslims suffer from Western stereotypes depicting them as backward, misogynists, violent, terrorists, anti-modernity, and anti-democracy, showing no respect to adherents of other religions, particularly Jews and Christians (Firestone, 2010; Gingrich, 2005; Gottschalk, 2019).

This monograph discusses the negative impact of stereotypes on the overall well-being of Muslim communities in North America, being racially segregated, economically disadvantaged, and socially stigmatized and marginalized (Crewe, 2016). There is an adverse impact of institutional and collective racism on the well-being of Muslims among other ethnic groups. Furthermore, many actors involved in the Islamophobic campaigns have built extensive international networks, and have long been sharing organizational models, market strategies (supply and demand), tactics, and resources. The deep concern of North American countries about the place of Islam in the West goes beyond national frontiers, moving to global horizons.

This monograph provides evidence showing that North American Muslims have experienced a negative sentiment caused by a number of interrelated quality-of-life factors triggered by Islamophobia. These factors include religious drivers, as evidenced by increased Western vilification of Islamic beliefs and values; cultural drivers, as reflected in the perceived indifference of Western culture and Western prejudice against Muslims; economic drivers, as manifested by disparities in economic resources between Muslims and Western or non-Muslim communities; political factors, as mirrored in the exclusion of Muslims from mainstream civil and political affairs; and globalization and media factors, as represented by the manipulation of national and international media against Muslims.

In brief, Islamophobia results in a negative impact on the well-being of Muslims and non-Muslims living in North America and beyond. Islamophobia prevents Muslims from contributing to social, economic, and political development of their North American communities.

Bloomfield Hills, MI   el-Sayed el-Aswad

Acknowledgment

A long history of conducting anthropological and sociological researches as well as serving tenure at universities in the USA, Egypt, Bahrain, and the United Arab Emirates have provided me with the opportunity to advance cross-cultural perspectives as evidenced in this monograph. I hope the reader finds reading this book as enlightening and enriching an experience as I have found this investigation into patterns of the Islamophobic industry impacting the quality of life and well-being of both Muslims and non-Muslims living in North America to be.

This book would not have come to fruition without the endorsement and inspiration of Richard J. Estes and M. Joseph Sirgy, editors of the Springer book series *Human Well-Being Research and Policy Making*. The comments and feedback of Richard J. Estes and M. Joseph Sirgy as well as of anonymous peer reviewers and scholars have enriched and deepened the scholarly discussion of this book.

I would like to thank my wife, Mariam, for providing editorial assistance. My son, Kareem, introduced me to a number of Muslim American/Canadian youths in both Dearborn, Michigan, and Windsor, Ontario. My son, Amir, aided in fashioning three maps of North America, the USA, and Canada by using Adobe Photoshop and Adobe Illustrator. He, also, benefiting from meticulous editing training at Chicago Law School, provided editorial insights.

I am grateful to the editorial team at Springer International Publisher, with special thanks to Shinjini Chatterjee, Aurelia Heumader, Ameena Jaafar, and Ramya Prakash, for their administrative assistance of this work.

With appreciation,

el-Sayed el-Aswad

About the Book

The book contains eleven chapters divided into four parts: Part I—*the Background*—includes the first three chapters; Part II—*Outcomes of Islamophobia*—includes Chap. 4; Part III—*Drivers of Islamophobia*—contains three chapters; and Part IV—*Policies to Combat Islamophobia*—includes the last four chapters.

Part I: Background

Chapter 1, the *Introduction*, presents the main approach of the study. It introduces the reader to a quality-of-life approach that identifies the causes or drivers of Islamophobia from which counter-Islamophobic programs can be construed. The chapter will discuss the negative impact of stereotypes on the overall well-being of Muslim communities in North America. Special focus will be placed on the economic, political, cultural, religious, and media drivers of Islamophobia. There is a negative impact of institutional and collective racism on the well-being of Muslims (among other ethnic groups)

Chapter 2, *Research Methods*, discusses multiple sources used for obtaining data for this monograph. Macro and micro research methods are applied. In addition to reports of Islamophobia provided by specialized governmental agencies within the USA and Canada, data will be collected from international agencies such as the *United Nations*, the *World Bank*, the *Pew Research Center*, the *Gallup Poll* (Gallup Organization), the *Transparency International* (*Corruption Perceptions Index*), and the UNESCO Institute for Statistics among other global data collection agencies. In addition, micro data are collected from informants belonging to two communities, Dearborn, Michigan, in the USA, and Windsor, Ontario, in Canada. The collected macro and micro data will be used for analytical and comparative purposes.

Chapter 3, *Brief History*, addresses the historical roots of Islam–Christian conflicts that go back to the middle ages and have continued into the present in the form of Islamophobia in the West, particularly North America. A brief description of the economic and demographic features of Canada and the USA is provided. Further, this chapter addresses the rise and spread of Islamophobic organizations before and after the tragic events of 9/11.

Part II: Outcomes of Islamophobia

Chapter 4, *Outcomes of Islamophobia*, uses reliable output indicators to trace and document the impact of increased negative sentiment toward Muslims or Islamophobia on the deterioration of the quality of life and well-being of North American Muslims. These negative outcomes are reflected in major domains of living, including economic inequality, political exclusion, religious discrimination, and media exploitation.

Part III: Drivers of Islamophobia

Chapter 5, *Economic and Political Drivers of Islamophobia*, applies a quality-of-life perspective to analyze the economic and political drivers of far-right and extremist groups who have targeted immigrants and refugees in North America. This chapter addresses the impact of government policies, political parties, and political leaders on the dissemination of Islamophobia in Canada and the USA.

Chapter 6, *Religious and Cultural Drivers of Islamophobia*, employs a quality-of-life approach to investigate religious drivers, represented in extreme religiosity of some Christians, particularly white evangelicals, and cultural drivers, displayed in discrimination against Muslims and ignorance of Islam. Religious and cultural drivers of Islamophobia also include far-right groups, white supremacists, and other radical organizations, instigating broader patterns of racial, cultural, and social inequality in North America.

Chapter 7, *Media Drivers of Islamophobia*, examines negative and biased factors of the media that embolden and help spread Islamophobic stereotypes. This chapter focuses on three core media drivers of Islamophobia including far-right conservative ideologies, media bias, and mediated politicization of Islamophobia. Biased media outlets have contributed to the rise of Islamophobia by normalizing voices of racism, prejudice, and hatred, in the name of augmenting public discourses. The problem of biased media is that they deal with Muslims as if they were forming a monolithic and homogenous community, which is erroneous.

Part IV: Policies to Combat Islamophobia

Chapter 8, *Policies Confronting Biased Media*, assesses the effectiveness of policies that counter biased media known for having long-standing traditions of misrepresentations and prejudicial depictions of Muslims in North America. The challenge facing policymakers is to engage media outlets to eradicate Islamophobia either by imposing bylaws that restrict freedom of expression or by espousing a competitive marketplace of ideas, assuring freedom of expression as well as the dissemination of information from diverse and opposing sources.

Chapter 9, *Education Policy*, focuses on two core objectives. The first one addresses the negative impact of Islamophobia and discrimination on students' academic achievement and overall well-being in North America. The second sheds light on the educational policies implemented in the USA and Canada to reform their education systems and counteract Islamophobia in schools and beyond.

Chapter 10, *Human Rights Policy*, discusses human rights policies institutionalized and implemented by the governments of the USA and Canada as well as NGO agencies or advocacy organizations. It also addresses the United Nations and North American policy initiatives of human rights that support the implementation of laws and law enforcement to safeguard Muslims and other minorities against perpetrators. This chapter tackles ways and mechanisms used by Muslim organizations and individuals in countering Islamophobia.

Chapter 11, *Concluding Thoughts: Projected Policies of Counter-Islamophobia*, reviews the principal findings of the study and provides ideas for long-term policies and recommendations aimed at reducing or eliminating the rising tide of racism and Islamophobia. The objective here is to show to what extent understanding the drivers of ideologies and activities of Islamophobia help governments and policymakers generate sociocultural plans aimed at implementing a set of policies and interventions designed to effectively counter Islamophobia and enhance the well-being of both Muslim and non-Muslim communities in North America.

References

Crewe, S. E. (2016, August 31). Stigmatization and labeling. *Encyclopedia of Social Work*. Oxford University Press. Retrieved from https://doi.org/10.1093/acrefore/9780199975839.013.1043

el-Aswad, el-S. (2013). Images of Muslims in western scholarship and media after 9/11. *Digest of Middle East Studies, 22*(1), 39–56.

Estes, R. J., Land, K. C., Michalos, A. M., Phillips, R., & Sirgy, M. J. (2017). Well-being in Canada and the United States. In R. J. Estes & M. J. Sirgy (Eds.), *The pursuit of human well-being: The untold global history* (pp. 257–299). Springer.

Firestone, R. (2010). Islamophobia & anti-Semitism: History and possibility. *Arches Quarterly, 4*(7), 42–51.

Gingrich, A. (2005). Anthropological analyses of Islamophobia and anti-Semitism in Europe *American Ethnologist, 32*(4), 513–515.

Gottschalk, P. (2019, June 03). Hate crimes associated with both Islamophobia and anti-Semitism have a long history in America's past. *The Conversation.*

Griggs, M. B. (2014, August 28). The first people to settle across North America's arctic regions were isolated for 4,000 years. *Smithsonian Magazine*. Accessed August 26, 2015, from http://www.smithsonianmag.com/smart-news/isolated-culturethrived-arctic-4000-years-180952505/?no-ist

Contents

About the Author

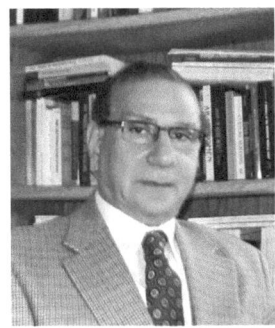

el-Sayed el-Aswad received his doctorate in anthropology from the University of Michigan, Ann Arbor. He has taught at Wayne State University (USA), Tanta University (Egypt), Bahrain University, and United Arab Emirates University (UAEU). He achieved the CHSS-UAEU Award for excellence in scientific research publication for the academic year 2013–2014. He served as Chairperson of the Sociology Departments at both the UAEU and Tanta University as well as the Editor-in Chief of the *Journal of Horizons in Humanities and Social Sciences: An International Refereed Journal* (UAEU). He has published widely in both Arabic and English and is the author of Rethinking knowledge and power hierarchy in the Muslim world (Brill 2021) in Alan. Fromherz and Nadav Samin (Eds.), *Knowledge, Authority and Change in Islamic societies: Studies in Honor of Dale F. Eickelman*, Oriental Images and Ethics: British Empire and the Arab Gulf (1727–1971)—A Perspective from Historical Anthropology, *Anthropos,* (2021, 116(2): 319–330), Global Jihad and International Media Use (coauthor-*Oxford Research Encyclopedia of Communication* 2020), The Quality of Life and Policy Issues among the Middle East and North African Countries (Springer 2019), Keys to al-Ghaib: A cross-cultural study. *Digest of Middle East Studies* (2019, *28(2): 277–295*), coauthor of *Combatting Jihadist terrorism through nation-building: A Quality-of-life perspective* (Springer, 2019), The Impact of Digital Technologies on the Promotion of the Emirates Intangible Cultural Heritage. *MEMORIAMEDIA*

Review (2019, 4. Art.3) https://review.memoriamedia.
net/index.php/emirates-digital-ich, Political Challenges
Confronting the Islamic World. In Habib Tiliouine and
Richard J. Estes (eds.) *The State of Social Progress of
Islamic Societies: Social, Economic, Political, and Ideo-
logical Challenges* (2016, pp. 361–377), *Muslim World-
views and Everyday Lives* (AltaMira Press, 2012),
Dreams and the Construction of Reality: Symbolic
Transformation of the Seen and Unseen in the Egyptian
Imagination," *Anthropos*, 2010), *Religion and Folk
Cosmology: Scenarios of the Visible and Invisible in
Rural Egypt* (Praeger Press, 2002; translated into Arabic
in 2005), *Symbolic Anthropology: A Critical Compara
tive Study of Current Interpretative Approaches of
Culture* (Munsh't al-Ma'raif, Alexandria, 2002), *The
Dynamics of Identity Reconstruction among Arab Com-
munities in the US,* Anthropos, 101(1), 111–121, and
*The Folk House: An Anthropological Study of Folk
Architecture and Traditional Culture of the Emirates
Society* (al-Bait al-Sha'bi) (UAE University
Press, 1996).

He has been awarded fellowships from various insti-
tutes including the Fulbright Program, the Ford Foun-
dation, the Egyptian government, and the United Arab
Emirates University. He is a member of Editorial Advi-
sory Boards of the Digest of Middle East Studies
(DOMES), Muslims in Global Societies Series, Tabsir:
Insight on Islam and the Middle East, and CyberOrient
(Online Journal of the Middle). He is a member of the
American Anthropological Association, the Middle
Eastern Studies of North America, the American Academy of Religion, and the International Advisory Council
of the World Congress for Middle Eastern Studies
(WOCMES). He has published nine books, over one
hundred papers in peer-reviewed and indexed journals,
and over forty book reviews.

List of Abbreviations

AMM	American Muslim Mission
AIC	Amnesty International Canada
ADC	Arab–American Anti-Discrimination Committee
AMSS	Association of Muslim Social Scientists in North America
BLM	Black Lives Matter
CAN	Canadian Anti-Hate Network
CMF	Canadian Muslim Forum
CMU	Canadian Muslim Union
CISNA	Council of Islamic Schools in North America
CAP	Center for American Progress
CPI	Corruption Perceptions Index
CAIR	Council on American–Islamic Relations
HRW	Human Rights Watch
ISP	Index of Social Progress
IT	Information technology
ISPU	Institute for Social Policy and Understanding
IIIT	International Institute of Islamic Thought
ISNA	Islamic Society of North America
ICD	Islamic Center of Detroit
ICI	Islamic Cultural Institute
ISSA	Islamic Social Services Association
ISNA	Islamic Society of North America
KKK	Ku Klux Klan
MAS	Muslim American Society
MAP	Muslims for American Progress
MPAC	Muslim Public Affairs Council
MSA	Muslim Students Association
NOI	Nation of Islam
NCCM	National Council of Canadian Muslims
NGO	Non-governmental organization

OCR	Office for Civil Rights (the U.S. Department of Education)
OHRC	Ontario Human Rights Commission
OSCE	Organization for Security and Cooperation in Europe
QOL	Quality-of-life
PRRI	Public Religion Research Institute
SCMS	Sister Clara Muhammad Schools
SPI	Social Progress Index
SPLC	Southern Poverty Law Center
START	Study of Terrorism and Responses to Terrorism
TI	Transparency International
UMA	United Muslims of America
UN	United Nations
UNDP	United Nation Development Programme
UNESCO	United Nations Educational, Scientific and Cultural Organization
UDHR	Universal Declaration of Human Rights
WCAI	Worldwide Coalition against Islam
WCIW	World Community of Al-Islam

List of Figures

List of Maps

List of Tables

Part I
Background

Chapter 1
Introduction

1.1 Introduction

This book contributes to the scholarly and public policy literatures on quality of life, human rights, and the understanding and countering of Islamophobia.

Researchers have studied the phenomenon of Islamophobia and have generated definitions based on their varying theoretical and ideological orientations. According to the Runnymede Trust Islamophobia refers to the "dread or hatred of Islam—and therefore, to fear or dislike of all or most Muslims" (1997, p. 1) the consequences of which are "unfounded prejudice and hostility" to the extent of "unfair discrimination against Muslim individuals and communities, and to the exclusion of Muslims from mainstream political and social affairs" (1997, p. 4). Some scholars, relying on this definition, focused on the irrational fear of Muslims as well as perceptions that Muslims are a threat or enemy that must be fought (Ciftci, 2012; Gottschalk & Greenberg, 2008; Green, 2015; Kunst et al., 2013). In terms of affective domains, Islamophobia has been defined as *"indiscriminate negative attitudes or emotions directed at Islam or Muslims"* (Bleich, 2011, p. 1582, italics in original) as well as to the suspicion and distrust exhibited toward Islam and consequently toward Muslims (Kazi, 2018; Lean, 2012; Love, 2017).

In addition to addressing private dimensions of Islamophobia, some researchers point out what they define as state-driven Islamophobia with reference to institutional and systemic discrimination against Muslims by the state (Bahdi & Kanji, 2018; Beydoun, 2018; Curtis, 2013). Other scholars have focused on the notion of the instrumentality of Islamophobia as presented in the political ideology and politics of fear, particularly with reference to western and American manipulation of Islamophobia for the purpose of dominating Muslims through colonialism and imperialism. Islamophobia is defined as a systematic, political, ideological or financial tool used by groups of people for their own benefit (Ekman, 2015; Joshi, 2018: Richardson, 2004; Semati, 2010; Tyrer, 2013). Combining race and politics, Tyrer has treated Islomphobia as a form of 'biopolitical racism' (2013). Other scholars

el-S. el-Aswad, *Countering Islamophobia in North America*, Human Well-Being Research and Policy Making, https://doi.org/10.1007/978-3-030-84673-2_1

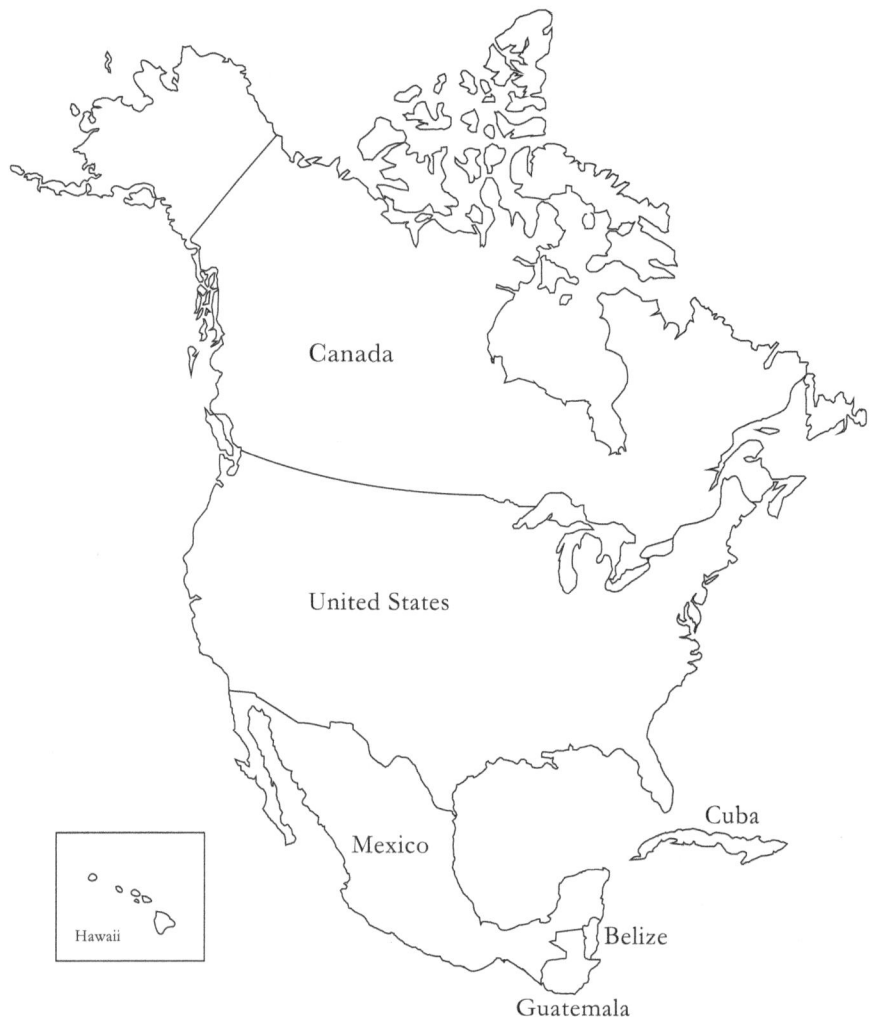

Map 1.1 North America (© Amir el-Aswad)

have viewed Islamophobia as a form of religious intolerance and a new form of racism. For example, a religious minority can be racialized and targeted by racism (Bravo López, 2011).

Within this book, Islamophobia will be concerned with these different aspects or defining elements. Most importantly, however, Islamophobia will be situated within the larger historical and social contexts of the major changes in the relationships within North America, mostly that between Muslims and Christians. It will undertake an elaborated discussion of the political, economic, social, religious and educational impact on the well-being of North American Muslims (See Map 1.1).

Countering Islamophobia "involves first recognizing anti-Muslim prejudice as a systematic, political, ideological or financial tool, and calling out those who seek to use it for their own benefit. To not to do so is to risk the stability and peace of our future" (Shaheen, 2017, xxii). To treat Islamophobia as an isolate without considering its relationship to historical events, imperialism, racism, globalization, and people's well-being is to fail not only in understanding its complexity, but also in responding to it. Specifically, this research is a grounded construction of the discourses that counter Islamophobic tropes in North America. One of its objectives is to make it possible for a range of policymakers to discuss anti-Muslim rhetoric and action in order to provide solutions to offset Islamophobic incidents. In other words, this monograph seeks to examine how public policies, new conceptualizations and social movements can transform from Islamophobia toward a more positive and healthy discourse. Surprisingly, and apart from selected media studies (Bleich et al., 2018; Said, 1981), empirical investigations about countering Islamophobia, racism and hate are rare. This book proposes effective means and mechanisms to help generate debate, dialogue and discussion concerning policy issues to help mitigate Islamophobia.

This study proposes that Islamophobia is both a cause and an outcome of the misunderstanding and prejudice that may evolve as a result of racism, ignorance, preconception, fear of different worldviews, and intolerance in dealing with Muslims. Muslims have experienced a variety of forms of discrimination and stigmatization based on such factors as religion, race, ethnicity, customs, language, Muslim names, and dress (Crewe, 2016; el-Aswad, el-S., 2012, 2013, 2016, 2019; Center for American Progress, 2011), attributes of being seen as the 'other.' One problem is that in 2014 the Pew Research Center (2014) found only 38% of Americans personally knew someone who was Muslim. Violence toward Muslims became evident and by 2015 the FBI reported 257 incidents of anti-Muslim hate crimes, a 67% increase from the previous year (Pew Research Center, 2016). On January 29, 2017, six people were killed and nineteen injured at a mosque in Quebec City, Canada. Adrienne Clarkson (2017), asked how one explains to the world that people were killed, shot in the back, while they were praying to the one God who created all people? Are there any explanations possible? What is happening in North America affects other parts of the world and vice versa. On June 8, 2021, in London, Ontario, a man ran over a Muslim family, killing 4 persons and injuring a 9-year-old boy, with his pickup truck because of their religion. Police said the terrorist attack was intentionally operated. London Mayor Ed Holder said this was a terrorist act of mass murder against Muslims, rooted in unspeakable hatred (ABC News, 2021). On March 15, 2019, a terrorist attack struck two mosques killing 51 persons and injuring over 40 people of a small Muslim minority in Christchurch, New Zealand. The shooter posted an online "manifesto" identifying Donald Trump supremacist supporters and right-wing American media agents who inspired him to commit acts of violence (Gambrell, 2019; Wankin, 2019).

Over the past two decades and following the tragic event of September 11, 2001, negative images of Muslims have been entrenched in North American media and scholarship. Scholars examining negative representations of Muslims in the two

largest countries of North America, the U.S. and Canada, known for their multiculturalism (Cader & Kassamali, 2012; Considine, 2017; Day, 2000; Estes et al., 2017;
Green, 2015; Love, 2017), have found Islam and Muslims often depicted by those
who endorse Islamophobia and anti-Muslim bigotry as militants, fanatics, and
terrorists (Kunst, 2012; Morey et al., 2019). Moreover, Muslims living in North
America have been accused of not assimilating or adapting to the mainstream life of
North America (Pew Research Center, 2017a, b). Muslims have been depicted as the
enemy within by North American Islamophobic advocates such Daniel Pipes (2001),
Mike Keegan (2007), and David Yerushalmi, among others (Gottschalk &
Greenberg, 2008; Musaji, 2007, 2012). In addition to economic, political, religious,
media and cultural drivers, Islamophobia among the North American population are
caused by other factors including ignorance, discrimination, propaganda and
misinformation. Briefly, Western depictions of Muslims as violent and aggressive
have generated fear, anxiety, xenophobia and Islamophobia, or the irrational fear of
Muslims (el-Aswad, el-S., 2013, 2016; Habib, 2016; Husain, 2015; Rendall et al.,
2008).

Islamophobia results in excessive inequities for Muslims in North American
communities threatening such domains of quality of life and well-being as health,
economic resources, education, employment, freedom of religion, free expression,
migration policy, and civil rights. For example, Islamophobia has been used to
justify immigration bans and border security measures (Esses & Abelson, 2017).
There has been a negative impact of institutional and collective racism on the well-
being of Muslims (among other ethnic groups) as several authors have linked higher
incidences of stress-related diseases to Muslims' recurring exposure to racism,
segregation and discrimination (Broman, 1997; Caldwell, 2009; Camarota, 2012;
DeNavas-Walt et al., 2012; Gingrich, 2005; Gongloff, 2014; Nazroo & Bécares,
2017).

Past and contemporary tragic events show that when religion is demonized, the
outcome is a religious-political extremism threatening people's well-being. Western
cultures are exhibiting an irrational and uninformed fear towards Islam (Gottschalk
& Greenberg, 2008). The discriminatory act may produce a sense of threat within the
victim that may cause various reactions, including fear, distress, anger, humiliation
and denial. These reactions could produce a physiological response (be it cardio-
vascular, endocrine, neurological, or immunological) that subsequently affects
health (Ablon, 2002; Buchanan, 2002; Nazroo & Bécares, 2017). Furthermore,
studies dealing with children reveal that ethnic minority children raised in a detrimental environment where experiences of racial discrimination are widespread are
more likely to suffer from socio-emotional problems as they grow up than their peers
from ethnic minority backgrounds whose families do not report experiences of racial
discrimination (Bécares et al., 2015).

Comparatively little work has been done that critically examines the underlying
drivers of racism and hate (Kazi, 2018; Kumar, 2012; Sheehi, 2011). The Council on
American-Islamic Relations (2018) reported that Islamophobic incidents have
increased and racist groups, white supremacists, anti-immigrant hate groups, and
far-right extremist groups as well as leftist groups (Beydoun, 2018; Considine, 2017;
Schafer et al., 2014) have intensified their use of propaganda to spread Islamophobic

messages at unprecedented rates (Al-Solaylee, 2017; Love, 2017). According to the Institute for Social Policy and Understanding (2019), Muslims are the most likely group to report experiencing religious discrimination (62%). Meanwhile, Muslim women report higher levels of discrimination (68%) than men (55%).

1.2   Features of Islamophobia

It is impossible to counter Islamophobia in the absence of clear conceptualization of its complex features. The term of Islamophobia emerged in the 1970s and "became popular for European anti-racist activists in the 1980s and 1990s" (Rana, 2007 p. 148). Islamophobia means unfounded hostility towards Islam as well as irrational fear of Muslims, indicating a form of biopolitical racism (Tyrer, 2013). Although "'Muslims' is a religious categorization, scholars have increasingly recognized the 'racialization' of Muslims in the United States, especially those of Arab and South Asian descent" (Fording & Schram, 2020, p. 6). Race here is understood in terms of attitudes, beliefs, religion, language, manners, ways of life and group identification (Omi & Winant, 1994). In this context, terms such as anti-Muslim racism, Islamophobia, anti-religious discrimination, anti-Muslim prejudice, and xenophobia are used interchangeably in this research.

The Runnymede Trust sums up eight core features of Islamophobia or closed-views of Islam as follows. 1—Islam is monolithic, static and unresponsive to new realities. 2—Islam is separate and viewed as an 'other', having neither shared values or aims with other cultures, nor impacting them or impacted by them. 3—Islam is viewed as inferior to the West as well as irrational, sexist and primitive. 4—Islam is seen as an enemy enticing aggressive, violent, threatening, and terrorist actions that lead a clash of civilizations. 5—Islam is manipulative and driven by political ideology, seeking to achieve political and military gains. 6—Criticisms made by Islam or Muslims of the of the West are totally rejected. 7—Discrimination and exclusion of Muslims from mainstream society are justified by hostility towards Islam. 8—Islamophobia is viewed as natural and anti-Muslim hostility is accepted as normal (Runnymede Trust, 1997).

1.3   Drivers of Islamophobia

It is imperative to divulge and reveal the underlying drivers of Islamophobia to be able to effectively understand and counter it within a quality-of-life approach. It is important for quality-of-life and well-being to be investigated holistically across critical drivers, mainly those related to social, economic, political, religious, health, education and media factors (el-Aswad, el-S., 2019). Notably, Islamophobia is viewed here as both a driver and outcome of negative sentiment toward Muslims. To reiterate, Islamophobia is an ideological viewpoint that endeavors to rationalize

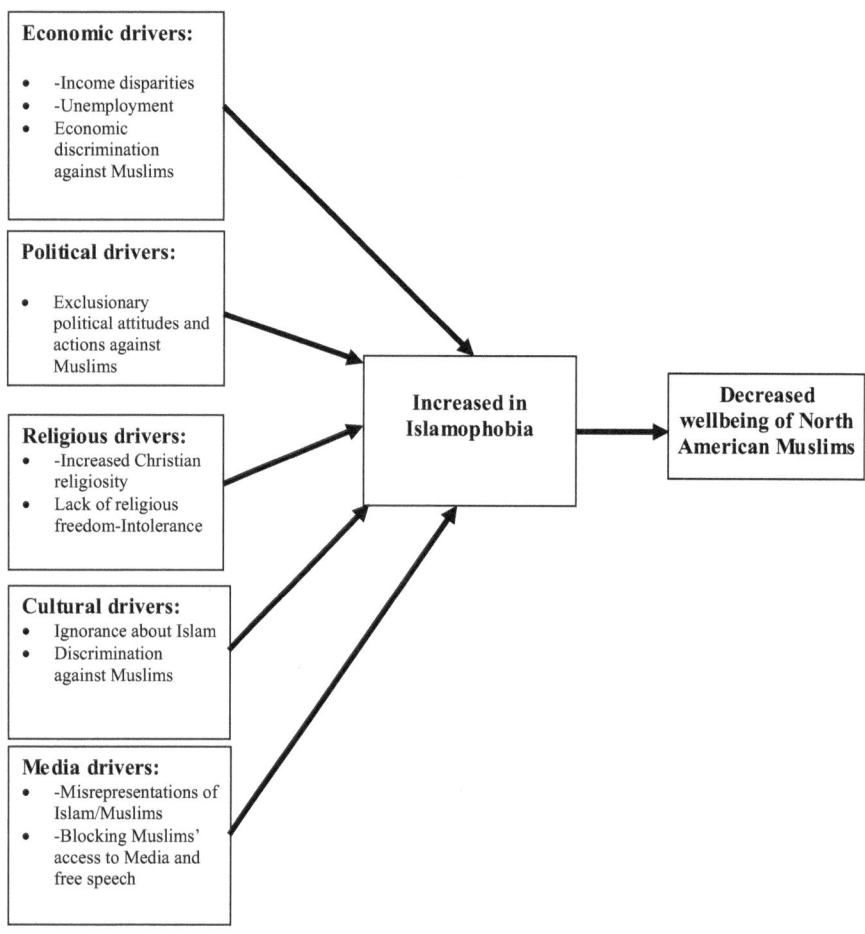

Fig. 1.1 Quality-of-life factors causing Islamophobia

"ills of the (global) society" by attributing them to Islam (Semati, 2010, p. 257). Applying a quality-of-life approach (Sirgy et al., 2019), this monograph provides evidence showing that North American Muslims have experienced a negative sentiment caused by a number of interrelated quality-of-life factors triggered by Islamophobia. These factors include religious drivers, as evidenced by increased North American vilification of Islamic beliefs caused by extreme religiosity of certain extreme white evangelicals; cultural drivers, as reflected in the ignorance of certain North American groups about Islam as well as in forms of prejudice and discrimination against Muslims; economic drivers, as manifested by disparities in economic resources between Muslims and non-Muslim communities living in North America; political drivers, as mirrored in the exclusion of Muslims from mainstream civil and political affairs; and media drivers, as represented by the provocation or manipulation of international media against Muslims (Fig. 1.1).

Racism is considered to be a key factor of ethnic inequalities in economic, political rights and health. Several scholars view Islamophobia as a form of racism (Garner & Selod, 2014; Massoumi et al., 2017). Racism can be defined "as invidious discrimination among differing social groups; generally, such beliefs and actions are based on assumption that social characteristics are fixed, genetically transmitted, and capable of hierarchical ranking on some scale of superiority and inferiority" (Ward, 2002, pp. xi–x). Living with a fear of experiencing racism may have an impact on people's well-being and health. There is strong evidence that anti-Muslim prejudice and discrimination directly harm both the mental and physical health of Muslim people. Racism increases exposure to the internalization of stigma and negative messages leading to decreased self-esteem and poorer mental health (Ablon, 2002; Garner & Selod, 2014; Goffman, 1959, 1963; Kunst, 2012 ; Passas & Agnew, 1997). Islamophobia or racism is a problem of the social psychology of race relations and the accumulation of exposure to racial discrimination over time is associated with increased risk of poor health (Nazroo & Bécares, 2017; Ward, 2002).

1.4 Objectives

This book seeks to provide a holistic understanding of Islamophobia, hate rhetoric and racism in challenging socio-political climates in North America. The monograph endeavors to examine the role played by the media and far right ideology in the depiction of Islam and Muslims in North America. A literature review shows that numerous studies have focused on derogatory anti-Muslim misinformation and stereotypes (Green, 2015; Lean 2012; Love, 2017).

Nevertheless, studies or books concerning the discourses and movements that counter such derogatory misinformation are sparse. One of the principal goals of this monograph is to help make accessible many of the academic concepts and findings that can be easily applied by policymakers and practitioners involved in countering hate rhetoric plans and operations. The objectives of the monograph can be summed as follows:

1. To present a critical and cross-cultural review of the discourses and trends of Islamophobia in North America.
2. To identify and describe the drivers of Islamophobia: economic, political, religious, cultural, and media.
3. To analyze the impact of Islamophobia on the quality of life and well-being of Muslims living in North America.
4. To understand how human rights are being conceptualized, practiced, attacked and defended.
5. To assess and contribute to action-oriented initiatives and policies implemented by governments, NGOs, and advocacy organizations in North America to counter Islamophobia and its major drivers, in addition to policies related to human rights, education, and media.

1.5   Key Questions

The book seeks to answer the following questions:

1. What is the historical context of Islamophobia in North America?
2. What are the major drivers of Islamophobia in North America?
3. To what extent does Islamophobia affect the well-being of Muslims in North America?
4. To what extent do social and public policies counter Islamophobia in North America?
5. How can Islamophobia tropes be countered through policymaking issues and practices?

1.6   Conclusion

This chapter has exposed the critical, serious and dangerous issue of Islamophobia, threatening Muslims' quality of life and well-being in North America and worldwide. Identifying the outcomes and drivers of Islamophobia within the historical context of prejudice and racism is a necessary step toward constructing plans and initiatives to counter all forms of discrimination against Muslim communities and minority groups. Another focus has been on the interplay between social policy paradigms and efforts of governments, NGOs, and advocate agencies in combating Islamophobia.

References

ABC News. (2021, June 8). *Four dead in 'terrorist attack' as driver runs over Muslim family in London*, Ontario. Retrieved from https://www.abc.net.au/news/2021-06-08/canada-attack-four-muslims-dead-ontario/100197174

Ablon, J. (2002). The nature of stigma and medical conditions. *Epilepsy and Behavior, 3*(6), 2–9.

Al-Solaylee, K. (2017, April 14). *Anti-Muslim hate has been in Canada - and our politics - long before the violence*. The Globe and Mail.

Bahdi, R., & Kanji, A. (2018). What is Islamophobia? *University of New Brunswick Law Journal, 69*, 325–363.

Bécares, L., Nazroo, J., & Kelly, Y. (2015). A longitudinal examination of maternal, family, and area-level experiences of racism on children's socioemotional development: patterns and possible explanations. *Social Science and Medicine, 142*, 128–135.

Beydoun, K. (2018). *American Islamophobia: Understanding the roots and rise of fear*. University of California Press.

Bleich, E. (2011). What is Islamophobia and how much is there? theorizing and measuring an emerging comparative concept. *American Behavioral Scientist, 55*(12), 1581–1600.

Bleich, E., Souffrant, J., Stabler, E., & Veen, A. M. (2018). Media coverage of Muslim devotion: A four-country analysis of newspaper articles, 1996–2016. *Religions, 9*(8), 247–262.

Bravo López, F. (2011). Towards a definition of Islamophobia: Approximations of the early twentieth century. *Ethnic and Racial Studies, 34*(4), 556–573.

Broman, C. L. (1997). Race-related factors and life satisfaction among African Americans. *Journal of Black Psychology, 23*(1), 36–49.

Buchanan, P. (2002). *The death of the West: How dying populations and immigrant invasions imperil our country and civilization*. St. Martin's Griffin.

Cader, F., & Kassamali, S. (2012, February 1). *Islamophobia in Canada: A primer. New Socialist: Ideas for radical change*. Retrieved from http://newsocialist.org/islamophobia-in-canada-a-primer/

Caldwell, C. (2009). *Reflections on the revolution in Europe: Immigration, Islam, and the West*. Doubleday.

Camarota, S. A. (2012). *Immigrants in the United States, 2010: A profile of America's foreign-born population*. Center for Immigration Studies.

Center for American Progress. (2011, August 26). *Fear, Inc. The roots of the Islamophobia network in America*. Retrieved from https://www.americanprogress.org/issues/religion/reports/2011/08/26/10165/fear-inc/

Ciftci, S. (2012). Islamophobia and threat perceptions: Explaining anti-Muslim sentiment in the West. *Journal of Muslim Minority Affairs, 32*(3), 293–309.

Clarkson, A. (2017, January 31). We must remember that Canadians are not immune to racism. The Globe and Mail. Retrieved from https://www.theglobeandmail.com/opinion/we-must-remember-that-canadians-are-not-immune-from-racism/article33852998/

Considine, C. (August 26, 2017). The Racialization of Islam in the United States: Islamophobia, hate crimes, and "flying while Brown" Religions 8 (165): 1-19. doi:https://doi.org/10.3390/rel8090165.

Council on American-Muslim Relations. (2018). *Report: Anti-Muslim bias incidents, hate crimes spike in second quarter of 2018*. Retrieved July 12, from https://www.cair.com/press_releases/cair-report-anti-muslim-bias-incidents-hate-crimes-spike-in-second-quarter-of-2018/

Crewe, S. E. (2016, August 31). *Stigmatization and labeling. Encyclopedia of Social Work*. Oxford University Press. doi:https://doi.org/10.1093/acrefore/9780199975839.013.1043.

Curtis, E. E. (2013). The Black Muslim scare of the twentieth century: The history of state Islamophobia and its post 9/11 variations. In C. W. Ernst (Ed.), *Islamophobia in America: The anatomy of intolerance* (pp. 75–106). Palgrave Macmillan.

Day, R. J. F. (2000). *Multiculturalism and the history of Canadian diversity*. University of Toronto Press.

DeNavas-Walt, C., Proctor, B. D., & Smith, J. C. (2012). *Income, poverty, and health insurance coverage in the United States: 2011: Current population reports*. : United States Census Bureau. Accessed August 27, 2015, from http://www.census.gov/prod/2012pubs/p60-243.pdf

Ekman, M. (2015). Online Islamophobia and the politics of fear: Manufacturing the green scare. *Ethnic and Racial Studies, 38*(11), 1986–2002.

el-Aswad, el-S. (2012). *Muslim Worldviews and everyday lives*. AltaMira Press.

el-Aswad, el-S. (2013). Images of Muslims in Western scholarship and media after 9/11. *Digest of Middle East Studies, 22*(1), 39–56.

el-Aswad, el-S. (2016). Political challenges confronting the Islamic world. In H. Tiliouine & R. J. Estes (Eds.), *The state of social progress of Islamic societies: Social, economic, political, and ideological challenges* (pp. 361–377). Springer.

el-Aswad, el-S. (2019). *The quality of life and policy issues among the Middle East and North African countries*. Springer.

Esses, V. M., & Abelson, D. E. (2017). *Twenty-first-century immigration to North America: Newcomers in turbulent times*. McGill-Queen's University Press.

Estes, R. J., Land, K. C., Michalos, A. C., Phillips, R., & Sirgy, M. J. (2017). Well-being in Canada and the United States. In R. J. Estes & M. J. Sirgy (Eds.), *The pursuit of human well-being: The untold human history* (pp. 257–299). Springer International Publishing.

Fording, R. C., & Schram, S. F. (2020). *Hard white: The mainstreaming of racism in American politics*. Oxford University Press.

Gambrell, J. (2019, 15 March). *Mosque killer's rifles bore white-supremacist references*. Associated Press. Retrieved from https://apnews.com/597933f5d8454f448db02d1fc077730d

Garner, S., & Selod, S. (2014). The racialization of Muslims: Empirical studies of Islamophobia. *Critical Sociology, 41*(1), 9–19. Retrieved from https://journals.sagepub.com/doi/abs/10.1177/0896920514531606

Gingrich, A. (2005). Anthropological analyses of Islamophobia and anti-Semitism in Europe. *American Ethnologist, 32*(4), 513–515.

Goffman, E. (1959). *The presentation of self in everyday life*. Doubleday.

Goffman, E. (1963). *Stigma: Notes on the management of spoiled identity*. Prentice-Hall.

Gongloff, M. (2014, September 16). 45 million Americans still stuck below poverty line: Census. *The Huffington Post*. http://www.huffingtonpost.com/2014/09/16/poverty-household-income_n_5828974.html

Gottschalk, P., & Greenberg, G. (2008). *Islamophobia: Making Muslims the enemy*. Rowman & Littlefield Publishers.

Green, T. H. (2015). *The fear of Islam: An introduction to Islamophobia in the West*. Fortress Press.

Habib, S. (2016). Islamophobia is on the rise in the US. But so is Islam. *The World*. Retrieved from https://www.pri.org/stories/2016-09-09/muslims-america-are-keeping-and-growing-faith-even-though-haters-tell-them-not

Husain, A. (2015, February 2). *Islamophobia. Oxford Research Encyclopedia of Social Work*. Oxford University Press. https://doi.org/10.1093/acrefore/9780199975839.013.964

Institute for Social Policy and Understanding. (2019). *American Muslim poll 2019 predicting and preventing Islamophobia*. Retrieved from https://www.ispu.org/american-muslim-poll-2019-predicting-and-preventing-islamophobia/

Joshi, K. Y. (2018, May 24). *Race and religion in U.S. public life. Oxford Research Encyclopedia of Religion*. New York: Oxford University Press. doi:https://doi.org/10.1093/acrefore/9780199340378.013.460.

Kazi, N. (2018). *Islamophobia, race, and global politics*. Rowman & Littlefiel.

Keegan, M. (2007, May 24). *Frontline America*. Retrieved from http://frontline-america.blogspot.com/2007/05/enemy-within.html

Kumar, D. (2012). *Islamophobia and the politics of empire*. Haymarket Books.

Kunst, J. R. (2012). Coping with Islamophobia: The effects of religious stigma on Muslim minorities' identity formation. *International Journal of Intercultural Relations, 36*(4), 518–532.

Kunst, J. R., Sam, D. L., & Ulleberg, P. (2013). Perceived Islamophobia: Scale development and validation. *International Journal of Intercultural Relations, 37*(2), 225–237.

Lean, N. (2012). *The Islamophobia industry: How the right manufactures fear of Muslims*. Pluto Press.

Love, E. (2017). *Islamophobia and racism in America*. New York University Press.

Massoumi, N., Mill, T., & Miller, D. (2017). Islamophobia, social movements, and the state: For a movement-centered approach. In N. Massoumi, T. Mill, & D. Miller (Eds.), *Islamophobia? Racism, social movements, and the state* (pp. 3–34). Pluto Press.

Morey, P., Yakin, A., & Forte, A. (2019). *Contesting islamophobia: Anti-Muslim prejudice in media, culture and politics*. I.B. Tauris.

Musaji, S. (2007, July 26). *Are Muslims "The Enemy Within?"* The American Muslim. Retrieved from http://theamericanmuslim.org/tam.php/features/articles/are_muslims_the_enemy_within1/

Musaji, S. (2012, October 15). *A who's who of the anti-Muslim/anti-Arab/Islamophobia industry*. The American Muslim. Retrieved from http://theamericanmuslim.org/tam.php/features/articles/a_whos_who_of_the_anti-muslimanti-arabislamophobia_industry

Nazroo, J., & Bécares, L. (2017). Islamophobia, racism and health. In F. Elahi & O. Khan (Eds.), *Islamophobia still a challenge for us all* (pp. 31–35). Runnymede.

Omi, W., & Winant, H. (1994). *Racial formation in the United States*. Routledge.

Passas, N., & Agnew, R. (1997). *The future of anomie theory*. Northeastern University Press.

Pew Research Center. (2014). *How many people of different faiths do you know?* Retrieved from https://www.pewresearch.org/fact-tank/2014/07/17/how-many-people-of-different-faiths-do-you-know/

Pew Research Center. (2016). *Anti-Muslim assaults reach 9/11-era levels, FBI data show*. Retrieved from https://www.pewresearch.org/fact-tank/2016/11/21/anti-muslim-assaults-reach-911-era-levels-fbi-data-show/

Pew Research Center. (2017a, November 15), *Assaults against Muslims in U.S. surpass 2001 level*. Retrieved from https://www.pewresearch.org/fact-tank/2017/11/15/assaults-against-muslims-in-u-s-surpass-2001-level/

Pew Research Center. (2017b, July 26), *U.S. Muslims concerned about their place in society, but continue to believe in the American Dream*. Retrieved from https://www.pewforum.org/2017/07/26/findings-from-pew-research-centers-2017-survey-of-us-muslims/

Pipes, D. (2001). The Danger within: Militant Islam in America. *Commentary, 112*, 19–24.

Rana, J. (2007). The story of islamophobia. *Souls: A Critical Journal of Black Politics, Culture, and Society, 9*(2), 148–162.

Rendall, S., Naureckas, J., Macdonald, I., Cassidy, V., Jacir, D. M., & Hollar, J. (2008). *Smearcasting: How Islamophobes spread fear, bigotry, and Misinformation*. Fairness and Accuracy in Reporting.

Richardson, J. E. (2004). *(Mis)representing Islam: The racism and rhetoric of British broadsheet newspapers*. John Benjamins.

Runnymede Trust. (1997). Islamophobia: A challenge for us all. *The Runnymede Commission on British Muslims and Islamophobia*. Retrieved from https://www.runnymedetrust.org/companies/17/74/Islamophobia-A-Challenge-for-Us-All.html

Said, E. W. (1981). *Covering Islam: How the media and the experts determine how we see the rest of the world*. Pantheon Book.

Schafer, J. A., Mullins, C. W., & Box, S. (2014). Awakenings: The emergence of white supremacist ideologies. *Deviant Behavior, 34*(3), 173–196.

Semati, M. (2010). Islamophobia, culture and race in the age of empire. *Cultural Studies, 24*(2), 256–275.

Shaheen, J. G. (2017). Introduction to the second edition. In N. Lean (Ed.), *The Islamophobia industry: How the right manufactures fear of Muslims* (pp. xix–xxiii). Pluto Press.

Sheehi, S. (2011). *Islamophobia: The ideological campaign against Muslims*. Clarity Press.

Sirgy, M. J., Estes, R., & el-Aswad, el-S., & Rahtz, D. (2019). *Combatting Jihadist terrorism through nation-building: A quality-of-life perspective*. Springer International Publishers.

Tyrer, D. (2013). *The politics of Islamophobia: Race, power and fantasy*. Pluto Press.

Wankin, J. (2019, March 15). *Alleged New Zealand Mosque mass shooter's manifesto praises Donald Trump as 'symbol of renewed white identity.'* Inquisitr. Retrieved from https://www.inquisitr.com/5343540/new-zealand-mass-shooter-trump-supporter-candace-owens-manifesto/

Ward, P. (2002). *White Canada forever: Popular attitudes and public policy toward Orientals in British Columbia*. McGill-Queen's University Press.

Chapter 2
Research Methods

2.1 Introduction

This monograph is based on ethnographic material from 'the field' as well as academic research from the 'library.' It does not rely solely on a theoretical synthesis of the literature on the topic of Islamophobia. It focuses on anti-Muslim racism in North America as expressed by individuals, maintained and reported by community resources, and addressed by government actions and policies. It also relies on ethnographic and empirical data collected from two Muslim communities: one from Dearborn, Michigan in the U.S, and the other from Windsor, Ontario in Canada. Personal narratives were used to reflect the issue of Islamophobia as experienced by Muslims. Previous ethnographic studies from Dearborn (el-Aswad, el-S., 2006, 2010, 2012, 2013) facilitated my fieldwork for the present study. Part of the ethnographic research was conducted directly with the informants before the spread of the COVID-19 pandemic, during which time I employed other communication means such as phone, e-mail, Skype and Zoom to converse and collect data. Before the spread of the Corona virus, I conducted twelve in-depth, in-person semi-structured interviews with individuals living in the aforementioned two Muslim communities. The interviews included members of local Muslim organizations.

The following is a brief description of the two communities in which I conducted ethnographic study. The city of Dearborn is located in the Detroit metropolitan area of Wayne County, Michigan (Map 2.1). As of the 2020 U.S. census (U.S. Census, 2021), it had a total population of 98,153. Despite the fact that the census did not include a count of religious groups, Dearborn has one of the largest Muslim (Sunni and Shi'a) populations in the United States. It is home to the Islamic Center of America, which is the largest mosque in North America (Fig. 2.1).

The city of Dearborn is composed of descendants from multiple, diverse cultural and ethnic groups from Lebanon, Palestine, Iraq, Syria, Yemen, Jordan, and Egypt (el-Aswad, el-S., 2010). It is also the place where the Arab American National Museum, the Ford Motor Company Headquarters, the Islamic Institute of

© The Author(s), under exclusive license to Springer Nature Switzerland AG 2021
el-S. el-Aswad, *Countering Islamophobia in North America*, Human Well-Being
Research and Policy Making, https://doi.org/10.1007/978-3-030-84673-2_2

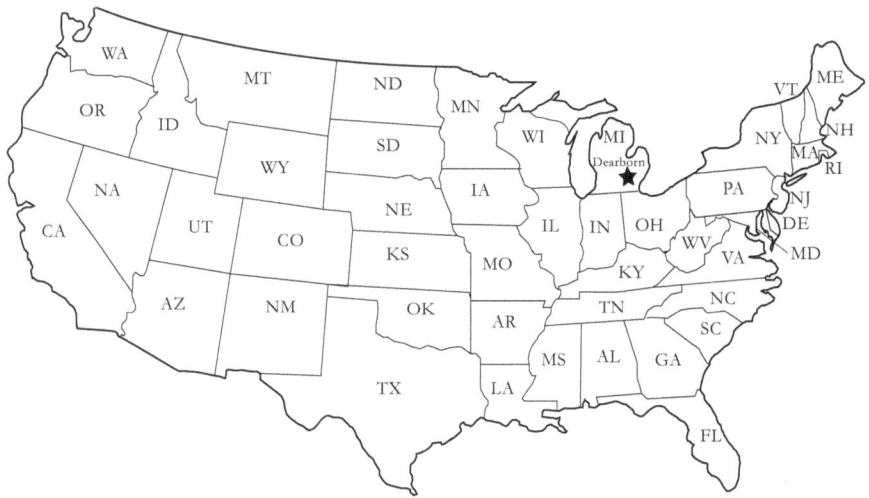

Map 2.1 The U.S. (© Amir el-Aswad)

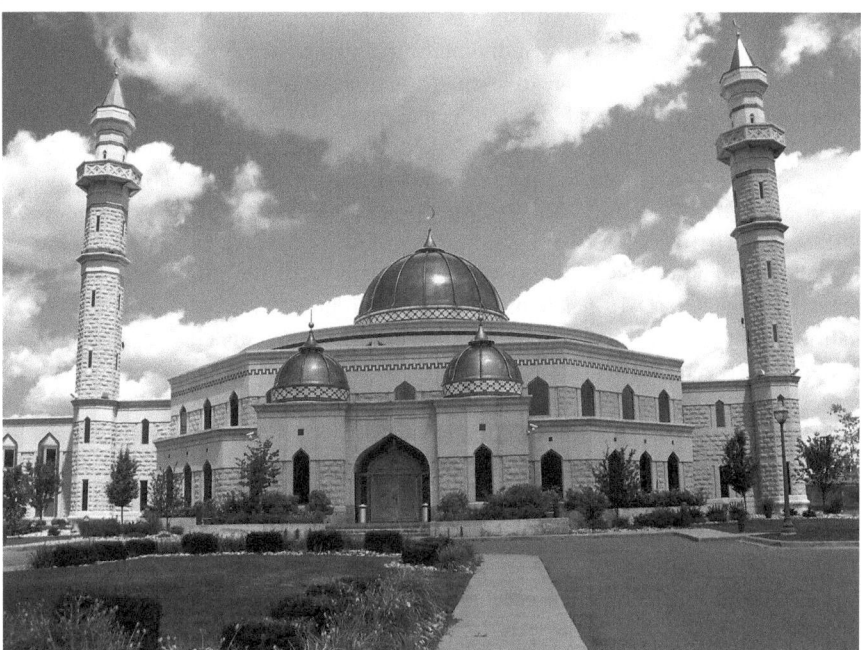

Fig. 2.1 Islamic Center of America, Dearborn, Michigan (© el-Sayed el-Aswad)

Knowledge, the Dearborn Community Center, and the Islamic Council of America (Fig. 2.2) are located. The city holds a satellite campus of the University of Michigan as well as the campus of the Henry Ford College. Additionally, Dearborn is the place

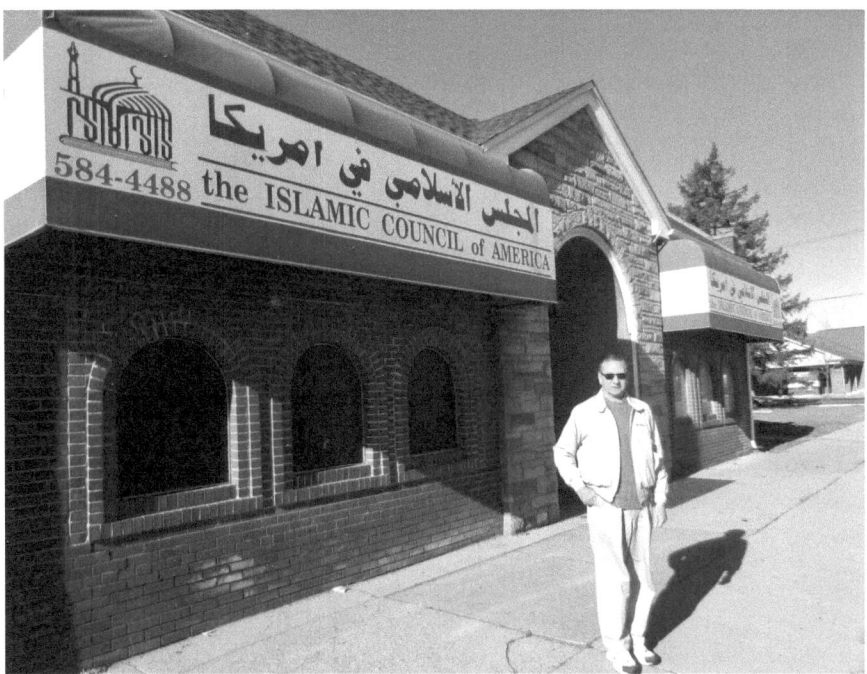

Fig. 2.2 The Islamic Council of America, Dearborn, Michigan (the author, © el-Sayed el-Aswad)

of the Arab Community Center for Economic and Social Services (ACCESS) (2014), a community-focused non-profit organization.

Windsor is a city located in Essex County in southwestern Ontario, Canada (Map 2.2). Windsor shares some significant common features with Dearborn, especially since it is a hub of the automotive industry in Canada (including two Ford Motor Company engine plants) and home to about 15,000 Muslims, or 7% of the population (Statistics Canada, 2016). Windsor is a place where Islamic associations and mosques, such as the Windsor Islamic Association and the United Islamic Trust: South Windsor, are located. Windsor is also culturally diverse and embraces academic institutions, including the University of Windsor and St. Clair College. The Ambassador bridge, an important border crossing, connects Detroit with Windsor (Government of Canada, 2020).

2.2 Methods

This research applies multiple macro-cross-cultural studies and micro-ethnographic inquiries, through conducting participant observations, in-depth interviews, and case studies.

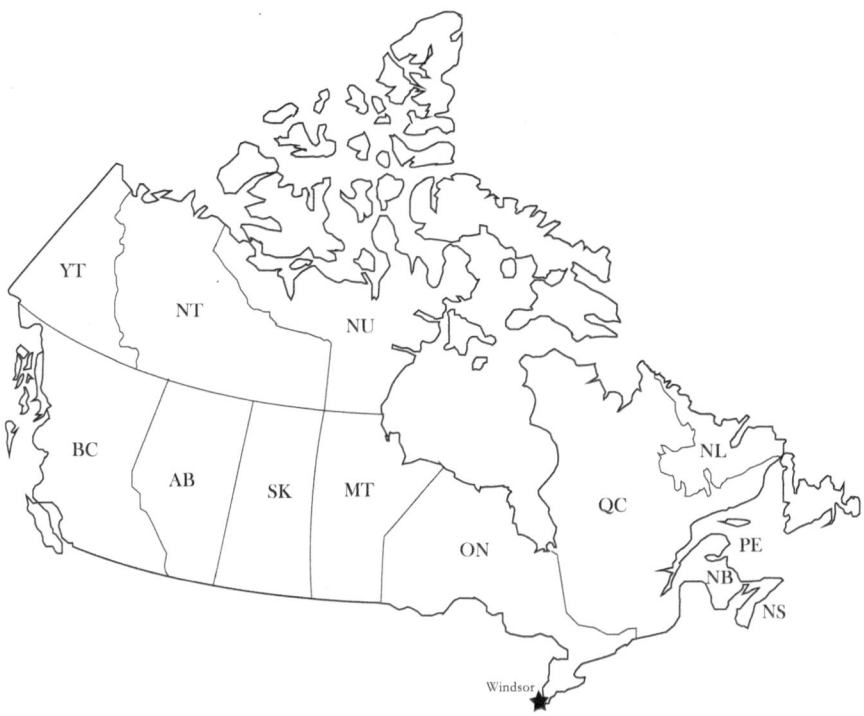

Map 2.2   Canada (© Amir el-Aswad)

Narratives drawn from individuals and members of local communities are not expected to be representative of views of all North American Muslims. Instead, the narratives serve as examples of how everyday Muslims express their experiences as victims of prejudice in their own words and what they think about the issue of Islamophobia.

In addition, this research uses the anthropological approaches of emic ('inside,' or of the participants' views) and etic ('outside," or of the researcher's analysis) perspectives. An emic approach refers to an internalized cultural perspective (Agar, 2007, 2011; Pike, 1967) that is used to understand interlocutors' subjective points of view which leads to revelation of their subjective well-being (Helliwell & Putnam, 2004). On the other hand, an etic method represents the researcher's analysis of the data gathered from ethnographic fieldwork as well as from national and global data collections. These two anthropological methods are relevant to the quality of life and well-being study that focuses on a variety of indicators that can be "viewed in terms of inputs (investments) and outputs (results)" (Sirgy et al., 2017, p. 136).

The outputs refer to conditions that can be viewed as subjective and objective indicators (Estes, 2019). Subjective outcome indicators reflect the personal voice of those in the direct line of experience that can be addressed by the emic method and generalized to the population as a whole, notwithstanding implicit personal biases.

Objective outcome indicators refer to objective information and data collected and disseminated by official government agencies (Sirgy et al., 2017) and resources. These objective outcome indicators will be addressed in this monograph through an etic analysis. For example, the author has gathered data including detailed statistics on events and incidents of Islamophobia reported in Canada and the US. In addition to reports of Islamophobia provided by specialized governmental agencies within Canada and the U.S., data were collected from international agencies such as the *United Nations*, the *Human Development Index* (HDI), the *UNESCO Institute for Statistics*, the *Social Progress Index*, the *World Bank*, the *Pew Research Center*, the *Gallup Poll* (Gallup Organization), the *Transparency International* (TI) (*Corruption perceptions index*), the *Values and Beliefs of the American Public Survey* (the Baylor Religion Survey, 2017), and the *Environics Institute for Survey Research*. The collected data have been used for analytical and comparative purposes. This helped provide the necessary statistical and primary data needed to understand and analyze the problem of Islamophobia.

Concerning input indicators, they refer to forces impacting the well-being of people individually and collectively. They encompass public and private investments in attaining certain outcomes and designing policies that urge people and organizations to act in a particular fashion. In brief, input indicators include factors in "*the social, cultural, political, technological, and physical environments* that impact the quality of life of individuals" (Sirgy et al., 2017, p. 143, italics original), belonging to a minority group, province, or country. They also impact both subjective output indicators and objective output indicators.

The quality of life approach also uses equity indicators with regard to the society's degree of equality or inequality with reference to the distribution of various resources accessible to the entire people of a specific country, particularly those who suffer from historical inequities, including disadvantaged groups such as minorities, women, and the disabled. This research focuses on Muslim minority groups that are marginalized and do not participate fully in the social, political, and economic mainstreams of North America. The monograph discusses the significant public policies countering Islamophobia provided by international organizations, North American governments and advocacy Muslim and non-Muslim organizations.

2.3 Theoretical Framework

This research is guided by multiple theories including the quality-of-life paradigm, the reference group theory, the social identity theory, and a market approach, each of which are relevant in dealing with Islamophobia.

A quality-of-life approach addresses the drivers of Islamophobia in North America from which a set of policies and strategies can be inferred and construed to counter vicious Islamophobic ideology. The overall "quality of life of a country is usually determined by assessing the levels of economic, social, educational, health, and environmental well-being of most people residing in that country" (Sirgy et al., 2019, p. viii). In this context, the concept of life satisfaction is "a pivotal concept in several quality-of-life (QOL) research streams capturing aspects of material well-being, consumer well-being, employee well-being, residential wellbeing, and community well-being" (Sirgy, 2020, p. vii).

Reference group theory refers to a group's collective view of its identity that impacts individuals' behavior, rejecting or vilifying other groups' identities or norms. Individuals use their reference group to make judgments comparing themselves to other individuals or other groups (Merton & Rossi, 1968). Ordinary people tend to view themselves as distinct or empowered as a result of belonging to a reference group (Dawson & Chatman, 2001)

Social identity theory stresses the centrality of an ingroup or reference group in which people attempt to maintain or augment their own cultural identity or self-esteem by viewing other socio-cultural groups or outgroups in negative or adverse terms reinforcing ingroup favoritism and outgroup bias (Dawson & Chatman, 2001; Merton & Rossi, 1968; Pettigrew, 1997). This specific concept of ingroup is akin to the term ethnocentrism; that one's culture or group is superior to that of another thereby denigrating the culture of the other (Baldwin, 2017).

Reference group is impacted by two important distinct concepts mainly worldview and ideology. Worldview, which is shared by a group or large groups of people, is generated by people's aspiration to reach a unified comprehension of the world, drawing together facts, principles, assumptions, generalizations, and answers to ultimate questions. It constitutes the common understanding that makes possible common practices and a widely shared sense of legitimacy (el-Aswad, el-S., 2012). The concept of worldview—comparable to "Weltanschauung," a perceptual framework or cognitive orientation—indicates belief systems and related symbolic actions, while ideology, a subcategory of worldview, implies certain economic and political orientations as well as asymmetrical relations of power aimed at attaining domination (el-Aswad, el-S., 2012). The foremost thrust here is not only related to the intellectual and cognitive aspects of worldview but also to the socio-cultural and subjective domains in which individuals locate and define themselves in their relations to others. The cultural dimension of this method helps researchers and readers understand the cultural and ideological orientations impacting people's views and attitudes. Within this context, Islamophobia is dealt with in this study as an ideology adopted and used by reference groups such as white supremacists, far-right, and extreme militant religious groups

It is important to identify the place of the Muslim group minority in relation to other minorities in North America. This research uses the classification of minority groups proposed by Kalkan et al. (2009) according to which there are two major minority groups or bands in the U.S. This classification, however, can be applied to Canada as well. On the one hand, there is a band that includes religious and racial minority groups, including, respectively, Jews and African Americans. On the other hand, there is a band that includes cultural minority groups (or the cultural 'other') such as illegal immigrants. But, Muslims in the U.S. are distinctive in that they belong to both bands; that is, "they are a religious minority group with cultural practices that are very different from mainstream conventions" (Kalkan et al., 2009, p. 2). Moreover, there are Arab Muslims, Asian Muslims, Black Muslims and White Muslims, all of which are targets of Islamophobia and discrimination.

This study also uses Goffman's work on stigma (Goffman, 1959) as well as theories related to deprivation and social anomie (Ablon, 2002; Major & O'Brien, 2005; Passas & Agnew, 1997; Pescosolido et al., 2010) to explore the socially-embedded nature of stigmatization related to Islamophobia. Stigma is described as the situation of persons who are disqualified from full social acceptance" (Goffman, 1963). Social scientists have recurrently used the concept of stigma to describe adverse experiences of individuals or groups, like Muslims, who are identified by negatively-connoted icons and signs such as race, religion, physical appearance and sexuality (Crewe & Guyot-Diangone, 2016; Hodge et al., 2016; Kunst, 2012; Lean, 2017; Rosenfeld, 2014). Researchers reveal that the custom of Islamic veiling is attacked and viewed as "a practice laden with stigmatization in the Western mindset" (Sandikci & Ger, 2010, p. 16). The World Health Organization affirms that "stigma is a major cause of discrimination and exclusion: it affects people's self-esteem, helps disrupt their family relationships and limits their ability to socialize and obtain housing and jobs. It hampers the prevention of mental health disorders, the promotion of mental well-being and the provision of effective treatment and care. It also contributes to the abuse of human rights" (World Health Organization, 2013).

The literature on countering Islamophobia is woefully scant. Although this monograph adopts a market approach and addresses supply domain concerns such as the shutting down of biased media outlets and the curtailing of financial or funding resources of Islamophobia organizations, it pays more attention to market demand components including, for example, racial discrimination, cultural prejudice, religious extremism, far-right ideology, white supremacy, violation of human rights, lack of political freedom, media bias, income disparities, and unemployment (Sergi et al., 2019). Jack Levin has argued that prejudice is beneficial to the dominant group and the minority group. For the dominant group, prejudice serves to demarcate the cultural borderlines between the in-group and the rest. For the minority group, prejudice encourages marginalized people to fight, to join forces with allies, and to challenge the dominant group (Levin, 1975).

As opposed to market-supply factors that rely on short-term strategies, market-demand factors necessitate long-term strategies to counter Islamophobia. This monograph proposes a set of policies designed to eliminate future Islamophobia market demand, reducing the risk of future Islamophobic hostilities and aggressions.

2.4 Conclusion

The chapter adopts broad and multiple research methods and theoretical perspectives encompassing macro and micro analyses of the complicated phenomenon of Islamophobia. Macro and micro research methods are represented, respectively, in objective information collected from official government agencies, and subjective ethnographic data collected from informants' points of views. To understand both the outcomes and drivers of Islamophobia, this study relied on multiple theoretical paradigms that included: quality-of-life approach, market approach, reference group theory, social identity theory, and Goffman's theory of social stigma.

References

Ablon, J. (2002). The nature of stigma and medical conditions. *Epilepsy and Behavior, 3*(6), 2–9.

Agar, M. (2007). Emic/etic. In G. Ritzer (Ed.), *The Blackwell encyclopedia of sociology*. Wiley-Blackwell. Retrieved from https://onlinelibrary.wiley.com/doi/abs/10.1002/9781405165518.wbeose035

Agar, M. (2011). Making sense of one other for another: Ethnography as translation. *Language and Communication, 31*, 38–47.

Arab Community Center for Economic and Social Services. (2014). *About: Annual reports*. Retrieved from https://www.accesscommunity.org/about/annual-reports-0

Baldwin, J. (2017, January 25). Culture, prejudice, racism, and discrimination. In *Oxford research encyclopedia of communication* (pp. 1–26). New York: Oxford University Press. Doi: doi: https://doi.org/10.1093/acrefore/9780190228613.013.164.

Baylor Religion Survey. (2017). *One nation, divided, under Trump: Findings from the 2017 American values survey*. Retrieved from https://www.prri.org/research/american-values-survey-2017/

Crewe, S. E., & Guyot-Diangone, J. (2016, August 31). Stigmatization and labeling. *Encyclopedia of Social Work*. Oxford University Press. doi:https://doi.org/10.1093/acrefore/9780199975839.013.1043.

Dawson, E. M., & Chatman, E. A. (2001). Reference group theory with implications for information studies: A theoretical essay. *Information Research, 6*(3) Retrieved from http://informationr.net/ir/6-3/paper105.html#ref4

el-Aswad, el-S. (2006). The dynamics of identity reconstruction among Arab communities in the United States. *Anthropos: International Review of Anthropology and Linguistics, 101*, 111–121.

el-Aswad, el-S. (2010). Narrating the self among Arab Americans: A bridging discourse between Arab tradition and American culture. *Digest of Middle East Studies, 19*(2), 234–248. https://doi.org/10.1111/j.1949-3606.2010.00032.x. Retrieved from https://onlinelibrary.wiley.com/doi/abs/10.1111/j.1949-3606.2010.00032.x

el-Aswad, el-S. (2012). *Muslim worldviews and everyday lives*. AltaMira Press.

el-Aswad, el-S. (2013). Images of Muslims in Western scholarship and media after 9/11. *Digest of Middle East Studies, 22*(1), 39–56. https://doi.org/10.1111/dome.12010. Retrieved from https://onlinelibrary.wiley.com/doi/abs/10.1111/dome.12010

Estes, R. J. (2019). The social progress of nations revisited. *Social Indicators Research, 144*, 539–574. https://doi.org/10.1007/s11205-018-02058-9

Goffman, E. (1959). *The presentation of self in everyday life*. Doubleday.

Goffman, E. (1963). *Stigma: Notes on the management of spoiled identity*. Prentice-Hall.

Government of Canada. (2020). *Canada border services agency: Ambassador bridge*. Retrieved from https://www.cbsa-asfc.gc.ca/do-rb/offices-bureaux/961-eng.html

Helliwell, J. F., & Putnam, R. D. (2004). The social context of well-being. *Philosophical Transactions of the Royal Society of London Series B: Biological Sciences, 359*(1449), 1435–1446. https://doi.org/10.1098/rstb.2004.1522

Hodge, D. R., Zidan, T., & Husain, A. (2016). Depression among Muslims in the United States: Examining the role of discrimination and spirituality as risk and protective factors. *Social Work, 61*(1), 45–52.

Kalkan, K. O., Layman, G. C., & Uslaner, E. M. (2009). 'Bands of others'? Attitudes toward Muslims in contemporary American Society. *Journal of Politics, 71*(3), 847–862.

Kunst, J. R. (2012). Coping with Islamophobia: The effects of religious stigma on Muslim minorities' identity formation. *International Journal of Intercultural Relations, 36*(4), 518–532.

Merton, R. K., & Rossi, A. S. (1968). Contributions to the theory of reference group behavior. In R. K. Merton (Ed.), *Social Theory and Social Structure* (pp. 279–334). Free Press.

Lean, N. (2017). *The Islamophobia industry: How the right manufactures fear of Muslims*. Pluto Press.

Levin, J. (1975). *The functions of prejudice*. Harper & Row.

Major, B., & O'Brien, L. T. (2005). The social psychology of stigma. *Annual Review of Psychology, 56*, 393–421.

Passas, N., & Agnew, R. (1997). *The future of anomie theory*. Northeastern University Press.

Pescosolido, B., Martin, J., Long, J., Medina, T., Phelan, J., & Link, B. (2010). "A disease like any other"? A decade of change in public reactions to schizophrenia, depression, and alcohol dependence. *The American Journal of Psychiatry, 167*(11), 1321–1330.

Pike, K. L. (1967). *Language in relation to a unified theory of human behavior*. The Hague, Mouton.

Pettigrew, T. (1997). Generalized intergroup conflict effects on prejudice. *Personality and Social Psychology Bulletin, 23*(2), 173–185.

Rosenfeld, J. (2014). Violence. In G. Laderman & L. León (Eds.), *Religion and American cultures: Tradition, diversity, and popular expression* (pp. 787–812). ABC-CLIO.

Sandikci, O., & Ger, G. (2010). Veiling in style: How does a stigmatized practice become fashionable? *Journal of Consumer Research, 37*, 15–35.

Sirgy, M. J., Estes, R. J., & Selian, A. N. (2017). How we measure well-being: The data behind the history of well-being. In R. J. Estes & M. J. Sirgy (Eds.), *The pursuit of human well-being: The untold global history* (pp. 135–157). Springer.

Sirgy, M. J., R. Estes, el-Aswad, el-S., & Rahtz, D. (2019). *Combatting Jihadist terrorism through nation-building: A quality-of-life perspective*. Springer International Publishers.

Sirgy, M. J. (2020). *Positive balance: A theory of well-being and positive mental health*. Springer Nature.

Statistics Canada. (2016). *Census profile, 2016 census: Windsor, City*. Retrieved from https://www12.statcan.gc.ca/census-recensement/2016/dp-pd/prof/details/page.cfm?Lang=E&Geo1=CSD&Code1=3537039&Geo2=CD&Code2=3537&Data=Count&SearchText=Windsor&SearchType=Begins&SearchPR=01&B1=All&TABID=1

U.S. Census. (2021). *Current Dearborn, Michigan population, demographics and stats in 2020, 2019*. Retrieved from https://suburbanstats.org/population/michigan/how-many-people-live-in-dearborn

World Health Organization. (2013). *Mental health priority areas: Stigma and discrimination*. Retrieved from http://www.euro.who.int/en/health-topics/noncommunicable-diseases/mental-health/priority-areas/stigma-and-discrimination

Chapter 3
Brief History of Islamophobia

3.1 Introduction

Though the actual term, Islamophobia, appeared most predominantly in the 1970s (Rana, 2007), contemporary manifestations of Islamophobia are viewed as a continuation or re-emergence of historical anti-Muslim racism or anti-Islamic prejudice (Allen, 2010; Runnymede Trust, 1997; Sardar, 1995). In other words, Islamophobia is a new concept for an antiquated phenomenon. The past is full of stories of savagery, exploitation, and violence carried out in the name of God. Anti-Muslim prejudice, fear, or Islamophobia is a complex phenomenon with deep historical roots as Islam-Christian conflicts predate the decades of the Crusades and historical discrimination has continued well into the present (Firestone, 2010; Green, 2015; Kazi, 2018; Shaheen, 2001). The phenomenon of Islamophobia or anti-Muslim racism has been considered a 'virus' that has existed inside Western bodies for centuries (Aked et al., 2019; Helly, 2004; Kolchin, 2003).

Several scholars have argued that Islamophobia can be understood by placing it within a long historical trajectory of racism in North America (Baldwin et al., 2011; Lean, 2017; Love, 2017). The "denial of Islamophobia's racism in turn naturalizes its racial politics based on the attempt to represent Muslims in terms of incomplete raciality" (Tyrer, 2013, p. 36). It is worthy to point out that Muslim Americans have been a part of North America since West African Muslims were brought as slaves after only a few years of the first European settlers. As Michael Gomez states (Gomez, 1994, p. 671),

> One of the belief systems introduced into the Americas by Africans was Islam. However, the dawn of Islam in the Americas and its association with Africans have yet to receive the scholarly attention that is merited. This is particularly true of North American historical studies, in which one rarely reads of the early existence of Islam in what would become the United States.

Without ignoring the broader reality and complexities of Islamophobia, this chapter traces old and new variants of Islamophobia in North America. The thrust

el-S. el-Aswad, *Countering Islamophobia in North America*, Human Well-Being Research and Policy Making, https://doi.org/10.1007/978-3-030-84673-2_3

here is that anti-Muslim discrimination goes beyond the Orientalists' theory proposing that the roots of Islamophobia and Orientalism, viewing the Oriental people and Muslims as inferior, can be traced back to the era of colonialism, which resulted in the fragmentation of nations and the rise of geopolitics based on economic interests (Said, 1978, 1981). This chapter seeks to answer the following key question: What is the historical context of Islamophobia in North America, particularly Canada and the U.S.?

3.2   North America: Canada and the United States

This monograph focuses on two large countries in North America: Canada and the U.S. The U.S. is located between Canada and Mexico, bordering both the North Atlantic Ocean and the North Pacific Ocean. Canada is located in northern North America, bordering the North Atlantic Ocean on the east, North Pacific Ocean on the west, and the Arctic Ocean on the north, north of the conterminous U.S. (Central Intelligence Agency, 2020). See Map. These two countries comprise more than 80% of the total land area of North America (Hardwick et al., 2013) in which more than 4,600,000 Muslims reside (Map 1.1).

Globally, the world's Muslim population is expected to increase from 1.9 billion in 2020 and to 2.2 billion by 2030. Muslims will make up 26.4% of the world's total projected population of 8.3 billion in 2030, up from 23.4% of the estimated 2010 world population of 6.9 billion (Pew Research Center, 2018).

In North America, most of the projected growth of the Muslim population takes place in the U.S. and Canada in which Muslims are a racially and ethnically diverse population. Historically, these two North American federations have been enriched by attracting great waves of immigrants (Esses & Abelson, 2017; Estes et al., 2017; Woodward, 2012; Migration Policy Institute, 2020). For instance, three-quarters of U.S. Muslims are immigrants or the children of immigrants (Pew Research Center, 2017a). The Pew Research Center (2018) estimates that there were about 3,450,000 Muslims living in the U.S. in 2017, and that Muslims made up about 1.1% of the total U.S. population. In 2018, other resources estimated the population to be between 5.5 and six million Muslims (Joshi, 2018). The Muslim population is projected to increase from 3.5 million in 2020 to 6.2 million by 2030 (1.7%), in large part because of immigrants, known for their higher-than-average fertility rate, and converts. By 2040, Muslims will be the U.S. nation's second-largest religious group after Christians. By 2050, the U.S. Muslim population is projected to reach 8.1 million, or 2.1% of the nation's total population of 438 million people, the majority of whom will be people of color and members of cultural minority groups (Pew Research Center, 2018).

The vast majority of Muslims living in the U.S. (82%) are American citizens, including 42% who were born in the U.S. and 40% who were born abroad but who have naturalized. The remainder are not U.S. citizens (18%) (Pew Research Center, 2017a). According to 2019 American Muslim poll conducted by the Institute for

Social Policy and Understanding (2019), American Muslims are the most ethnically diverse faith group in the U.S., composed of Black or African American (28%), Asian/Chinese/Japanese (23%), White (19%), Arab (14%), Hispanic (8%), Native American/American Indian/Alaska Native (2%) and Other (5%). Muslims who are Black experience the same systemic racism that all Black Americans face in their day to day lives, in addition to the religious discrimination faced by many Americans who are Muslim. In the same 2019 American Muslim poll, 66% of Muslims who identify as Black or African American and 75% of Black Americans in the general public report experiencing racial discrimination (Institute for Social Policy and Understanding, 2019).

Despite the large amount of land available to Canada, it is affected by especially challenging and difficult winters, and its population is therefore substantially smaller than that of the United States. Canada's population ranks 37th worldwide. According to Canada's 2011 National Household Survey, there were 1,053,945 Muslims in Canada, or about 3.2% of the total population of 35.9 million people, making Islam the second largest religion in the country after Christianity (Statistics Canada, 2017). The number of Muslims in Canada is expected to reach 2.7 million in 2030, making up 6.6% of Canada's total population (Pew Research Center, 2011). Almost seven in ten (68%) Muslims in Canada are foreign-born, and they come from many countries, principally in Asia and Africa. Those who identify themselves as South Asians (e.g., Pakistanis, Indians) constitute 36%, while those who identify themselves as Arabs make up 25%. Smaller percentages identify themselves as West Asian (Iranian, Afghan), Black, and East Asian (Chinese, Japanese, Korean) (Environics, 2016; Hamdani, 2015). In 2011, there were also more than 1000 Muslims who identified as Aboriginal, known as First Nation or Métis (Environics, 2016). Canadian Muslims are younger on average than other Canadians. The median age of Canadian Muslims "is 28.1 years, compared to the overall Canadian population average age of 37 years" (Hanniman, 2008, p. 272).

Scholars observe that Canada's proximity to the U.S. has played a part in undermining the citizenship of Canadian Muslims. In redefining its global reach, particularly after the tragic event of 9/11, the U.S. has declared the right to question the citizenship of Muslims in other states, including Canada. Since their first entry into Canada to the present day, Muslims have been subjected to discrimination and Orientalist negative portrayals (Anderson, 1991; Helly, 2004; Nagra, 2011).

3.3 Anti-Muslim Prejudice in the Medieval Era

The historical conflict and clash between Islam and Western Christianity "left on both sides a legacy of misunderstanding, fear, prejudice, and, in some cases, hatred" (Smith, 2010, p. xi). The main driver of anti-Muslim bigotry or Islamophobia is not just a history of weakness and minority survival, but also a history of progress and enormous success. The Golden Age of Islam coincided with the period of the European Dark Ages (500 CE–1000 CE). During the Middle Ages, Islamic civilization was far ahead of its Christian rival, offering enticing advances in architecture, law, literature, philosophy, and, indeed, in most areas of cultural activity (Renima et al., 2016).

While addressing the historical background of Islamophobia, this study stresses that "social environment plays a significant role in the make-up of well-being" of people (Sirgy, 2020, p. 155). Discrimination against Muslims is in part due to what Robert Merton (1968) calls a reference group theory, referring to a group's collective view of its identity group impacting individuals' behavior and rejecting or vilifying outgroups' identities as expressed in 'we-they' or 'us-them'. An ingroup's prejudice against an outgroup is part of a tendency to degrade that outgroup, the 'other,' more generally (Dawson & Chatman, 2001; Kalkan et al., 2009). It is worth pointing out that new religions often suffer from the hostility of establishment religions that inevitably consider them threatening "others." The roots of Islamophobia go back to the Christian denunciation of Islam as a religion in the eighth century, particularly when Islam was perceived by Christians as a theological and political threat to Christianity (Firestone, 2010; Kalin, 2009). (Table 3.1).

For hundreds of years, great Islamic armies threatened Europe, reaching Spain and France in the eight-century (Polk, 2018; Said, 1981; Southern, 1978). After defeating Byzantium, the Muslim empire stretched from the Atlantic Ocean to India in a short period of time while the Christian domains were confined to Anatolia and a few provinces west of the Bosporus. Christian theology and supremacy were questioned by Muslims' success in overpowering the Christian West. It was therefore from a military position, associating Islam with violence and aggression and, perhaps more importantly, cultural weakness that Christian Europe developed negative images about Islam, some of which survive to the present day (Blanks, 1999; Daniel, 1960). In part, "this hostility was the result of continued political and military conflict, but it likewise ensued from a Western sense of cultural inferiority" (Blanks & Frassetto, 1999, p. 3).

The Christian response to the great success of Islam was to embrace an unfathomable xenophobia or fear that became entrenched in "the Christian self-concept and view of the Muslim 'other.' This is Islamophobia, even if no special word had yet been coined to describe the sentiment" (Firestone, 2010, p. 47). One of the earliest reactions to Islamic progress was expressed by Theophanes, an eighth century Byzantine priest, who allegedly claimed that Muhammad was a fraud, not a real prophet (Firestone, 2010). In the twelfth century, while living in Spain, Peter of Toledo, who made the first translation of the Qur'an into Latin, viewed Islam to be a product of satanic scheming. Further, in the thirteenth century, Riccoldo da Monte di Croce, an Italian Dominican monk, claimed that Muhammad was chosen not by God but by the devil (Firestone, 2010; Tolan, 2019).

The Christian Crusades in the eleventh and thirteenth centuries (1095–1291) were motivated by political ideology with the goal of returning control of the Holy Lands from Islamic control (Kalin, 2009; Sirgy et al., 2019). In his book *White Supremacy*, George Fredrickson (1981, pp. 7–8) states:

Table 3.1 The Modern History of Anti-Muslim Racism and Islamophobia in North America

Year	World	United States	Canada
1605			The establishment of the first permanent European settlement by French colonists
1607		The British Empire in America	
1731	Anglo-Americans	Transatlantic slave trade brought African Muslims to Maryland (including Muslim slave Ayuba Suleiman Diallo)	
1763		Britain established colonies in America following victory over France ended by signing of the Treaty of Paris	The French colony of Canada became a part of the British empire (the Treaty of Paris)
1774		Colonists form First Continental Congress	
1775		American Revolution: George Washington leads Continental army to fight against British rule.	
1776 (July 4th)		Declaration of independence endorsed by Congress. New nation of the United States of America. "all men are created equal", but racism has been a core element in American society.	
Seventeenth–eighteenth centuries		Hundreds of thousands of Africans (including Muslims) brought over and sold into slavery to work on cotton and tobacco plantations	
1783		Treaty of Paris: Britain accepts loss of colonies	
1787–1788		New constitution for United States of America	
1800–present		Muslim immigrants coming from different countries	Muslim immigrants coming from different countries
1808	Atlantic slave trade abolished		
1861–65		U.S. Civil War: Opponents of slavery against advocates of slavery	

(continued)

Table 3.1 (continued)

Year	World	United States	Canada
1867 (July 1)			Union of British North American colonies (Self-governing dominion of Canada)
1896–1914			Canada received more than three million immigrants
1913		Moorish Science Temple	
1914	Outbreak of World War I	US enters into World War I	Canada fights on the side of Britain and France
1916	Sykes-Picot Agreement dividing and controlling MENA countries		
1917	Balfour Declaration		
1918	End of World War I Collapse of Ottoman Empire	Hollywood film industry and negative depiction of Arabs and Muslims	
1921		Muslims founded a mosque in the Highland Park area of metropolitan Detroit (Michigan)	
1922	USSR established		
1924	The Ottoman caliphate was abolished by the Turkish Grand National Assembly		
1928	Foundation of Muslim Brotherhood		
1929		The Great Depression	
1930		Nation of Islam	
1934			First Muslim organization in Canada registered by immigrants
1938			First Canadian mosque was constructed in Edmonton, Canada
1939	Outbreak of World War II		
1945	End of World War II		
1947	United Nations recommends partition of Palestine into separate Jewish and Arab states		Canada is declared to be of equal status with Great Britain within the Commonwealth
1948	First Arab-Israeli war		

(continued)

Table 3.1 (continued)

Year	World	United States	Canada
1950s		Racism was widespread and explicit in the United States	
1952		Federation of Islamic Associations in the United States and Canada (FIA)	Federation of Islamic Associations in the United States and Canada (FIA)
1956	Israel, Britain and France invaded Egypt	US objected the invasion of Egypt by Israel, Britain and France	
1963		Muslim Student Association of the U.S. & Canada (MSA National)	Muslim Student Association of the U.S. & Canada (MSA National)
1967	Six-Day War: A pre-emptive attack on Egypt, Syria and Jordan launched by Israel. Israel seized Sinai and Gaza Strip from Egypt, the Golan Heights from Syria and the West Bank and East Jerusalem from Jordan	The impact of 1967 war on the relationship between the U.S. and Egypt	
1968		The establishment of the Islamic Circle of North America (ICNA)-umbrella organization	
1970s 1971	Islamophobia scholarship (writing)		Canada's adoption of multiculturalism policy
1973	October War with Israel (The Yom Kippur War) in which parts of Sinai were restored		
1979	Egypt and Israel signed a peace treaty	U.S. President Jimmy Carter effectively participated in Egypt and Israel peace treaty	
1979	Islamic Revolution (Iran)	Negative impact on Iran-US relationship: Islamophobia	
1980s		The rise of the Christian right	
1980	Start of Iran-Iraq war	Arab–American Anti-Discrimination Committee (ADC)	
1981	Foundation of Gulf Cooperation Council (GCC)		

(continued)

Table 3.1 (continued)

Year	World	United States	Canada
1982	• Israel invades Lebanon in order to expel Palestine Liberation Organization (PLO). Massacre of Palestinians in the Sabra and Shatila camps in Beirut • Egypt restored the last occupied portion of Sinai	Islamic Society of North America (ISNA): Anti-Islamophobia	The UK transfers final legal powers over Canada. Canada becomes completely free with a new constitution
1987	• Al-Qaeda, a global network of Islamic extremists designated by the United Nations Security Council as a terrorist group • Intifada uprising begins in Occupied Territories	Increase of Islamophobia	Increase of Islamophobia
1988	End of Iran-Iraq war	Muslim Public Affairs Council (MPAC): Anti-Islamophobia	
1990		American Muslim Council (AMC): Ant-Islamophobia	
1991	Gulf War –US led coalition liberating Kuwait from Iraqi occupation		
1993		• Muslim American Society (MAS): Ant-Islamophobia • The first Islamist-terrorist attack on America, destroying the World Trade Center and killing six and wounding 1500 people	
1994	Israel withdraws from most of Gaza and West Bank. Israel and Jordan sign a peace treaty	Council on American-Islamic Relations (CAIR): Anti-Islamophobia	
1995		Oklahoma bomb by far-right advocates killing more than 160 people	
2001	Increase of islamophobia (post-9/11)	Sept. 11 attack destroying New York World Trade Center killing at least 3044 people	

(continued)

Table 3.1   (continued)

Year	World	United States	Canada
2002		Iran. Iraq, and North Korea are viewed by US as an "axis of evil"	Canadian multicultural-ism Day (June 27) was designated
2003		United States attacked Iraq	
2007		Economic depression	
2008	Global economic crisis	Global economic crisis	Global economic crisis
2010	Fourth round of sanctions against Iran imposed by UN Security Council	Islamophobia	Islamophobia
2011	Arab Spring in 5 MENA countries		
2013	Islamic State or IS (for-mer ISIS) a global- ter-rorist group aiming at creating a caliphate across Iraq, Syria and beyond	The U.S. reaction to the Islamic State terrorism (Islamophobia)	
2015	Iran's nuclear deal with world powers (5 + 1)		
2017	Another wave of Islamophobia	Donald Trump (Republi-can) becomes the 45th President of the US (January 20) Increase of Islamophobia On January 27, Trump issued an executive order which banned Muslim nationals of Iran, Iraq, Libya, Somalia, Sudan, Syria and Yemen. This was the first iteration of the Muslim Ban Unite the Right (white supremacists) racist rally in Charlottesville (August 12)	Increase of Islamophobia
2018	Global tension—increase of Islamophobia	The US announced its withdrawal from the Joint Comprehensive Plan of Action (JCPOA) or the Iran's nuclear deal (May 8). Regional and global tension	
2020	COVID-19 (Corona virus) pandemic	COVID-19 impacting economy, health and equality Black Lives Matters anti-	

(continued)

Table 3.1 (continued)

Year	World	United States	Canada
		racism protest triggered by the brutal slaying of George Floyd by a police officer in Minneapolis, Minnesota (in May 25)	
2021	The discriminatory travel ban has been revoked Israel-Gaza/Palestine conflict (Al-Aqsa mosque) and attack of Israel on Gaza	Attack on the U.S Capitol (January 6) by far-right terrorists and white supremacists incited by D. Trump Joseph Biden (Democrat) becomes the 46th President of US (January 20)	

Source: Compiled by the author using multiple resources cited in the references of Chap. 3

there were two crucial distinctions that allowed Europeans of the Renaissance and Reformation period to divide the human race into superior and inferior categories. One was between Christian and heathen, the other between 'civil' and 'savage'. The first reflected in the religious militancy nurtured by the long and better struggle for supremacy in the Mediterranean between Christian and Islamic civilizations. The crusade had applied the principle that a war conducted in the name of the Church against infidels is *ipso facto* a just war.

During the Crusades, enduring stereotypes about Muslims crystallized and Muslims became entrenched as the enemy of Christian people (Kumar, 2012). Hundreds of thousands of Muslims and Christians were slaughtered in the name of each other's religion during this long and devastating period that ended with the dismemberment of the Ottoman Empire. In brief, Islam conjured notions of fear throughout the Crusades during which negative images of Muslims were stringently constructed and arguably remain in operation to this day (Gottschalk & Greenberg, 2008; Sha'ban, 1991).

3.4 Anti-Muslim Discrimination in Modern History

The following sections address anti-Muslim sentiment and discrimination represented in orientalism, colonialism and other racist movements.

3.4.1 Orientalism, Racism, Colonialism and Eurocentrism

The end of the Crusades was followed by the era of colonialism that started in the late 15th and early sixteenth centuries. There is a preoccupation with the distinctiveness or uniqueness of the West in its relation to the Orient, Islam or the non-west (el-Aswad, el-S., 2008). The relationship between colonialism, racism, and Islamophobia is historically documented (Bhattacharya, 2021; el-Aswad, el-S., 2021b). The European colonization of Muslim and non-Muslim societies was driven by economic, political, and religious (missionary) factors as well as by what colonialists call civilizing the other so as to justify racial discrimination. Colonialism, carried out exclusively in the Eastern societies, was backed by Orientalism, referring to a "Western style for dominating, restructuring, and having authority over the Orient" (Said, 1978, p. 3).

Orientalist misrepresentations of Islam were used to rationalize and justify absolute and unqualified domination over subjugated Muslims. Besides, Orientalism can be regarded as "a manner of regularized (or Orientalized) writing, vision, and study, dominated by imperatives, perspectives, and ideological biases ostensibly suited to the Orient" (Said, 1978, p. 202). Orientalism has a robust impact on the images of Muslims presented in literature, scholarship, and other domains of culture. For example, Humphrey Prideaux, an Orientalist, depicted Islam as a fraud and violent religion that spread by force (Kidd, 2009). During the colonial period and the nineteenth century, the Roman church associated "Islam with Antichrist" (Kidd, 2009, p. 8). In addition, administrators of British colonialism showed antipathy towards Islam and Muslims, viewing them in derogatory terms as a backward, fanatical, irrational, and intolerant people, a common orientalist trope (Abdel-Malek, 1963; Satia, 2008; Watt, 2019). This was a part of the complex legacy of Orientalism that "early Americans adopted from Europe and then developed within the specific matrices of their cultural imagination" (Marr, 2006, p. 7). In brief, eighteenth- century-Anglo-Americans attributed all these negative characteristics to Islam. (Table 3.1).

Historically, "Americans have utilized Islam as a rhetorical device for articulating various understandings of American identity from the time of the earliest Anglo-American settlers" (Sherrard, 2017, p. 1). Historians contend the "two main sources from which early Americans derived their impressions of Islam were the enslavement of Europeans and North Americans in North Africa, and widely circulated books and sermons related to Islam" (Kidd, 2009, p. 2). North American countries have been deeply impacted by imperial and colonial forces that spread anti-Muslim stereotypes. European or Anglo-American roots of anti-Muslim racism continue to influence American Islamophobia today. Richard Drayton (2005) argues that Britain was the principal slaving nation of the modern world. During the Atlantic slave trade, Muslims began arriving in the New World as slaves at the end of the sixteenth century when European explorers and colonists crossed the Atlantic in search of new trading routes (Drayton, 2005).

In "colonial and antebellum America, African Muslims, enslaved, were perceived as backward and luminal figures through whom Anglo-Americans rationalized existing racial and religious boundaries of their community primarily for commercial and evangelizing purposes" (el-Aswad, el-S., 2011, p. 113). Some enslaved Muslims were literate in Arabic (Omi & Winant, 2015). In 1731 the African Muslim, Ayuba Suleiman Diallo, was brought to North America (Maryland) as a slave by the transatlantic slave trade (Austin, 1984; Curtis, 2009; Diouf, 1998). Examples of other enslaved African American Muslims in the eighteenth and nineteenth century are "Omar ibn Said, Abdr-Rahman Ibrahim, Mahommah Gardo Baquaqua, Lamine Kebe, Mohammad Ali ben Said (Nicolas Said) and Bilali Muhammad (Ben Ali)" (Al Badaai, 2017, p. vii).

Colonial North Americans were able to acquire some information about Muslims because the wording of their printed treaties allowed them to believe that they "had legitimate 'knowledge' about Islam" (Kidd, 2009, p. 2). Thomas Kidd wrote:

> Anglo-American colonists used their knowledge of Islam to reinforce the superiority of their brand of Protestantism over their challengers, such as Deism and Catholicism, and to de-legitimize Islam religiously, morally, and racially (Kidd, 2009, p. 2).

Throughout the seventeenth and eighteenth centuries, the British established colonies in North America. Thousands of Muslim African slaves were working on colonial American plantations (Kolchin, 2003; Taylor, 2001). During the eighteenth and nineteenth century, "Muslims may have come to America by the thousands, if not tens of thousands" as slaves (Gomez, 1994, p. 682). In Canada, Muslims arrived during the period of 1850s and 1870s (Kazemipur, 2014). Other historians reported that more than 29,000 enslaved Muslims were living in America (Austin, 1984). The number of Muslims, due to immigration, has gradually increased over the twentieth and twenty first centuries, particularly since the 1960s (el-Aswad, el-S., 2013b).

Melissa Gismondi (2017) argues that a critical difference between the U.S. and Canada is that white settlers in the U.S., as in Canada, invaded Indigenous lands. But unlike in Canada, those people in the U.S. settled that land with a significant population of enslaved Africans and African-Americans (Gismondi, 2017). Racism has been a core element in American society. By 1776, when the phrase, "all men are created equal" was written into the Declaration of Independence by Thomas Jefferson, a slaveholder, a democratic country was born with a profound contradiction about race at its heart (Goodman et al., 2012). It is be noted here that most of the "Founding Fathers were large-scale slave owners, including George Washington, 'father of his country'" (Kolchin, 2003, p. 3). When slavery ended in 1865, the image of the Muslim as a hostile and unfriendly foreigner was crystalized (Curtis, 2013).

It is worth pointing out that in a recent interview with the Arkansas Democrat-Gazette, Arkansas Senator Tom Cotton said that slavery was the necessary evil upon which the Union was built (Carlson, 2020). And advocates of the far-right movement and white supremacists, based on an ideology of white nationalism, state that whiteness or Whites alone defined America as a European society and political order because the founding population of the United States was primarily Anglo-Saxon and Protestant. Other races inhabited the continent and were often set in conflict or subservience to Whites or white civilization (Fredrickson, 1981; Kiernan, 1980; Spencer, 2017; Thobani, 2007). Here, the notion of American exceptionalism goes back to the arrival of Puritan settlers in Massachusetts in 1620s who promoted the idea of a white American settlement, impacting evangelical Protestants, particularly in the eighteenth century (Bebbington, 1993; Gismondi, 2017). It is noteworthy that "Colonial Americans inherited English views that mostly rejected Islam" (Sherrard, 2017, p. 1).

Additionally, most Americans and Canadians, being descendants of European immigrants, have grown up with traditions in which negative images of Muslims persist. Put differently, for more than two centuries, North Americans have been influenced by the prejudice and attitudes of Europe regarding the Islamic world (Sha'ban, 1991). In both Canada and the U.S., anti-Muslim racism has been incorporated within the settler logic of white supremacy (Dossa, 2008). Descended from Baptists who settled in the American colonies in the seventeenth century, the Southern Baptist Convention, the largest Protestant denomination in Antebellum America, came into being in 1845 as the church of Southern slaveholders. The founding fathers of this school were deeply involved in slavery and deeply complicit in the defense of slavery (Gjelten, 2018; Jones, 2020). Following the Civil War in mid-nineteenth century in America, the "theologically backed assertion of the superiority of both 'white race' and Protestant Christianity undergirded a century of religiously sanctioned terrorism" in forms of ritualized lynching, extortion and public violence (Jones, 2020, p. 6).

Racist organizations such as white supremacist hate groups, including the Ku Klux Klan (KKK) among other racist bands spread in North America in the eighteenth and nineteenth centuries (Backhouse, 1999; Fredrickson, 1981; Jones, 2020). Jeffrey Ross stated that "Right-wing violence in Canada can be traced back as far as 1784 when Canada's first race riot took place in the Nova Scotian towns of Shelburne and Birchtown" (Ross, 1992, p. 77). During the nineteenth and twentieth centuries, Orientalists sought to assess the compatibility of Islam with European modernity (Gottschalk, 2019). In the twentieth century, particularly since the 1930s, the Nation of Islam (NOS) appeared in the U.S. as a strong domestic voice of the rising tide of civil rights concerning people of color and African American Muslims (Curtis, 2013). Under "Elijah Muhammad's leadership, and with the help of Malcolm X, the Nation of Islam in the 1950s and 1960s grew to become the most successful Black Nationalist movement in the United States" (el-Aswad, el-S., 2013b, p. 1525).

Canada has been impacted by conservative Christian beliefs handed down from British and European cultures as the life-blood of previously dominant United, Anglican, Presbyterian, and Lutheran denominations was immigration from Britain and Europe (Angus Reid Institute, 2015). Elspeth Cameron (2004) stated that Canada' early racist ideology, as an anglophone/francophone country, impacted its immigration policy as being ethnically selective accepting only American and European, particularly British immigrants. However, despite this racial immigration policy, people of many different origins entered British North America during the eighteenth and nineteenth centuries. During the period from 1896 to 1914, Canada received more than three million immigrants. As is the case of the US, Muslim immigrants who settled in Canada came from many nationalities, included Arabs, Black, South Asians, and South-East Asian Muslim communities. Recently, Canada has changed from an anglophone/francophone country to a Multicultural nation (Cameron, 2004).

In 1920, Muslim immigrants in Detroit initiated the Detroit Chapter of the Red Crescent and purchased plots for Muslim burials. They also founded a mosque in the Highland Park area of metropolitan Detroit in 1921. Another mosque was established in Cedar Rapids, Iowa in 1934 (el-Aswad, el-S., 2011). The first Canadian mosque was constructed in Edmonton, Canada in 1938. In that same year of 1938, there were approximately 700 European Muslims in Canada. In 1934, Muslim immigrants from Lebanon living in Regina, the capital city of the province of Saskatchewan, established the first Muslim organization in Canada (Habib & Habib, 2015; Kazemipur, 2014).

In Canada, the national policy on immigration accepted European and American immigrants during the 1940s. Small quotas of immigrants from such Muslim countries as Pakistan, India, and Ceylon (currently Sri Lanka) were accepted in the 1950s. After the removal of European immigration preferences in the late 1960s and early 1970s Muslims began to migrate to Canada in significant numbers. However, the most populous provinces and cities of Canadian Muslims are Ontario, Quebec and Alberta (Cameron, 2004; Henry & Tator, 2006) as well as Montreal, which attracted "immigrants from former French colonies in the Middle East and North Africa (Environics, 2016).

3.4.2   Islamophobia Challenges Since 1920

This section focuses on external and internal factors that have contributed to the rise of Islamophobia in North America.

3.4.2.1   External Factors

Despite some external factors occurring outside North American territories, they have had a great impact regionally and globally. For instance, during the First World War, the Sykes-Picot Agreement was made in 1916 between the British and French Allies, mandating and colonizing Middle East countries: the British would acquire Iraq, the French would control Syria and Lebanon, and Palestine would become an international territory. But, the Balfour declaration of 1917, proclaiming the establishment of a National Jewish Home in Palestine, triggered an ongoing Israeli–Palestinian conflict (Khalidi, 2020; el-Aswad, el-S., 2019). Subsequently two Arab-Israeli wars—one in 1948 and another in 1967—were fought which resulted in the Israeli military occupation of Palestinian territories and the denial of civil rights to Palestinians. The U.S. "provides economic and military aid to Israel and oppressive regime, policies that cause anger against America in many Muslim countries" (Nimer, 2002, p. 17). In a word, the "double standard of U.S. policy in the Middle East arising from its strategic relationship with Israel is also a factor" (Johnston, 2016, p. 169).

The Israeli–Palestinian conflict has impacted the view of American people, particularly political decision makers, toward Arabs and Muslims as being depicted in negative terms (el-Aswad, el-S., 2013c; Salaita, 2006). According to the Pew Research Center (2016), more Americans continue to sympathize more with Israel (54%) than with the Palestinians (19%) in the Middle East dispute. Many people in North America refer to Islam as a way of understanding the causes of tension and conflict between Muslims and non-Muslims not only in the Middle East, but also in the West.

During the 1960s, there was the beginning of heavy Muslim/Arab immigration to North America; however, the rise of Islamist movements in the 1970s along with the Iranian Revolution (1978–79) and the subsequent American hostage crisis drove Americans to view Muslims as a threat. This negative view of Muslims was fortified by the increase of terrorist attacks by Islamist jihadists in the 1980s and 1990s, evidencing a connection between extreme Jihadism and Islamophobia (el-Aswad, el-S., 2021a).

The American foreign policy towards Islam has changed since the end of the Cold War. The anti-Islam campaigns aimed at both policy makers and public opinion have increased in the US. There has been discontent among the Muslims in the US who feel they are being viewed as disloyal and as enemies (Hussain, 2018, Lowrie, 1995). Many radical jihadist organizations, supported by the US, were formed during the Soviet–Afghan War (1979–1989). The anti-Soviet Afghan jihad in the 1980s gave birth to many radical jihadi organizations (el-Aswad, el-S. et al., 2020). The intervention of the US in the Iraqi-Kuwait crisis (the Gulf War 1990–1991), which pushed Saddam's forces to withdraw from Kuwait triggered al-Qa'ida to carry out terrorist attacks against U.S. diplomatic and military targets. The 1993 World Trade Center bombing increased prejudice and violence against American Muslims (GhaneaBassiri, 2010, 2013). Additionally, a former U.S. defense secretary stated that al-Qa'ida was behind the 1996 terrorist attack on an American military base located in the city of Al Khobar, Kingdom of Saudi Arabia, in which a robust truck bomb was used to kill 19 and injure 372 members of the U.S. Air Force (Archive. today, 2007). Other sources claim that Iran was responsible for the Khobar Towers bombing (Leonnig, 2006). Attacks carried out by Muslim terrorists have increased discrimination against resident Muslims in North America. Since 1995 to the present, the U.S. has imposed unilateral sanctions against Iran, accusing it of aiding Islamist terrorists (Fayazmanesh, 2003). Meanwhile, the declaration of jihad on the alleged "American's occupation of Saudi Arabia"—the country of two of the most sacred places, Mecca and Medina—was issued in August 1996 (el-Aswad, el-S. et al., 2020). It was Osama bin Laden's first call to global jihad against the United States (bin Laden, 2008) that led to the tragic events of September 11, 2001.

3.4.2.2   Internal Factors

By the 1920s, the federal government of the US, particularly the FBI started targeting "Muslim American groups such as the Moslem Welfare Society of Sunni

Muslim missionary of Satti Majid, the NOI, and the Moorish Science Temple [established in 1913]," examining the growth of Islam in various organizations during the interwar period (Curtis, 2013, p. 77).

During the 1950s, racism was widespread and explicit in the United States. When the large number of Muslim immigrants came to the U.S. in the 1960s–1980s and managed to establish themselves in different American cities, the negative coverage of Muslims and Islam in the national media worked to alienate Muslims from their local communities (GhaneaBassiri, 2013; Morey et al., 2019; Powell, 2011; Semati, 2010). Even North American schools and textbooks on Islam were full of misconceptions during 1970s and 1980s as one "could compose an extensive rouges' gallery of errors in the description of Islam, its origins, beliefs, and practices to which entries might be added to each textbook cycle. For example, misconstrue names of the founding individuals and even the name of 'Islam' itself could then still be found occasionally represented as 'Mohammedanism'" (Douglass, 2009, p. 87).

The negative image of Muslims played a crucial role in conspiracy theory, targeting American Muslims. For instance, two hundred and twenty-two hate crimes against Muslims in the U.S. were reported in the days immediately following the terrorist attack on the Federal Building in Oklahoma City on April 19, 1995 though no Arabs or Muslims were involved (el-Aswad, el-S., 2005). Although the term Islamophobia began to appear in the 1970s (Rana, 2007), it has become common and widespread since the 9/11 terrorist attack on New York and the Pentagon (Allen, 2010; el-Aswad, el-S. 2012, 2013a; Love, 2017). Because fifteen of the nineteen high jackers had grown up in Saudi Arabia, worldwide attention has been focused on Arabs and Muslims, generating hostility and fear of Islam itself. This external terrorist attack has had profound consequences impacting the internal factors of Islamophobia from within the U.S. For instance, although George W. Bush "himself took pains to repeat the mantra 'Islam means peace' several times, his administration defined itself by means of 'war on terror,' both globally and domestically ... U.S. war policy targeted Muslims, Arabs, and South Asians both around the world and domestically" (Omi & Winant, 2015, p. 227). Several authors argue that the 9/11 attack has negatively impacted the American public psyche as Americans became worried about another overwhelming attack by Muslim extremists (Steinback, 2011). New Orientalists have initiated military attacks and invasions of Muslim countries in their call for a global war on terror (el-Aswad, el-S., 2008).

Muslims living in North America have suffered economically and politically, particularly following the terrorist attack of the 9/11 and the declaration of the global war on terror after which the U.S. led coalition invaded two Muslim countries, Afghanistan and Iraq, in 2001 and 2003, respectively. The U.S. war against Afghanistan and Iraq provided justifications for creating negative images about Muslims as well as for maintaining U.S. political and economic hegemony and power abroad (Berger et al., 2008; Kumar, 2012; Pluralism Project, 2020). The internal factors of racism were reflected in the cumulative legislative and political proceedings targeting Muslims' immigration and scrutiny. On October 26, 2001, the Congress passed the USA PATRIOT Act, which provided enforcement and immigration authorities, along with the Treasury, enormous power of surveillance and regulation to obstruct terrorism (USA Congress, 2001).

Surveillance and the threat of terrorism became a much more routine part of Americans' lives (GhaneaBassiri, 2013). As is the case in the United Kingdom, Muslims in North America experience racist patterns of behavior and attitudes represented in being treated with suspicion, or being ignored, avoided, turned down and ridiculed (Sheridan, 2006). Muslim Americans are not the first religious or ethnic group considered a threat to North America. At the turn of the twentieth century, Jewish, Italian, Hispanic, Asian, and Middle Eastern immigrants were denigrated in the mainstream as racially inferior to other Americans (Read, 2008). However, Muslims have suffered more than any other minority before and after 9/11 tragic attacks. In 1996, Muslims experienced 240 acts of discrimination, violence and harassment, a threefold increase over the previous year. These discriminatory acts "ranged from Muslim women being fired or denied jobs because of their religious garb, to harassment of Muslims at the nation's airports, other public facilities, schools, and government agencies because of the persons' apparent religious affiliation" (Council on American-Islamic Relations, 1997, p. vi). The number of assaults against Muslims in the United States rose from 93 incidents in 2001, the year of the September 11 terrorist attacks, to 127 in 2016 (Pew Research Center, 2017b). All of these discriminatory practices severely limit people's capacity for attaining the level of well-being that they seek (Estes, 2017).

Islamophobia appears as an ideological phenomenon extensively used by white supremacists, nationalists, and the far-right in both the U.S. and Canada as the rising tide of conservative Christian attacks on Islam (Geddes, 2013; Perry & Scrivens, 2019; Ward, 2002). For instance, in the decade since 9/11, there has been a significant increase in distrust and prejudice towards Muslims in Canada (Hanniman, 2008; National Council of Canadian Muslims, 2013; Yousif, 1953). In 2009, 46% of Canadians held an unfavorable view of Islam, but that figure has risen sharply to 54% in 2013 (Geddes, 2013). Six in ten in Canada can identify at least one group whom they believe are targeted for discrimination due to race. As Charmaine Nelson (2017) states, Canada is a country that was built on large-scale racism. In Canada, the "racial groups most commonly identified as affected include Indigenous or Aboriginal Peoples, Black or African people, and Muslims or people from the Middle East" (Environics, 2019, p. 4). Additionally, recent polls indicate that 69% of people living in Quebec have biases towards Islam, while 54% of Canadians, as a whole, have a negative opinion of the faith (Bakali, 2015). In the U.S. anti-Islam groups received more than $119 million in funding between 2008 and 2011. In 2013, the inner core of the US-based Islamophobia network was comprised of 37 organizations whose primary purpose was to promote prejudice against or hatred of Islam and Muslims (Council on American-Islamic Relations, 2013; Ryder & Umut, 2009).

3.5 Conclusion

Although Islamophobia is a recently coined term, it refers to a multilayered history of fear and hatred of Muslims in the West, in general, and North America in particular. This chapter has provided a brief historical overview of Islamophobia in North America. Islamophobia has deep historical roots that go back to early periods of the Middle Ages and Christian Crusades. To be more specific, historical periods of the development of negative images of Islam and Muslims go back to the conflict between Christianity and Islam when Prophet Muhammad began to convey his message to people in seventh century Arabia. Christian supremacy was challenged by the success of Muslims. The new religion encountered resistance and prejudice from the Christian establishment where negative stereotypes of Muslims were intensified in Europe during the Crusade. In the sixteenth century, North American colonies were founded and impacted by negative European stereotypes of Muslims and Islam. After the end of the Crusades and the beginning of the West's ascendancy, followed by colonialism, negative attitudes toward Muslims were further exacerbated. During the last two decades, particularly after the 9/11 terrorist attacks, advocates of far-right movements and white supremacists, allied with extreme evangelicals, have been key drivers of Islamophobia in North America. More recently, during the presidency of Donald Trump, supremacists and right-wing groups along with media and conspiracy theorists carried on extensive anti-Muslim bigotry messages and Islamophobic agendas in both the U.S. and Canada.

References

Abdel-Malek, A. (1963). Orientalism in Crisis. *Diogenes, 11*(44), 104–112.

Aked, H., Jones, M., & Miller, D. (2019). *Islamophobia in Europe: How governments are enabling the far-right "counter-jihad" movement*. Public Interest Investigations. Retrieved from https://research-information.bris.ac.uk/files/192414854/Aked_Jones_Miller_Counterjihad_report_2019.pdf.

Al Badaai, M. S. N. (2017). *Situating African American Muslim slave narratives in American literature*. PhD thesis, College of Humanities and Social Sciences, United Arab Emirates University. Retrieved from https://scholarworks.uaeu.ac.ae/cgi/viewcontent.cgi?article=1643&context=all_theses

Allen, C. (2010). *Islamophobia*. Ashgate.

Anderson, K. (1991) *Vancouver's Chinatown: Racial discourse in Canada, 1875-1980*.

Angus Reid Institute. (2015, March 26). *Religion and faith in Canada today: Strong belief, ambivalence and rejection define our views*. Retrieved from http://angusreid.org/faith-in-canada/

Archive.today. (2007, July 29). Security and terrorism – Briefing. Washington, DC: United Press International. Retrieved from https://archive.vn/20070729234432/http://www.upi.com/Security_Terrorism/Briefing/2007/06/06/perry_us_eyed_iran_attack_after_bombing/7045/#selection-1027.25-1027.39

Austin, A. D. (1984). *African Muslims in Antebellum America: A sourcebook*. Garland.

Backhouse, C. (1999). *Colour-coded: A legal history of racism in Canada, 1900–1950*. University of Toronto Press.

Bakali, N. (2015). Challenging anti-Muslim racism through a critical race curriculum in Quebec secondary schools. *Critical Intersections in Education, 3*, 19–24.

Baldwin, A., Cameron, L., & Kobayashi, A. (2011). *Rethinking the great white north: Race, nature, and the historical geographies of whiteness in Canada*. UBC Press.

Bebbington, D. W. (1993). *Evangelicalism in modern Britain: A history from the 1730s to the 1980s*. Routledge.

Berger, P., Davie, G., & Fokas, E. (2008). *Religious America, secular Europe?* Ashgate Publishing Company.

Bhattacharya, K. (2021, March 25). De/colonizing educational research. *Oxford Research Encyclopedia of Education*. Oxford University Press. Retrieved from. https://doi.org/10.1093/acrefore/9780190264093.013.1386

bin Laden, O. (2008). Declaration of jihad against Jews and Crusaders. In M. Perry & E. N. Howard (Eds.), *The theory and practice of Islamic terrorism: An anthology* (pp. 41–48). Palgrave Macmillan.

Blanks, D. R. (1999). Western views of Islam in the premodern period: A brief history of past approaches. In D. R. Blanks & M. Frassetto (Eds.), *Western views of Islam in medieval and early modern Europe* (pp. 11–54). St. Martin's Press.

Blanks, D. R., & Frassetto, D. R. (1999). Introduction. In D. R. Blanks & M. Frassetto (Eds.), *Western views of Islam in medieval and early modern Europe* (pp. 1–10). St. Martin's Press.

Cameron, E. (2004). The historical background: From 'The contributions of other ethnic groups' (Report of the Royal Commision on Bilingualism and Biculturalism, Book IV). In E. Cameron (Ed.), *Multiculturalism and immigration in Canada: An introductory reader* (pp. 3–16). Canadian Scholars Press.

Carlson, A. (2020, July 27). Arkansas Sen. draws backlash after arguing Founding Fathers saw slavery as "Necessary Evil." *People*. Retrieved from https://people.com/politics/tom-cotton-founding-fathers-slavery-necesary-evil/

Central Intelligence Agency. (2020). *The world fact book*. Central Intelligence Agency. Retrieved from https://www.cia.gov/library/publications/the-world-factbook/geos/us.html

Council on American-Islamic Relations. (1997). *The state of Muslim civil rights in the United Sates: Unveiling prejudice*. Retrieved from https://www.cair.com/wp-content/uploads/2020/08/1997-The_Status_of_Muslim_Civil_Rights_in_the_United_States_1997.pdf

Council on American-Islamic Relations. (2013). *Islamophobia network funded with $119 million 2008 to 2011*. Retrieved from https://ca.cair.com/sandiego/updates/cair-report-islamophobia-network-funded-with-119-million-2008-to-2011/

Curtis, E. E. (2009). *Muslims in America: A short history*. Oxford University Press.

Curtis, E. E. (2013). The Black Muslim scare of the twentieth century: The history of state Islamophobia and its post 9/11 variations. In C. W. Ernst (Ed.), *Islamophobia in America: The anatomy of intolerance* (pp. 75–106). Palgrave Macmillan.

Daniel, N. (1960). *Islam and the West: The making of an image*. Edinburgh University Press.

Dawson, E. M., & Chatman, E. A. (2001). Reference group theory with implications for information studies: A theoretical essay. *Information Research, 6*(3). Retrieved from http://informationr.net/ir/6-3/paper105.html#ref4

Diouf, S. A. (1998). *Servants of Allah: African Muslims enslaved in the Americas*. New York University Press.

Dossa, S. (2008). Lethal Muslims: White-trashing Islam and the Arabs. *Journal of Muslim Minority Affairs, 28*(2), 225–236.

Douglass, S. L. (2009). Teaching about religion, Islam, and the world in public and private schooling curricula. In Y. Y. Haddad, F. Senzai, & J. I. Smith (Eds.), *Educating the Muslims of America* (pp. 85–108). Oxford University Press.

Drayton, R. (2005, August 20). *The wealth of the west was built on Africa's exploitation*. The Guardian. Retrieved from https://www.theguardian.com/politics/2005/aug/20/past.hearafrica05

el-Aswad, el-S. (2005). Review of Islam in urban America: Sunni Muslims in Chicago. *Digest of Middle East Studies, 14*(1), 78–81.

el-Aswad, el-S. (2008). *al-istishrāq al-jadīd: Jadaliyyat al-thunā'iyya al-thaqāfiyya bayn al-gharb/ al-sharq wa al-gharb/al-islām* (New Orientalism: A dialect of cultural dualism between West/ East and West/Islam). *Thaqafat, 21*, 204–233.

el-Aswad, el-S. (2011). Review of a history of Islam in America: From the new world to the new world order. *Digest of Middle East Studies, 20*(1), 113–116.

el-Aswad, el-S. (2012). *Muslim worldviews and everyday lives.* AltaMira Press.

el-Aswad, el-S. (2013a). Images of Muslims in western scholarship and media after 9/11. *Digest of Middle East Studies, 22*(1), 39–56.

el-Aswad, el-S. (2013b). Muslim Americans. In C. E. Cortés (Ed.), *Multicultural America: A multimedia encyclopaedia* (pp. 1525–1530). Sage.

el-Aswad, el-S. (2013c). Arab Americans. In C. E. Cortés (Ed.), *Multicultural America: A multimedia encyclopedia* (pp. 265–270). Sage.

el-Aswad, el-S. (2019). *The quality of life and policy issues among the Middle East and North African countries.* Springer.

el-Aswad, el-S. (2021a). Oriental images and ethics: British empire and the Arab Gulf (1727–1971) – A perspective from historical anthropology. *Anthropos, 116*(2), 319–330.

el-Aswad, el-S. (2021b). Oriental images and ethics: British empire and the Arab Gulf (1727–1971) – A perspective from historical anthropology. *Anthropos, 116*(2), 319–330.

el-Aswad, el-S., Sirgy, M. J., Estes, R., & Rahtz, D. R. (2020). Global Jihad and international media use. *Oxford research encyclopedia of communication.* New York and Oxford: Oxford University Press. doi:https://doi.org/10.1093/acrefore/9780190228613.013.1151.

Environics. (2016). *Survey of muslims in Canada 2016. Environics Institute for Survey,* Toronto, ON. Retrieved from https://nsiip.ca/wp-content/uploads/survey_of_muslims_in_canada_2016_final_report.pdf

Environics. (2019). *Race relations in Canada 2019: A survey of Canadian public opinion and experience.* Toronto, ON: Environics Institute for Survey. Retrieved from https://www.environicsinstitute.org/docs/default-source/project-documents/race-relations-2019-survey/race-relations-in-canada-2019-survey%2D%2D-executive-summary-english.pdf?sfvrsn=10442386_2

Esses, V. M., & Abelson, D. E. (2017). *Twenty-first-century immigration to North America: Newcomers in turbulent times.* McGill-Queen's University Press.

Estes, R. J. (2017). The search for well-being: From ancient to modern times. In R. J. Estes & M. J. Sirgy (Eds.), *The Pursuit of human well-being: The untold global history* (pp. 3–30). Springer.

Estes, R. J., Land, K. C., Michalos, A. M., Phillips, R., & Sirgy, M. J. (2017). Well-being in Canada and the United States. In R. J. Estes & M. J. Sirgy (Eds.), *The pursuit of human well-being: The untold global history* (pp. 257–299). Springer.

Fayazmanesh, S. (2003). The politics of the U.S. Economic sanctions against Iran. *Review of Radical Political Economics, 35*(3), 221–240. https://doi.org/10.1177/0486613403254535

Firestone, R. (2010). Islamophobia & Anti-Semitism: History and possibility. *Arches Quarterly, 4* (7), 42–51.

Fredrickson, G. M. (1981). *White supremacy: A comparative study in American and South African history.* Oxford University Press.

Geddes, J. (2013, October 03). *Canadian anti-Muslim sentiment is rising, disturbing new poll reveals.* Maclean's. Retrieved from https://www.macleans.ca/politics/land-of-intolerance/

GhaneaBassiri, K. (2010). *A history of Islam in America: From the new world to the new world order.* Cambridge University Press.

GhaneaBassiri, K. (2013). Islamophobia and American history: Religious stereotyping and out-grouping of Muslims in the United States. In C. W. Ernst (Ed.), *Islamophobia in America: The anatomy of intolerance* (pp. 53–74). Palgrave Macmillan.

Gismondi, M. J. (2017, August 15). *Don't tell me Canadians are less racist than Americans. We're just quieter about it. The Conversation.* Retrieved from https://theconversation.com/quiet-canadian-ugly-american-does-racism-differ-north-of-the-border-81388

Gjelten, T. (2018, December 13). *Southern Baptist Seminary confronts history of slaveholding and 'deep racism'.* NPR. Retrieved from https://www.npr.org/2018/12/13/676333342/southern-baptist-seminary-confronts-history-of-slaveholding-and-deep-racism

Gomez, M. A. (1994). Muslims in early America. *The Journal of Southern History, 60*(4), 671–710.

Goodman, A. H., Moses, Y. H., & Jones, J. L. (2012). *Race: Are we so different?* Wiley-Blackwell.

Gottschalk, P. (2019, June 03). *Hate crimes associated with both Islamophobia and anti-Semitism have a long history in America's past.* The Conversation. Retrieved from https://theconversation.com/hate-crimes-associated-with-both-islamophobia-and-anti-semitism-have-a-long-history-in-americas-past-116255

Gottschalk, P., & Greenberg, G. (2008). *Islamophobia: Making Muslims the enemy.* Rowman & Littlefield Publishers.

Green, T. H. (2015). *The fear of Islam: An introduction to Islamophobia in the West.* Fortress Press.

Habib, M. N., & Habib, N. (2015). *History of the Muslims of Regina, Saskatchewan, and their organizations: Islamic association, Canadian council of Muslim women, Muslim for peace and justice a cultural integration.* Indiana University.

Hamdani, D. (2015). *Canadian Muslims: A statistical review.* The Canadian Dawn Foundation.

Hanniman, W. (2008). Canadian Muslims, Islamophobia and national security. *International Journal of Law, Crime and Justice, 36*, 271–285.

Hardwick, S. W., Shelley, F. M., & Holtgrieve, D. G. (2013). *The geography of North America: Environment, culture, economy.* Pearson Education.

Helly, D. (2004). Are Muslims discriminated against in Canada since September 2001? *Canadian Ethnic Studies Journal, 36*(1), 24–48.

Henry, F., & Tator, C. (2006). *The colour of democracy: Racism in Canadian Society.* Thomson Nelson.

Hussain, A. (2018). *Islam in North America.* Oxford Bibliographies. Retrieved from https://www.oxfordbibliographies.com/view/document/obo-9780195390155/obo-9780195390155-0057.xml

Institute for Social Policy and Understanding. (2019). *American Muslim poll 2019: Predicting and preventing Islamophobia.* Retrieved from https://www.ispu.org/american-muslim-poll-2019-predicting-and-preventing-islamophobia/#4t

Johnston, D. M. (2016). Combating Islamophobia. *Journal of Ecumenical Studies, 51*(2), 165–173. https://doi.org/10.1353/ecu.2016.0022

Jones, R. P. (2020). *White too long: The legacy of white supremacy in American Christianity.* Simon & Schuste.

Joshi, K. Y. (2018, May 24). Race and religion in U.S. public life. In *Oxford Research Encyclopedia of Religion.* New York: Oxford University Press. doi:https://doi.org/10.1093/acrefore/9780199340378.013.460.

Kalin, I. (2009). Roots of misconception: Euro-American perceptions of Islam before and after September 11. In J. E. B. Lumbard (Ed.), *Islam, fundamentalism, and the betrayal of tradition: Essays by western Muslim scholars* (pp. 149–193). World Wisdom, Inc.

Kalkan, K. O., Layman, G. C., & Uslaner, E. M. (2009). 'Bands of others'? Attitudes toward Muslims in contemporary American Society. *Journal of Politics, 71*(3), 847–862.

Kazemipur, A. (2014). *The Muslim question in Canada: A story of segmented integration.* University of British Colombia (UBC) Press.

Kazi, N. (2018). *Islamophobia, race, and global politics.* Rowman & Littlefield.

Kidd, T. S. (2009). *American Christians and Islam: Evangelical culture and Muslims from the colonial period to the age of terrorism.* Princeton University Press.

Khalidi, R. (2020). *The hundred years' war on Palestine: A history of settler colonialism and resistance, 1917–2017.* Metropolitan Books, Henry Holt and Company.

Kiernan, V. G. (1980). *America: The new imperialism from white settlement to world hegemony.* Zed Press.

Kolchin, P. (2003). *American slavery: 1619–1877.* Hill and Wang.

Kumar, D. (2012). *Islamophobia and the politics of empire.* Haymarket Books.

Lean, N. (2017). *The Islamophobia industry: How the right manufactures fear of Muslims*. Pluto Press.

Leonnig, C. D. (2006). Iran held liable in Khobar attack. *Washington Post*. Retrieved form https://www.washingtonpost.com/wp-dyn/content/article/2006/12/22/AR2006122200455.html

Love, E. (2017). *Islamophobia and racism in America*. New York University Press.

Lowrie, A. L. (1995). The campaign against Islam and American foreign policy. *Middle East Policy, 4*(1/2), 210–219.

Marr, T. (2006). *The cultural roots of American Islamicism*. Cambridge University Press.

Merton, R. K. (1968). *Social theory and social structure*. Free Press.

Migration Policy Institute. (2020). North America. Retrieved from https://www.migrationpolicy.org/regions/north-america

Morey, P., Yakin, A., & Forte, A. (2019). *Contesting Islamophobia: Anti-Muslim prejudice in media, culture and politics*. I.B. Tauris.

Nagra, B. (2011). *Unequal citizenship: Being Muslim and Canadian in the post 9/11 era*. PhD thesis, University of Toronto. Retrieved from https://tspace.library.utoronto.ca/bitstream/1807/29823/1/Nagra_Baljit_201106_PhD_thesis.pdf

Nelson, C. A. (2017, July 21). *The Canadian narrative about slavery is wrong*. Walrus. Retrieved from https://thewalrus.ca/the-canadian-narrative-about-slavery-is-wrong/

Nimer, M. (2002). *The North American Muslim resource guide: Muslim community life in the United States and Canada*. Routledge.

Omi, W., & Winant, H. (2015). *Racial formation in the United States*. Routledge.

Perry, B., & Scrivens, R. (2019). *Right-wing extremism in Canada*. Palgrave.

Pew Research Center. (2011). *The future of the global Muslim population*. Retrieved from https://www.pewforum.org/2011/01/27/thefuture-of-the-global-muslim-population/

Pew Research Center. (2016, May 5). *Public uncertain, divided over America's place in the world*. Retrieved from https://www.pewresearch.org/politics/2016/05/05/public-uncertain-divided-over-americas-place-in-the-world/

Pew Research Center. (2017a, July 26), *U.S. Muslims concerned about their place in society, but continue to believe in the American Dream*. Retrieved from https://www.pewforum.org/2017/07/26/findings-from-pew-research-centers-2017-survey-of-us-muslims/

Pew Research Center. (2017b, November 15), *Assaults against Muslims in U.S. surpass 2001 level*. Retrieved from https://www.pewresearch.org/fact-tank/2017/11/15/assaults-against-muslims-in-u-s-surpass-2001-level/

Pew Research Center. (2018, January 3). *New estimates show U.S. Muslim population continues to grow*. Retrieved from https://www.pewresearch.org/fact-tank/2018/01/03/new-estimates-show-u-s-muslim-population-continues-to-grow/

Pluralism Project. (2020). *Muslims and American politics*. Harvard University. Retrieved from https://pluralism.org/muslims-and-american-politics

Polk, W. R. (2018). *Crusade and jihad: The thousand-year war between the Muslim world and the global north*. Yale University Press.

Powell, K. A. (2011). Framing Islam: An analysis of US media coverage of terrorism since 9/11. *Communication Studies, 62*(1), 90–112.

Rana, J. (2007). The history of Islamophobia. *Souls, 9*(2), 148–161.

Read, J. G. (2008). Muslims in America. *Contexts, 7*(4), 39–43. Retrieved from https://journals.sagepub.com/doi/pdf/10.1525/ctx.2008.7.4.39

Renima, A., Tiliouine, H., & Estes, R. J. (2016). The Islamic golden age: A story of the triumph of the Islamic civilization. In H. Tiliouine & R. J. Estes (Eds.), *The state of social progress of Islamic societies: Social, economic, political, and ideological challenges* (pp. 25–52). Springer International Publishing.

Ross, J. I. (1992). Contemporary radical right-wing violence in Canada: A quantitative analysis. *Terrorism and Political Violence, 4*(3), 72–101.

Runnymede Trust. (1997). Islamophobia: A challenge for us all. *The Runnymede Commission on British Muslims and Islamophobia*. Retrieved from https://www.runnymedetrust.org/uploads/publications/pdfs/islamophobia.pdf

Ryder, N., & Umut, T. (2009). Islamophobia or an important weapon? An analysis of the US financial war on terrorism. *Journal of Banking Regulation, 10*(4), 307–320.

Said, E. W. (1978). *Orientalism: Western conceptions of the Orient*. Pantheon Books.

Said, E. W. (1981). *Covering Islam: How the media and the experts determine how we see the rest of the world*. Pantheon Book.

Salaita, S. G. (2006). *Anti-Arab racism in the USA: Where it comes from and what it means for politics today*. Pluto Press.

Sardar, Z. (1995). Racism, identity and Muslims in the West. In S. Z. Abedin & Z. Sardar (Eds.), *Muslim minorities in the West* (pp. 1–17). Grey Seal.

Satia, P. (2008). *Spies in Arabia: The Great War and the cultural foundations of Britain's covert empire in the middle east*. Oxford University Press.

Semati, M. (2010). Islamophobia, culture and race in the age of empire. *Cultural Studies, 24*(2), 256–275.

Sha'ban, F. (1991). *Islam and Arabs in early American thought: The roots of orientalism*. The Acorn Press.

Shaheen, J. G. (2001). *Reel bad arabs: How hollywood vilifies a people*. Olive Branch Press.

Sheridan, L. P. (2006). Islamophobia pre- and post-September 11th, 2001. *Journal of Interpersonal Violence, 21*(3), 317–336.

Sherrard, B. (2017, December 19). Islam and the Middle East in the American imagination. In *Oxford Research Encyclopedia of Communication*. Oxford University Press. Doi: doi:https://doi.org/10.1093/acrefore/9780199340378.013.508.

Sirgy, M. J. (2020). *Positive balance: A theory of well-being and positive mental health*. Springer Nature.

Sirgy, M. J., Estes, R., el-Aswad, el-S., & Rahtz, D. (2019). *Combatting Jihadist terrorism through nation-building: A quality-of-life perspective*. Springer International Publishers.

Smith, J. I. (2010). *Islam in America*. Columbia University Press.

Southern, R. W. (1978). *Western views of Islam in the middle ages*. Cambridge, MA.

Spencer, R. (2017). *What it means to be alt-right*. Alt-Right com. Retrieved from https://altright.com/2017/08/11/what-it-means-to-be-alt-right/

Statistics Canada. (2017). *Census profile, 2016 census*. Retrieved from https://www12.statcan.gc.ca/census-recensement/index-eng.cfm?MM=1

Steinback, R. (2011). *Jihad against Islam. Southern Poverty Law Center: Intelligence report*, issue 142. Retrieved from http://www.splcenter.org/get-informed/intelligence-report/browse-all-issues/2011/summer/jihad-against-islam

Taylor, A. (2001). *American colonies: The settling of North America*. Penguin Books.

Thobani, S. (2007). *Exalted subjects: Studies in the making of race and nation in Canada*. University of Toronto Press.

Tolan, J. V. (2019). *Faces of Muhammad: Western perceptions of the prophet of Islam from the Middle Ages to today*. Princeton University Press.

Tyrer, D. (2013). *The politics of Islamophobia: Race, power and fantasy*. Pluto Press.

USA Congress (2001). *Public law 107–56—OCT. 26, 2001*. Retrieved from https://www.congress.gov/107/plaws/publ56/PLAW-107publ56.pdf

Ward, P. (2002). *White Canada forever: Popular attitudes and public policy toward Orientals in British Columbia*. McGill-Queen's University Press.

Watt, J. (2019). *British orientalisms, 1759–1835*. Cambridge University Press.

Woodward, B. (2012). *The price of politics*. Simon & Schuster.

Yousif, A. (1953). *Muslims in Canada: A question of identity*. Legas.

Part II
Outcomes of Islamophobia

Chapter 4
Outcomes of Islamophobia

4.1 Introduction

Backed by reliable outcome indicators, this chapter investigates the impact of Islamophobia on the economic-political, religious and social well-being of Muslims residing in North America by employing a quality-of-life approach (Sirgy et al., 2019). It examines the relationship between Islamophobia and overall well-being and life satisfaction of Muslims living in North America.

The peoples of Canada and the United States share extensive social histories as exhibited by their experiences as former European colonies, the size and richness of their economies and natural resource base, the depth of their human resources, and the diversity of their social, political, cultural, religious, racial, and ethnic makeup. The residents of both countries easily cross borders into one another's country (Estes et al., 2017). Economically, Canada and the U.S. enjoy the world's most comprehensive bilateral trade and investment relationship, with goods and services trade totaling more than $680 billion in 2017, and two-way investment stocks of more than $800 billion (Central Intelligence Agency, 2020). Canada and the United States "are each other's largest economic partners, with a combined trading level exceeding 25.9% of the world's total economic output of USD74,555 billion in 2015" (Estes et al., 2017, pp. 258–259).

Notwithstanding the economic prosperity of North America, race has negatively impacted people's economic, cultural, educational, social and political spaces (Allen, 2012; Lean, 2017; Love, 2017). Islamophobia is entwined in a wider racial politics and becomes "an emblematic expression of contemporary biopolitical racism" (Tyrer, 2013, p. 21). As a contemporary domain of racism, Islamophobia is composed of an array of postulates, images, and practices which serve not to differentiate and dominate but also "to deny full participation in economic, social, political and cultural life by the essence that they posit" (Anthias & Davis, 1992, p. 15). The institutionalized apprehension of Muslims is both a driver and an outcome of Islamophobia leading to negative consequences reflected in economic disparities and political inequalities between Muslims and non-Muslim communities in North America. Put differently, Islamophobia harms the North American economy as it excludes Muslims from mainstream social, economic and political affairs. Moreover, Islamophobia is designed and intended to prevent Muslims from making positive contributions to civil society and their communities or countries in which they live (Hayoun, 2013).

4.2 Economic-Political Outcomes

Immigrant populations and minorities are expected to participate in the economic-political activities of the host country. They are also expected to equally share in the economic outcome and prosperity enjoyed by the majority of that country. Islamophobia is not merely an adverse aspect of social problems, but is a structural and industrial phenomenon reflected in economic-political systems, legislation, and law enforcement practices. The Islamophobia industry, at that, is driven by networks of individuals and institutions that have managed to attach Islamophobia permanently to the banner of the right-wing populism, opposing immigration, particularly from Muslim countries (Lean, 2017; Spencer, 2017). Islamophobia, as a form of racism (Anthias & Davis, 1992; Grosfoguel, 2012; Tyrer, 2013), is considered a system of structuring opportunity and delegating values to people and groups, based on phenotypic, religious and cultural characteristics, that results in economic advantages of some individuals and communities at the expense of others (Jones, 2000; Love, 2017).

Economic inequality has been one of the defining issues of the Islamophobic phenomenon to put the well-being of Muslim minorities at risk. Evidence indicates that people from ethnic minority groups have lower incomes and are concentrated in economically and environmentally poorer geographic areas, live in overcrowded accommodations, and have higher rates of unemployment than their ethnic majority counterparts (Nazroo & Bécares, 2017). This statement is applicable to North American Muslims, especially since 9/11, despite the fact that since 1871, the U.S., has maintained its position as the world's largest economy. The size of the U.S. economy was at $20.58 trillion in 2018 and $22.32 trillion in 2020, and is expected to reach $24.88 trillion by 2023 (Investopedia, 2020). However, "the United States is not among the group of most socially developed countries. This unfortunate reality results from the country's wide spread poverty (1:5 children are officially classified as poor), the country's very high crime and violence rates—especially that associated with gun violence" (Estes, 2019, p. 565, footnote 4). The problem is that racism and inequality, durable and dynamic stratifying elements in U.S. society and culture, are imbedded in American institutions and everyday lives as well as in the interests of wealthiest elites, who, as the top 1% of the population, make 40% of the country's wealth, having greater wealth than the bottom 90% of households combined (Ingraham, 2017). The daily language in the U.S. reflects the continuing racialization hierarchy, with white at the top (Goodman et al., 2012).

The following subsections address, in detail the economic outcomes in the U.S. and Canada.

4.2.1 The U.S.

Prior to September 11, 2001, many Muslim Americans "achieved prosperity in business, academia, engineering, and other fields and as such were successful and mainstreamed in U.S. society and politics" (el-Aswad, el-S., 2006, p. 113). However, the image of Muslim Americans', particularly Arab Muslims', success changed dramatically after 9/11/2001 (el-Aswad, el-S., 2013a, b, c). Though some were and continue to be successful entrepreneurs and doctors, since 9/11 Muslims have faced greater scrutiny, greater discrimination in the work place, and greater difficulty getting hired if their social media platforms reveal their religious preference (Lakhani, 2017).

Even before 9/11 discriminatory actions against Muslims included, for example, the firing of Muslim women from jobs because of their religious garb, and the harassment of Muslims at the nation's airports, public facilities, and government agencies because of their apparent religious affiliation (Council on American Islamic Relations, 1997).

In spite of the wealth the U.S. enjoys, Muslim Americans overall suffer from economic inequality (DeSilver, 2013; Gongloff, 2014). In its poll about Muslim Americans' place in U.S. society, the Pew Research Center (2017a) indicated that 40% of Muslim American household incomes fell under $30,000 as compared with 32% of the U.S. population as a whole. While 35% of Muslim households fell into the middle range of income (between $30,000 and $99,999), 45% of the general population of American households did so. The share of Muslims who reported owning a home (37%) was substantially lower than that of other Americans (57%). Furthermore, 44% of Muslim adults said they were employed full time, as compared with 49% of other Americans. Overall, 29% of Muslims were underemployed compared with 12% of other American adults.

The findings of the Pew Research Center (2017a) were similar to those of the Institute for Social Policy and Understanding (ISPU) (2017) according to which Muslim Americans reported far lower incomes as compared with those of other faith communities. The percentage of Muslim Americans whose annual income was less than $30,000 in 2017 was 35%, compared with Protestants (14%), Catholic (15%), Jewish (17%), non-affiliated groups (18%) and the general public (14%). Similar economic indicators were evident regarding the annual income indicator of $30,000–50,000 according to which Muslims rated the highest (18%) as compared with other faith communities and the general public (11%). Concerning the annual income indicator of $50,000–$100,000, Catholic groups (at 27%) ranked higher than Jewish (25%), Muslim (23%) and Protestant groups (21%). On the other hand, the percentage of Muslim Americans with a greater than $100,000 annual income rated 14%, lower than other faith communities (Table 4.1).

Table 4.1 Economic indicators of Muslim Americans' income compared to other faith groups

Annual Income	Less than $30,000	$30,000–50,000	$50,000–$100,000	More than $100,000
Muslim	35%	18%	23%	14%
Protestant	14%	13%	21%	20%
Catholic	15%	11%	27%	21%
Jewish	17%	11%	25%	29%
Non-affiliated	18%	13%	22%	24%
General Public	14%	11%	23%	21%

Source: Adapted with modification from the Institute for Social Policy and Understanding (2017)
Note: Numbers do not add up to 100% because remaining respondents did not provide a response to this question

Table 4.2 Economic indicators of the income among American Muslim ethnic groups

Annual income	Less than $30,000	$30,000–50,000	$50,000–$100,000	More than $100,000
Black	44%	14%	23%	7%
White	28%	15%	28%	19%
Asian	30%	16%	25%	20%
Arab	37%	21%	17%	16%
General Public-Black	19%	15%	23%	14%
General Public-White	12%	12%	24%	24%

Source: Adapted with modification from the Institute for Social Policy and Understanding (2017)
Note: Numbers do not add up to 100% because remaining respondents did not provide a response to this question

Indicators of economic disparities were also found among Muslim American minorities, according to the ISPU (2017). For those whose annual income was less than $30,000 in 2017, Black Muslims ranked the lowest (44%), followed by Arabs (37%), Asians (30%), and White (28%) as compared to the general public-Black (19%) and general public-White (12%) populations. Regarding the annual income of $30,000–50,000 indicator, Arab Americans, ranked 21%, ranking higher than Asian (16%), White (15%) and Black (14%) as compared to the general public-Black (15%) and general public-White (12%) populations. For the annual income of $50,000–$100,000 indicator, White Muslim Americans (28%) ranked higher than Asian (25%), Black (23%) and Arab (17%) as compared to the general public-Black (23%) and general public-White (24%) populations. Black Muslims (7%) ranked the lowest regarding the more than $100,000 annual income indicator, while Asian Muslims (20%) ranked the highest, followed by White Muslims (19%), and Arab Muslims (16%) as compared to the general public-Black (14%), which was also low, and the general public-White (24%), which was the highest (Table 4.2).

Islamophobia has created a sort of socio-economic anxiety. For instance, in 2010, Muslim workers in the U.S. reported that they were victims of employment

Table 4.3 American faith groups' views of Muslims as committed to America's well-being

	Muslim	Jewish	Catholic	Protestant	White Evangelical	Non-affiliated	General Public
Most Americans believe that Muslims are committed to Well-being of America	81%	66%	64%	50%	30%	65%	**55%**

Source: Adapted with modification from the Institute for Social Policy and Understanding (2018)

discrimination. Workers reported being called names (such as 'terrorist' or 'Osama') by co-workers, and complained that the employers barred them "from the headscarf or participating in prayer times" (Moore, 2012, p. 93). In 2018, more than 80% of Muslim Americans reported that Muslims were committed to the well-being of America. Table 4.3 shows how U.S. major faith groups and the non-affiliated view Muslims as committed to America's well-being. It is to be noted that white evangelicals provided Muslims with the lowest rating (30%), followed by Protestants (50%) (Institute for Social Policy and Understanding, 2018). Despite economic inequality and disparity, most Muslims continue to hold the view that immigrants strengthen the U.S. because of their hard work and talents (Pew Research Center, 2017a).

Political outcomes of Islamophobia are mirrored in the marginalization and exclusion of Muslims from mainstream civil and political affairs in North America. Islamophobia is understood not only as a fear of the "other", but as a political campaign that is tied to political power subjecting Muslims to the power of the state and the interests of others (Tutt, 2013). Islamophobia implies the perception that Muslims are people who encourage violence and extremism and are not able to execute important public and government tasks or make necessary decisions without being influenced by their religion. In a poll conducted by the Arab American Institute (2014), Republicans (75%), more than triple that of Democrats (23%), revealed that they think religion would influence Muslims' decision-making if they were to attain important positions of influence in the U.S. government.

After 9/11, fear of government surveillance created a chill over freedom of expression and freedom of association on college campuses and congregations for American Muslims (U.S. Commission on Civil Rights, 2014). According to the Pew Research Center (2017a), 59% of Muslims began to think their communications, particularly phone calls and emails, were monitored by the U.S. government. Muslim American women (70%) are more apt to think their communications were subject to government monitoring than men (48%). Negative policies upheld by the U.S. government, including surveillance of Muslims (in mosques, on the Internet, and through library records, bank accounts, and places of employment) and a travel ban, have lead to the increase in Islamophobia (Institute for Social Policy and Understanding, 2018). Such biased attitudes and practices by the U.S. government have negative impact on the well-being and life satisfaction of Muslim Americans.

Table 4.4   Cases of hate crimes against Muslims in the U.S. 2014–2016

Year	2014	2015	2016
Crime against Muslims	Incidents	Incidents	Incidents
	154	257 (increased 67%)	307 (increased 19%)

Source: Adapted with modification from Pew Research Center (2017b)

In 2018, only 27% of Muslims reported being satisfied with the way things were going in the U.S. as compared to the general public (29%). This is a marked decrease from the score in 2017 when 41% of Muslims were satisfied, and from the score in 2016 when 63% of Muslims were satisfied.

In 2016, 75% of Muslim American adults complained that discrimination and hate crimes against Muslims in the U.S. were increasing, a view shared by 69% of adults in the general public (Pew Research Center, 2017b). The total number of anti-Muslim incidents increased from 154 in 2014 to 257 in 2015, reflecting an increase of 67%. In 2016, there were 307 incidents, marking a 19% increase from 2015 (Table 4.4). Even Muslim congresswomen have faced Islamophobia and racism by the former President Donald Trump and his administration (Choi, 2020; NPR, 2019; Stewart, 2019).

The outcomes of these policies devastate the relationship between the Muslim community and the U.S. Government. Muslim organizations maintain that these governmental policies create feelings of anxiety, and isolation that separate Muslims from the American mainstream. Additionally, 78% of Muslims agree that the negative things politicians say regarding Muslims is harmful not only to the Muslim community, but to the U.S. as a whole (Institute for Social Policy and Understanding, 2018). It is to be noted that anxiety, isolation and stress include mental, cognitive, emotional, social, and somatic difficulties (Akram-Pall & Moodley, 2016).

4.2.2   Canada

Canada's nominal GDP, ranking tenth worldwide, was about $1.774 trillion in 2017 and is expected to reach $2.13 trillion by 2023. Canada's per capita GDP of $46,260.71, ranked 16th globally (Central Intelligence Agency, 2020; Investopedia, 2020). However, limited economic opportunities, unemployment and discrimination are aspects of the everyday lives of Muslims in Canada. Although Muslims are on average younger and better educated than Canadian-born citizens, they experience higher rates of unemployment and lower incomes. Between 2002 and 2016, Canadian Muslims and those with no religious affiliation were almost tied for the lowest reported income. In 2002, Muslims had the lowest income, earning less than $30,000 annually. By 2016, Muslims earned $53,800 on average, compared with an average employment income of $63,000 for people in all other religiously affiliated categories (Statistics Canada, 2019). Unemployment, underemployment, and low-income

Table 4.5 Human Development Index (HDI) and Inequality-adjusted (IHDI) of Canada and the U.S.

Country	HDI value	HDI rank (out of 189 countries)	IHDI value	Loss (percent)
Canada	0.922	13	0.841	8.8
US	0.921	15	0.797	13.4

Source: Adapted with modification form United Nation Development Programme (2019)

rates are some of the main contributors to stress among Muslims in Canada (Jisrawi & Arnold, 2018). In 2016, when asked to identify what they considered to be the most critical problem facing them, 34% of Canadian Muslims stated the economy, followed by 18% who cited unemployment (as compared with 33% and 13% of non-Muslims, respectively) (Environics Institute for Survey Research, 2016).

Broadly, inequalities in economic resources lead to social and political dominance, resulting in discrimination, decline of development, and violation of human rights (Jones, 2000). To show the relationship between economic inequalities and decline of human development in both Canada and the U.S., this study refers to the Human Development Index (HDI). The HDI shows the average measure of basic human development achievements in a country. For instance, the United States' HDI value for 2018 was 0.920, which situated the country in the very high human development category, with a global rank of 15 out of 189 countries. However, there is also the Inequality-adjusted HDI (IHDI), which is basically the HDI discounted for inequalities. As the inequality in a country increases, the loss in human development also increases. For the U.S., when the value was discounted for inequality, the IHDI was calculated at 0.797, a loss of 13.4% (due to inequality in the distribution of the HDI dimension indices). The same observation is applicable to Canada. In 2018, Canada's HDI value was 0.922, and Canada achieved a global rank of 13 out of 189 countries; however, due to inequality, the IHDI fell to 0.84, a loss of 8.8% (United Nations Development Programme, 2019) (Table 4.5).

Inequality is considered as both a cause and outcome of corruption, lack of political rights, discrimination, and violence against minorities. When coupled with weak government systems and elites looking to take advantage of their power, corruption prevents the average citizen from accessing quality public goods and services like education, health care, or protection by the police (Transparency 2019). Despite the apparent economic advances of both Canada and the U.S., they have fallen in their global rank with regard to the global indicator of corruption. According to the Corruption Perceptions Index (CPI) conducted by Transparency International (2018, 2019), in 2018, Canada scored 81 (out of 100) and ranked 9 worldwide; however, in 2019, Canada lost 3 points, achieved a score of 77 and ranked 12 worldwide. Canada, though, was less corrupt than the U.S. whose score in 2018 was 71 and global ranking 22. Subsequently, in 2019, with a score of 68, the US ranked 23 worldwide (Table 4.6).

It is to be noted that the Social Progress Index (SPI) (2020) reached almost the same results concerning the indicator of corruption in both Canada and the U.S. For

Table 4.6 2018–2019 Corruption Perceptions Index (Canada and the U.S.)

	Score (100 = less corruption)		Global rank (out of 180 countries)	
Country	2018	2019	2018	2019
Canada	81	77	9	12
U.S.	71	68	22	23

Source: Adapted with modification from Transparency International (2018, 2019)

instance, in 2020, Canada scored 77 out of 100 and ranked 12 (out of 163 countries) on the indicator of corruption, while the U.S scored 69 out of 100 and ranked 22.

Comparable to the U.S. government, the Canadian government is known for its history of slavery and Muslim rights abuses. Troubled race relations and associated violence have long been a part of Canadian society (Parent & Ellis, 2014). In Canada, discriminatory political policies and practices by government agencies fortify anti-Muslim sentiment. Official use of profiling sends a message to the larger community that a person who fits a certain physical or religious description might be suspect (Perry & Poynting, 2006). Discrimination against Muslim Canadian communities have been detected "in organizational and government policies, practices, and procedures and normal ways of doing things" (Hanniman, 2008, p. 273).

Concerning the indicator of "political rights", in 2020, with a score of 40 out of 40, Canada outperformed the U.S., which achieved a score of 33 out of 40 and ranked globally 64 out of 163 countries. Furthermore, the U.S. underperformed on the indicator of "discrimination and violence against minorities", scoring 6.20 out of 10 and ranked 100 out of 163 countries, while Canada performed within the expected range of 2.50 out of 10 and ranked 11 out of 163 countries. Regarding the indicator of "equality of political power by socioeconomic position," Canada, with a grade of 3.22 out of 4, performed within the expected range, while the U.S., with a grade of 2.19 out of 4, did not. Finally, with reference to the indicator of "equality of political power by social group," Canada, with a score of 2.65 out of 4 and a global rank of 54 underperformed when compared to the U.S. which, with a score of 2.75 out of 4 and a global rank of 49, fell within the expected range (Social Progress Index, 2020) (Table 4.7).

Ethnographically, there is a tendency for Islamophobia to be exacerbated by the human crisis found in conditions such as that of the Covid-19 pandemic. For example, the widespread impact of the coronavirus has revealed that discrimination against minorities, including Muslims, plays a hidden role in people's economic and political lives. The following story was shared by Adam, a young Arab-American man living in Dearborn, Michigan. He narrated how he had worked diligently for a company dealing with sanitation and waste disposal. However, his employer began to lay off employees due to the Covid-19 pandemic. Adam reported that he felt sad and powerless to be among the first people to lose their jobs. It was low-paying job but his only source of likelihood. Adam expressed his suspicion that there was a sort of discrimination against Arab/Muslim employees as he heard that other Arab/Muslims were laid off. Adam was unable to find a new job and had to coast on unemployment benefits since the epidemic hit. Unfortunately the Michigan state

Table 4.7 Political rights and discrimination against minorities in Canada and the U.S. (2020)

Country	Political rights		Discrimination and violence against minorities		Equality of political power by socioeconomic position		Equality of political power by social group	
	Score (40 = full rights)	Global rank (out of 163)	Score (10 = high)	Global rank (out of 163)	Score (4 = equal power)	Global rank (out of 163)	Score (4 = equal power)	Global rank (out of 163)
Canada	40	1	2.50	11	3.22	6	2.65	56
U.S.	33	64	6.20	100	2.19	84	2.75	49

Source: Adapted with modification from Social Progress Index (2020)

government suspended his unemployment benefits. He is not sure what he is going to do or where he is going to live in the near future.

His story resonates in a similar narrative recounted by Adnan, a 35-year-old man who commuted between Windsor (Canada) and Dearborn looking for jobs. Adnan graduated with a B.A. from the University of Windsor in environmental engineering in 2010. After graduating, he was not able to find a job in his major. He said that he had to make a living working a few different gigs including construction work and landscaping. In December of 2019, he moved to the metro-Detroit area anticipating to begin an apprenticeship as an electric lineman which was supposed to begin in March of 2020. But, because of Covid-19, he was informed that the program was cancelled. He said, "my economic problem was always bad, but it became worse after the spread of Corona virus." Adnan spent almost all of his free time surfing the internet and spending time on conspiracy sites like Q-Anon and Infowars. He believed that there were plots against Arab and Muslims aimed at making it hard for them to find or have decent jobs. This troubling theory affected him psychologically. Compounded with the financial insecurity of his situation, he went back to Windsor where he attempted suicide.

Both the U.S. and Canada face the economic and political challenges of meeting public demands for quality improvements in health care, education, social services, and economic competitiveness (Central Intelligence Agency, 2020). Anti-Muslim racism and discrimination affect the full range of social and economic outcomes experienced by Muslim people (Nazroo & Bécares, 2017). The social and economic inequalities associated with racism and discrimination have negative impact on the health of Muslim minorities living in North America and other western countries.

4.3   Religious-Cultural Outcomes

The Runnymede Trust (1997, p. 4) defines Islamophobia as "unfounded prejudice and hostility. It refers also to the practical consequences of such hostility in unfair discrimination against Muslim individuals and communities, and to the exclusion of Muslims from mainstream political and social affairs."

Although race and religion are independent concepts, they interact in multifaceted ways, impacting the racial marking of religious identities. When religion is racialized, specific phenotypical features come to be associated in the popular mind with a given religion (Joshi, 2018; Pew Research Center, 2018). This is reflected in Islamophobia, which is a form of both racism and religious discrimination (Tyrer, 2013). Muslim organizations, mosques, and Muslims and their leaders are consistently subjected to a campaign of defamation and vilification by groups of neoconservative ideologists, Christian nationalists, evangelical Protestants, white supremacists, and influential think-tanks, among others. The following subsections address the religious-cultural outcomes in the U.S. and Canada.

4.3.1 The U.S.

Minorities with diverse religious, racial and cultural backgrounds are challenged by the vision of American belonging that is tightly linked to white Protestant identity as well as to individualist notions of a good religious citizen. This, in turn, complicates the perception that American nationhood is rooted in civic rather than ethnic membership, which reveals an intricate interplay between civic and ethnic drives of discrimination and exclusion (Braunstein, 2017). Researchers argue that because of their religious identity, Muslims, seemingly incompatible with American identity, are denied cultural citizenship (Garner & Selod, 2015). Culturally, prejudice is associated with the mainstream society's attitudes towards certain minority groups (Allport, 1979). For instance, Table 4.8 shows that Arabs and Muslims have the lowest favorable and highest unfavorable ratings among the ethnic/religious groups in the U.S.

Most conspicuous is the relatively higher regard Americans extend to Jews and evangelical Protestants, while Islam and its followers are assessed most unfavorably (Angus Reid Institute, 2015).

The negative impact of discrimination on the overall well-being of Muslims in North America is detectable and measurable. For instance, 82% of American adults say Muslims are subject to at least some discrimination in the United Sates (Masci, 2019). Asked about the extent to which being black, white, evangelical, or Muslim helps or hurts one's ability to get ahead in American society, Muslims are more likely than other racial or religious groups to say being Muslim hurts *a lot* (30%), followed by blacks (25%), evangelicals (5%), and whites (4%). On the contrary, Muslims are less likely than other racial or religious groups to say being Muslim helps *a lot* (3%), as compared with whites (38%), evangelicals (11%), and blacks (7%) (Pew Research Center, 2019) (Table 4.9).

Table 4.8 Americans' favorable/unfavorable attitudes toward ethnic/religious groups (2014)

Religion/Group		Total	Dem.	Rep.	Ind.	Young 18–29	Old 65+	White	Non-White
						Generations			
Arab	Favorable	32	38	28	27	42	32	30	38
	Unfavorable	39	30	54	34	38	50	40	27
Born Again Christians (evangelical)	Favorable	57	50	72	51	62	58	57	58
	Unfavorable	23	26	17	26	17	30	25	18
Hindus	Favorable	44	47	45	41	50	52	45	44
	Unfavorable	23	18	35	17	16	23	24	20
Jews	Favorable	66	64	75	62	63	84	71	56
	Unfavorable	12	10	13	14	16	5	11	17
Muslims	Favorable	27	35	21	22	38	23	25	32
	Unfavorable	45	33	63	39	25	58	50	33

Source: Adapted with modification from Arab American Institute (2014)

Table 4.9 Views of being one of a racial/religious group helps/hurts one's ability to get ahead in American society

Being ...	Hurts a lot %	Hurt little %	Helps little %	Helps a lot %	Neither help nor hurt %
White	4	7	21	38	28
Evangelical Christian	5	10	19	11	54
Black	25	30	10	7	26
Muslim	30	32	5	3	27

Source: Adopted with modification from Pew Research Center (2019)

American Muslims face a rising tide of religious discrimination in U.S. communities, workplaces and schools (Maygers, 2017). New America, a thinktank working with the American Muslim Institution, conducted 1165 interviews in four U.S. metropolitan areas in November 2018. According to the survey, a majority of non-Muslim Americans (71%) agree that there is a lot of illegal discrimination against Muslim Americans, compared to Black Americans (67%) (McKenzie, 2018). The rise of Islamophobia and the targeting of Muslims relates to religious stigma, causing depression, exasperation and a lack of well-being among Muslims (Crewe & Guyot-Diangone, 2016; Schormans, 2014). Stigma is described as the situation of persons who are "disqualified from full social acceptance" (Goffman, 1963).

White supremacists, targeting people of color and immigrants, are involved in anti-Muslim hate crimes and the spread of racist, anti-Islam messages. According to FBI data, during the period from 2001 to 2009, 1552 incidents of anti-Islamic hate crimes were reported resulting in 1785 offenses. In 2010, the FBI reported that hate crimes committed against Muslims accounted for 13.2% of all religion-motivated hate crimes in the U.S. (U.S. Commission on Civil Rights, 2014). In 2018, there were 1187 incidents instigated by white supremacists in the U.S., up from 421 incidents in 2017 (De Avila, 2019).

4.3.2   Canada

Despite the relatively better status of Muslims in Canada, when Muslims are compared with other immigrants in the country, they fall behind in many different areas (Kazemipur, 2014). In 2016, a survey conducted by the Angus Reid Institute (2017), found that Catholicism was viewed by 35% of Canadians as benefitting Canada through its presence in public life, followed by Protestantism (26%) and evangelical Christianity (24%). The survey declared that only one religion, Islam, was widely seen by 46% of Canadians to be harmful and damaging to Canada, which is double what Canadians say about any other religion. Only 30% of Canadians had a favorable opinion of Islam (Angus Reid Institute 2017). Although "Race, and

Table 4.10 Cases of hate crimes against Muslims in Canada, 2015–2017

Year	2015		2016		2017	
Crime against Muslims	Incidents	Percentage of all hate crimes	Incidents	Percentage of all hate crimes	Incidents	Estes
	159	12%	139	10%	349	17%

Source: Adapted with modification from Statistics Canada (2018)

whiteness in particular, supposedly are not very *relevant* in Canada" (Sullivan, 2019, p. 4, emphasis added), Muslim religious practices in Canada, as is the case in the U. S., take place in a dominantly white Christian country.

In Canada, there has been a startling rise in religious-based hate crimes and social hostilities. Hate crimes targeting Muslim communities in Canada numbered 99 incidents in 2014. That number swelled to 159 in 2015, an increase of 61%. During 2017, there were 349 incidents of police-reported hate crimes against Muslims in Canada, an increase of 210, or 151% from the previous year of 2016, which recorded 139 such cases. Hate crimes targeting the Muslim population accounted for 17% of all hate crimes in Canada (Statistics Canada, 2018) (Table 4.10).

Moreover, in May and June 2020, incidents of vandalism took place at a mosque in Toronto (Muslim Association of Canada, 2020) and on September 12, 2020, a member of the Canadian Muslim community, Mohamed-Aslim Zafis, was ruthlessly killed (his throat slit) in front of the International Muslims Organization (IMO) Mosque by an individual with apparent links to a neo-Nazi group. This attack, driven by hate and fear, did not happen in isolation as it was one in a chain of horrifying attacks on racialized communities in Canada (National Council of Canadian Muslims, 2019).

4.4   Media Outcomes

In North America, several media outlets, media platforms and the Internet have facilitated online Islamophobia, providing a virtual space where racist attitudes towards Muslim communities are easily disseminated into the public debate, intensifying hatred and animosity against Muslims (Ekman, 2015). All these negative features associated with Islamophobia are products of stigmatization and stereotypes.

According to Lawrence Blum (2004, p. 251), "Stereotypes are false or misleading generalizations about groups held in a manner that renders them largely, though not entirely, immune to counterevidence." Stereotypes are characteristics imposed upon groups of people because of their race, nationality, and sexual orientation. Lawrence Blum (2004, p. 277) further stated, "Muslims are stereotyped as terrorists and as fundamentalists. Although both characteristics are negative, obviously it is a much greater moral fault to be a terrorist than a fundamentalist." Media images generate stereotypes which distance Muslims from the rest of North America, inciting fear among Americans and Canadians and causing cultural polarization in which Muslims are depicted as aliens and threatening 'others.' Mediated stereotypes remain a tenacious part of the media operation (Dixon et al., 2019).

Fake media presentations generate fear, hate, mistrust, and anxiety (Kalsnes, 2018). Yet, media is to be blamed when fake news goes viral and turns to be harmful. For instance, repeated exposure to the Muslim terrorist stereotype may lead news viewers to conclude that all Muslims are terrorists. This cognitive linkage, in turn, might support punitive policies, such as a Muslim ban on entry to the United States (Dixon et al., 2019). The following subsections address media outcomes of Islamophobia in the U.S. and Canada.

4.4.1   The U.S.

In the U.S., Fox News, Breitbart News and other far right media and radio shows such as those of Sean Hannity, Rush Limbaugh and Glenn Beck are known for disseminating Islamophobic and misleading information about Muslim. About 93% of Fox News consumers identified as Republican or lean toward the party (Gramlich, 2020). And, the majority of Republicans are known for their unfavorable attitudes toward Islam (Smith & Haberman, 2010).

News is considered a form of political and ideological discourse through which politicians often use misinformation for achieving different political goals (Wei & Xu, 2019). Media portrayals of Muslims in America affect their well-being as well as their perception about being accepted or rejected in the mainstream cultures. Additionally, "Arab" and "Muslim" are manipulated interchangeably, and the politics and maneuvers of terrorists are labeled as "Islamic" by biased media and misguided political leaders (Joshi, 2018).

Many aspects of American and global media, driven by far-right groups and neoconservatives, have focused on what is known as fear of the other and the war on terror, rendering all Muslims a suspect community (el-Aswad, el-S., 2006, 2013a; el-Aswad, el-S. et al., 2020; Resnick, 2017). Media often falsely frame Muslims as felons, criminals, terrorists, and killers, overstating criminal attacks committed by Muslim extremists (Media Matters, 2017). According to a new research, terrorist attacks committed by Muslim extremists receive 357% more U.S. media coverage than those committed by non-Muslims. Attacks carried out by Muslims received 105 headlines on average, while attacks by non-Muslim receive 15 headlines, creating fear (Chalabi, 2018).

4.4.2   Canada

In Canada, conservative and right-wing advocates acquire their daily information through right-wing news outlets such as the Rebel News or The Rebel, the National

Post, and the Toronto Sun (Bothwell, 2017). Several Canadian media outlets are involved in the dissemination of Islamophobic and anti-Muslim imagery. For instance, newspaper photographs show "veiled women holding guns or supporting causes defined as fundamentalist" (Bullock & Jafri, 2000, p. 36). Such stereotypic images are so widespread that they constitute a reality for many media consumers (Watt, 2008). A survey of Canadian Muslims found that 56% of respondents indicated increased media bias against Muslims. And 55% of Canadian Muslims thought "the Canadian media were more biased since 9/11" (Perry & Poynting, 2006, p. 5). Many media commentators in Canada have suggested that Arabs generally and Muslims specifically may represent broad subjects of defamatory imagery and stereotypes.

As is the case in the U.S., far-right extremists in Canada use Facebook and Twitter to engage in anti-Muslim conversation. A recent study identified more than 6600 online channels — pages, accounts or groups — in which Canadians were involved in spreading white supremacist, misogynistic and other radical views targeting Muslims (Davey et al., 2020, p. 5). For example, a hate-motivated woman is seen in a video at a Mississauga Islamic center (in Canada) tearing the pages of a Qur'an and placing the pages on cars while shouting and designating the religious text as satanic (Patton & Westoll, 2018).

4.5   Conclusion

This chapter has addressed economic-political, cultural-religious and media outcomes and indicators that identify and show the negative impact of Islamophobia on the lives of Muslims living in the U.S. and Canada. Islamophobia in North America can be described as the suspicion and hostility towards Muslims, Islam, and those perceived as members of Islamist groups. Islamophobia is heightened and expedited by stereotypes portrayed in various forms of North American political platforms that have resulted in the exclusion of Muslims and denial of their economic-political and civil rights.

This study has highlighted the fact that for North American Muslims the outcomes and consequences of Islamophobia are serious and detrimental to their quality of life and well-being within major domains of living including economy, political rights, religion and media.

In the wake of the 9/11 attacks, the U.S. and Canadian governments cracked down on immigration policy and national security measures targeting Muslims. Muslim communities, already facing routine vilification, racial intimidation and violence would potentially face even greater monitoring and harassment by the state's government. The institutionalized Islamophobia has produced negative economic-political, religious-cultural and media outcomes reflected in undeniable and wide-ranging inequalities between Muslims and non-Muslim communities residing in North America.

References

Akram-Pall, S., & Moodley, R. (2016). "Loss and fear": Acculturation stresses leading to depression in South Asian Muslim immigrants in Toronto. *Canadian Journal of Counselling and Psychotherapy* 50(3-S), S137–S155. Retrieved from http://cjc-rcc.ucalgary.ca/cjc/index.php/rcc/article/view/2794

Allen, T. W. (2012). *The invention of the white race: Racial oppression and social control* (Vol. 1). Verso.

Allport, G. W. (1979). *The nature of prejudice*. Addison-Wesley Pub. Co.

Angus Reid Institute. (2015, March 26). *Religion and faith in Canada today: Strong belief, ambivalence and rejection define our views*. Retrieved from http://angusreid.org/faith-in-canada/

Angus Reid Institute. (2017, March 23). *M-103: If Canadians, not MPs, voted in the House, the motion condemning Islamophobia would be defeated*. Retrieved from http://angusreid.org/islamophobia-motion-103/

Anthias, F., & Davis, N. Y. (1992). *Racialized boundaries: Race, nation, gender, colour, and class and the anti-racist struggle*. Routledge.

Arab American Institute. (2014, July 29). *American attitudes toward Arabs and Muslims*. Retrieved from https://b.3cdn.net/aai/3e05a493869e6b44b0_76m6iyjon.pdf

Blum, L. (2004). Stereotypes and stereotyping: A moral analysis. *Philosophical Papers, 33*(3), 251–289.

Bothwell, R. (2017, November 8). Toronto Star. *The Canadian Encyclopedia*. Retrieved from https://www.thecanadianencyclopedia.ca/en/article/toronto-star

Braunstein, R. (2017). Muslims as outsiders, enemies, and others: The 2016 presidential election and the politics of religious exclusion. *American Journal of Cultural Sociology, 5*(3), 355–372. https://doi.org/10.1057/S41290-017-0042-X

Bullock, K. H., & Jafri, G. J. (2000). Media (mis)representations: Muslim women in the Canadian nation. *Canadian Women Studies, 20*(2), 35–40.

Central Intelligence Agency. (2020). *The world fact book*. Central Intelligence Agency. Retrieved from https://www.cia.gov/library/publications/the-world-factbook/geos/us.html

Chalabi, M. (2018, July 20). Terror attacks receive 357% more press attention, study finds. *The Guardian*. Retrieved from https://www.theguardian.com/us-news/2018/jul/20/muslim-terror-attacks-press-coverage-study

Choi, M. (2020, September 22). 'She's telling us how to run our country': Trump again goes after Ilhan Omar's Somali roots. *Politico*. Retrieved from https://www.politico.com/news/2020/09/22/trump-attacks-ilhan-omar-420267

Council on American Islamic Relations. (1997). *The state of Muslim civil rights in the United Sates: Unveiling prejudice*. Retrieved from https://www.cair.com/wp-content/uploads/2020/08/1997-The_Status_of_Muslim_Civil_Rights_in_the_United_States_1997.pdf

Crewe, S. E., & Guyot-Diangone, J. (2016, August 31). Stigmatization and labeling. In *Encyclopedia of social work*. Oxford University Press. https://doi.org/10.1093/acrefore/9780199975839.013.1043

Davey, J., Hart, M., & Guerin, C. (2020). *An online environmental scan of right-wing extremism in Canada: Interim report*. Institute for Strategic Dialogue. Retrieved from https://www.isdglobal.org/wp-content/uploads/2020/06/An-Online-Environmental-Scan-of-Right-wing-Extremism-in-Canada-ISD.pdf

De Avila, J. (2019, March 5). Hateful propaganda from white supremacists spreads. *Wall Street Journal*. Retrieved from https://www.wsj.com/articles/spread-of-hateful-propaganda-by-white-supremacists-climbs-11551783601

DeSilver, D. (2013). *U.S. income inequality, on rise for decades, is now highest since 1928*. Pew Research Center. Retrieved from http://www.pewresearch.org/fact-tank/2013/12/05/u-s-income-inequality-on-risefor-decades-is-now-highest-since-1928/

Dixon, T. L., Weeks, K. R., & Smith, M. A. (2019, May 23). Media constructions of culture, race, and ethnicity. In *Oxford research encyclopedia of communication*. Oxford Press. Retrieved from doi:https://doi.org/10.1093/acrefore/9780190228613.013.502

Ekman, M. (2015). Online Islamophobia and the politics of fear: Manufacturing the green scare. *Ethnic and Racial Studies, 38*(11), 1986–2002.

el-Aswad, el-S. (2006). The dynamics of identity reconstruction among Arab communities in the United States. *Anthropos: International Review of Anthropology and Linguistics, 101*, 111–121.

el-Aswad, el-S. (2013a). Images of Muslims in Western scholarship and media after 9/11. *Digest of Middle East Studies, 22*(1), 39–56.

el-Aswad, el-S. (2013b). Muslim Americans. In C. E. Cortés (Ed.), *Multicultural America: A multimedia encyclopaedia* (pp. 1525–1530). Sage.

el-Aswad, el-S. (2013c). Arab Americans. In C. E. Cortés (Ed.), *Multicultural America: A multimedia encyclopedia* (pp. 265–270). Sage.

el-Aswad, el-S., Sirgy, M., Estes, R., & Rahtz, D. (2020, December 17). Global jihad and international media use. In *Oxford research encyclopedia of communication*. Oxford University Press. doi: https://doi.org/10.1093/acrefore/9780190228613.013.1151

Environics Institute for Survey Research. (2016). Survey of Muslims in Canada 2016. https://nsiip.ca/wp-content/uploads/survey_of_muslims_in_canada_2016_final_report.pdf

Estes, R. J. (2019). The social progress of nations revisited. *Social Indicators Research*, 144, 539–574. Retrieved from doi:https://doi.org/10.1007/s11205-018-02058-9

Estes, R. J., Land, K. C., Michalos, A. M., Phillips, R., & Sirgy, M. J. (2017). Well-being in Canada and the United States. In R. J. Estes & M. J. Sirgy (Eds.), *The pursuit of human well-being: The untold global history* (pp. 257–299). Springer.

Garner, S., & Selod, S. (2015). The racialization of Muslims: Empirical studies of Islamophobia. *Critical Sociology, 41*(1), 9–19.

Goffman, E. (1963). *Stigma: Notes on the management of spoiled identity*. Englewood Cliffs.

Gongloff, M. (2014, September 16). 45 million Americans still stuck below poverty line: Census. *The Huffington Post*. http://www.huffingtonpost.com/2014/09/16/poverty-household-income_n_5828974.html

Goodman, A. H., Moses, Y. H., & Jones, J. L. (2012). *Race: Are we so different?* Wiley-Blackwell.

Gramlich, J. (2020, April 8). *5 facts about Fox News. Pew Research Center*. Retrieved from https://www.pewresearch.org/fact-tank/2020/04/08/five-facts-about-fox-news/

Grosfoguel, R. (2012). The multiple faces of Islamophobia. *Islamophobia Studies Journal, 1*(1), 9–33.

Hanniman, W. (2008). Canadian Muslims, Islamophobia and national security. *International Journal of Law, Crime and Justice, 36*, 271–286.

Hayoun, M. (2013, January 16). Islamophobia is bad for business: Anti-Arab and anti-Muslim sentiment has cost the United States and the West a number of business opportunities. *Boston Review: Political and Literary Forum*. Retrieved from http://bostonreview.net/world/islamophobia-bad-business

Ingraham, C. (2017, December 8). Nation's top 1 percent now have greater wealth than the bottom 90 percent. *Seattle Times*. Retrieved from https://www.seattletimes.com/business/economy/nations-top-1-percent-now-have-greater-wealth-than-the-bottom-90-percent/#:~:text=The%20wealthiest%201%20percent%20of,federal%20Survey%20of%20Consumer%20Finances

Institute for Social Policy and Understanding. (2017). *American Muslim poll 2017: Muslims at the crossroads*. Retrieved from https://www.ispu.org/american-muslim-poll-2017/

Institute for Social Policy and Understanding. (2018). *American Muslim Poll (2018): Pride and prejudice featuring the first-ever national American Islamophobia Index*. Retrieved from https://www.ispu.org/american-muslim-poll-2018-full-report/

Investopedia. (2020). The top 20 economies in the world. Retrieved from https://www.investopedia.com/insights/worlds-top-economies/

Jisrawi, A., & Arnold, C. (2018). Cultural humility and mental health care in Canadian Muslim communities. *Canadian Journal of Counselling and Psychotherapy, 52*(1), 43–64. Retrieved from https://cjc-rcc.ucalgary.ca/article/view/61133

Jones, C. (2000). Levels of racism: A theoretic framework and a gardener's tale. *American Journal of Public Health, 90*, 1212–1215.

Joshi, K. Y. (2018, May 24). Race and religion in U.S. public life. In *Oxford research encyclopedia of religion*. Oxford University Press. https://doi.org/10.1093/acrefore/9780199340378.013.460

Kalsnes, B. (2018, September 26). Fake news. In *Oxford research encyclopedia of communication*. Oxford Press. https://doi.org/10.1093/acrefore/9780190228613.013.809

Kazemipur, A. (2014). *The Muslim question in Canada: A story of segmented integration*. University of British Colombia (UBC) Press.

Lakhani, K. (2017, February 15 Workplace discrimination against Muslims. *On Labor*. Retrieved from https://onlabor.org/workplace-discrimination-against-muslims/

Lean, N. (2017). *The Islamophobia industry: How the right manufactures fear of Muslims*. Pluto Press.

Love, E. (2017). *Islamophobia and racism in America*. New York University Press.

Masci, D. (2019). Many Americans see religious discrimination in U.S. – Especially against Muslims. *Pew Research Center*. Retrieved from https://www.pewresearch.org/fact-tank/2019/05/17/many-americans-see-religiousdiscrimination-in-u-s-especially-against-muslims/

Media Matters. (2017, September 2). *When discussing Trump's Muslim ban, cable news excluded Muslims*. Retrieved from https://www.mediamatters.org/donald-trump/when-discussing-trumps-muslim-ban-cable-news-excluded-muslims

Maygers, B. (2017, December 6). Muslim discrimination cases disproportionately high in U.S. *Huffpost*. Retrieved from https://www.huffpost.com/entry/muslim-discrimination-cas_n_842076?guccounter=1

McKenzie, R. L. (2018). *Survey examines perceptions of Muslim (Muslim Diaspora Initiative)*. New America. Retrieved from https://www.newamerica.org/muslim-diaspora-initiative/press-releases/survey-examines-perceptions-muslim-americans/

Moore, A. (2012). American Muslim minorities: The new human rights struggle. *Human Rights & Human Welfare: An Online Journal of Academic Literature Review*, 91–99. Retrieved from http://www.du.edu/korbel/hrhw/researchdigest/minority/Muslim.pdf

Muslim Association of Canada. (2020, June 4). *Graffiti and vandalism incidents at masjid Toronto*. Retrieved from https://www.macnet.ca/2020/06/04/vandalism-at-masjid-toronto-dundas-missis sauga-june-4-2020/

National Council of Canadian Muslims. (2019). *Helping students deal with trauma related to geopolitical violence & Islamophobia*. Retrieved from https://www.toronto.ca/wp-content/uploads/2019/04/97e4-Geopolitical-Violence-and-Islamophopia.pdf

Nazroo, J., & Bécares, L. (2017). Islamophobia, racism and health. In F. Elahi & O. Khan (Eds.), *Islamophobia still a challenge for us all* (pp. 31–35). Runnymede.

NPR (National Public Radio). (2019, July 17). *Trump attacks congresswomen at N.C. rally, as crowd chants 'send her back'*. Retrieved from https://www.npr.org/2019/07/17/742896827/trump-attacks-congresswomen-at-n-c-rally-as-crowd-chants-send-her-back

Parent, R. B., & Ellis, J. O. (2014). Right-wing extremism in Canada. *The Canadian Network for Research on Terrorism, Security, and Society*. Retrieved from https://www.publicsafety.gc.ca/lbrr/archives/cnmcs-plcng/cn31894-eng.pdf

Patton, J., & Westoll, N. (2018, March 25). Police investigating after Ontario woman rips Qur'an, puts pages on cars outside of Islamic center. *Global News*. Retrieved from https://globalnews.ca/news/4103314/peel-police-investigating-hate-motivated-incident-islamic-centre/

Perry, B., & Poynting, S. (2006). *Inspiring Islamophobia: Media and state targeting of Muslims in Canada since 9/11*. Paper presented at TASA conference, University of Western Australia & Murdoch University, 4–7 December. Retrieved from https://web.archive.org/web/20180417175416/https://tasa.org.au/wp-content/uploads/2015/02/PerryPoynting.pdf

Pew Research Center. (2017a, July 26), *U.S. Muslims concerned about their place in society, but continue to believe in the American Dream.* Retrieved from https://www.pewresearch.org/wp-content/uploads/sites/7/2017/07/U.S.-MUSLIMS-FULL-REPORT.pdf

Pew Research Center. (2017b, November 15). *Assaults against Muslims in U.S. surpass 2001 level.* Retrieved from https://www.pewresearch.org/fact-tank/2017/11/15/assaults-against-muslims-in-u-s-surpass-2001-level/

Pew Research Center. (2018, June 13). *The age gap in religion around the world.* Retrieved from https://www.pewforum.org/2018/06/13/the-age-gap-in-religion-around-the-world/

Pew Research Center. (2019, April 9). *Race in America 2019.* Retrieved from https://www.pewsocialtrends.org/2019/04/09/race-in-america-2019/

Resnick, B. (2017, November 30). All Muslims are often blamed for single acts of terror. Psychology explains how to stop it. *Vox.com.* Retrieved from https://www.vox.com/science-and-health/2017/11/30/16645024/collective-blame-psychology-muslim

Runnymede Trust. (1997). Islamophobia: A challenge for us all. *The Runnymede Commission on British Muslims and Islamophobia.* Retrieved from https://www.runnymedetrust.org/companies/17/74/Islamophobia-A-Challenge-for-Us-All.html).

Schormans, A. F. (2014). Stigmatization. In A. C. Michalos (Ed.), *Encyclopedia of quality of life and well-being research.* Springer. https://doi.org/10.1007/978-94-007-0753-5_2871

Sirgy, M. J., Estes, R., el-Aswad, el-S., & Rahtz, D. (2019). *Combatting Jihadist terrorism through nation-building: A quality-of-life perspective.* Springer.

Smith, B., & Haberman, M. (2010, August 15). GOP takes harsher stance toward Islam. *Politico.* Retrieved from http://www.politico.com/news/stories/0810/41076.html

Social Progress Index. (2020). *Social progress imperatives.* Retrieved from https://www.socialprogress.org

Spencer, R. (2017, August 11). What it means to be alt-right. *Alt-Right com.* Retrieved from https://altright.com/2017/08/11/what-it-means-to-be-alt-right/

Statistics Canada. (2018). *Uniform crime reporting survey.* Retrieved from https://www23.statcan.gc.ca/imdb/p2SV.pl?Function=getSurvey&SDDS=3302

Statistics Canada. (2019). *Insights on Canadian society: The role of social capital and ethnocultural characteristics in the employment income of immigrants over time.* Retrieved from https://www150.statcan.gc.ca/n1/pub/75-006-x/2019001/article/00009-eng.htm

Stewart, E. (2019, December 4). The attacks on Ilhan Omar reveal a disturbing truth about racism in America. *Vox.* Retrieved from https://www.vox.com/policy-and-politics/2019/12/4/20995589/ilhan-omar-racism-attacks-twitter-danielle-stella-minnesota

Sullivan, S. (2019). *White privilege.* Polity.

Transparency International. (2018). *Corruption perceptions index.* Retrieved from https://www.transparency.org/en/cpi/2018

Transparency International. (2019). *Corruption perceptions index.* Retrieved from https://www.transparency.org/en/cpi/2019

Tutt, D. (2013). How should we combat Islamophobia? *Huffpost.* Retrieved from https://www.huffingtonpost.com/daniel-tutt/how-should-we-combat-islamophobia_b_3149768.html

Tyrer, D. (2013). *The politics of Islamophobia: Race, power and fantasy.* Pluto Press.

U.S. Commission on Civil Rights. (2014). *Federal civil rights engagement with Arab and Muslim American communities.* U.S. Commission on Civil Rights. Retrieved from https://www.usccr.gov/pubs/docs/ARAB_MUSLIM_9-30-14.pdf

United Nations Development Programme. (2019). *Human development report. Beyond income, beyond averages, beyond today: Inequalities in human development in the 21st century.* Retrieved from http://hdr.undp.org/sites/default/files/hdr2019.pdf

Watt, D. (2008). Challenging islamophobia through visual media studies: Inquiring into a photograph of Muslim women on the cover of Canada's National News magazine. *Studies in Media & Information Literacy Education, 8*(2), 1–14.

Wei, R., & Xu, L. Z. (2019, May 23). New media and politics: A synopsis of theories, issues, and research. In *Oxford research encyclopedia of communication.* Oxford University Press. https://doi.org/10.1093/acrefore/9780190228613.013.104

Part III
Drivers of Islamophobia

Chapter 5
Economic and Political Drivers of Islamophobia

5.1 Introduction

Notions of market supply and demand, as used in the examination of terrorist organizations (Krueger, 2003, 2007; Stern, 2003; Sirgy et al., 2019), are similarly used here in the analysis of economic and political drivers of Islamophobia. The marketing discipline can contribute significantly to the growing scholarly discourse on Islamophobia. Hence, Islamophobia can be viewed as a product like a consumer good or service provided by Islamophobes or politico-religious extremists who hold negative views of Islam and Muslims.

Several economic and political organizations espousing Islamophobia are run in ways similar to that of a firm embracing supply and demand domains. The supply side includes economic charges, expenses, finance, Islamophobic campaigns, and strategic management. For example, individuals or groups of people offer their services to Islamophobia organizations, promoting their ideology, as well as to those who demand them. The demand side of the Islamophobia market includes multiple components such as economic, political, religious, cultural, ideological, and media drivers, among other factors.

The following sections address economic and political drivers of Islamophobia in the U.S and Canada.

5.2 Economic Drivers

Despite the economic prosperity of North America, Islamophobia has negatively impacted Muslims' economic activities (Lean, 2017; Love, 2017). As Jack Levin (1975) has argued, prejudice is beneficial to both the dominant group and minority groups. For the dominant group, prejudice serves to delineate the cultural borderlines between the ingroup and the out-group. For the minority group, prejudice encourages marginalized people to fight, to join forces with allies, and to challenge the dominant group. However, it seems that the dominant group, including business tycoons and far-right politicians, benefit more by subjugating minorities (Levin, 1975). This statement fits the notion of Islamophobia which is an ideology used by politicians and right-wing extremist groups who seek to achieve economic-political gains by promoting hatred against Islam and Muslims.

The Islamophobia industry is driven by a small network of individuals and institutions, but the extent of their reach and consequences of their programs engenders anti-Muslim hate within vulnerable groups of people who, once adopting their Islamophobic propaganda, join their ranks. Islamophobes have managed to attach Islamophobia, which has become similar to other systematic organizations of hatreds, to the designation of right-wing populism (Lean, 2017).

Islamophobia can be viewed within a market framework. Right-wing groups and think tanks working to spread Islamophobia are viewed as the demanders, while those who financially or economically support them are considered the suppliers. This is to say that certain groups of conservative foundations and wealthy donors (for example, the Donors Capital Fund, the Richard Mellon Scaife foundations, the Lynde and Harry Bradley Foundation, the Newton D. & Rochelle F. Becker foundations and charitable trust, the Russell Berrie Foundation, the Anchorage Charitable Fund, the William Rossenwald Family Fund, and the Fairbrook Foundation, among others) serve as major financial resources or suppliers that feed Islamophobia organizations in the U.S. These foundations

> provide critical funding to a clutch of right-wing think tanks and misinformation experts who peddle hate and fear of Muslims and Islam—in the form of books, reports, websites, blogs, and carefully crafted talking points, which dedicated anti-Islam grassroots organizations and some right-wing religious groups use as propaganda for their constituency (Center for American progress, 2011, p. 13).

There is a U.S.-based Islamophobia network that was comprised of 74 groups in 2015, an increase from 69 in 2013. About 33 of these 74 organizations are tightly linked with one another and have engaged in marketing their Islamophobic campaigns and systematic operations of hatred against Islam. These Islamophobia organizations received at least $205,838,077 between 2008 and 2013 (Council on American-Islamic Relations & University of California, 2016), up from $119,662,719 between 2008 and 2011 (Council on American-Islamic Relations, 2013). The Donors Capital Fund is one of the top suppliers because it contributed $21,318,600 to organizations promoting Islamophobia from 2007 to 2009. In 2008, Donors Capital contributed more than $17 million to the Clarion Fund to help produce and freely distribute millions of copies of the DVD, "Obsession: Radical Islam's War Against the West," in order to persuade average Americans of an Islamist threat (Center for American progress, 2011).

Additional Islamophobia organizations include *ACT! for America* (Brigitte Gabriel, director), *Stop Islamization of America* (Pamela Geller and Robert Spencer, co-founders), *Society of Americans for National Existence* (David Yerushalmi, manager), *Campus Watch* (Daniel Pipes, founder), *Jihad Watch* (Robert Spencer, director), *Center for Security Policy* (Frank Gaffney, founder), and *Understanding the Threat* (John Guandolo, founder), to mention a few. These organizations receive millions of dollars annually from various donors and foundations (Council on American Islamic Relations, 2013; Saylor, 2014; Southern Poverty Law Center, 2011) to promote Islamophobia. Between 2001 and 2009, Richard Mellon Scaife's foundations contributed $7,875,000 to Islamophobic groups including the Center for Security Policy ($2,900,000), the Counterterrorism & Security Education and Research Foundation ($1,575,000), and the David Horowitz Freedom Center ($3,400,000) (Center for American progress, 2011, 2015). Between 2014 and 2016, DonorsTrust and Donors Capital Fund provided nearly $4 million to the Middle East Forum, over $400,000 to the Center for Security Policy, and over $300,000 to the David Horowitz Freedom Center (Council on American-Islamic Relations, 2018). These funds have been used to promote Islamophobic agendas and hate toward Muslims.

Further financing was provided to author and journalist Steven Emerson who declared that he had received a large share of the $325,000 financing for his work, *Jihad in America*, a documentary misrepresenting Islam and Muslims, from the Bradley Foundation of Milwaukee. This foundation also funded authors such as Robert Kaplan who, in his book (1993) *The Arabists: The Romance of an American Elite*, depicted Arab and Muslim American experts in incongruous and anti-Islamic terms (Lowrie, 1995). Kaplan (1993, p. 48) stated, "Islam was an exotic woman redolent of perfume, within breathing range of the British: meaning that she should have to be mastered." By the same token, David Horowitz has been targeting universities and academic freedom since 1980s. In his book, Horowitz (2006) erroneously designated what he called the 101 most dangerous academics in America, many of whom were prominent professors advocating Muslim and Palestinian rights.

Islamophobic organizations had strong connections with members of the far-right administration of former President Trump. Early, openly Islamophobic members of the Trump Cabinet (Steven Bannon, Michael Flynn and Sebastian Gorka) had ties with Gaffney's Center for Security Policy (Patel, 2017).

In Canada, a steady increase in Islamophobic organizations, like Pegida (an anti-Islam, far-right political organization), Storm Alliance (an ultranationalist group), and Soldiers of Odin (a white supremacist group), among others, have had opposition to what they call radical Islam as their sole raison d'être (Russell & Bell, 2019). The growth "from below" of such organizations and the nature of their racist fixations were an inevitable result of the racist fearmongering and maneuvering "from above" that significant sections of the economic-political establishment had been engaging in for years (Montréal Antifasciste, 2017; Schafer et al., 2014; Smith, 2020). In March 2019, a far-right and anti-Islamization group in Toronto organized protests chanting against Islam and Canadian Muslims (Global News, 2019).

5.3   Political Driver

The following sections focus on four major political elements and their support of or relation to Islamophobia: government, political parties, far-right groups and white supremacists.

5.3.1   Government

Politically, the United States is a federal republic with 50 distinct state governments, 1 federal government, and 1 special administrative government unit that governs the affairs of the District of Colombia, the territory in which the country's central government is located (Central Intelligence Agency, 2020; Estes et al., 2017).

In addition to economic drivers, in the U.S. "Islamophobia is also the product of the state's legal and extralegal attempts to control, discipline, and punish Muslim American individuals and organizations" (Curtis, 2013, p. 76). In response to the 9/11 attacks, the federal governments of both Canada and the U.S. engaged in sweeping anti-terror operations focused on individuals of Arab or Muslim descent. Racial profiling was used by enforcement officials in their anti-terrorism efforts (el-Aswad, el-S., 2013; Kumar, 2012). In the U.S., the Department of Homeland Security was established, and collaborated with several government agencies such as the Federal Emergency Management Agency, the U.S. Immigration and Customs Enforcement, the U.S. Citizenship and Immigration Services, the U.S. Customs and Border Protection, the U.S. Coast Guard, and the Transportation Security Administration (Bazian, 2014; Curtis, 2013) in identifying Muslim terrorists. Additionally, Congress passed the USA PATRIOT Act (in October 2001), which empowered enforcement and immigration authorities, along with the Treasury Department and the Clear Law Enforcement for Criminal Alien Removal Act, to increase surveillance and arrest of persons suspected of terrorism, including Muslims, without a warrant (Bazian, 2014).

Like the United States, Canada has a federal system of government. However, unlike the U.S., the country is a constitutional monarchy with a Westminster-style parliament containing a bicameral legislature consisting of a Senate whose members are appointed by the Prime Minister and a House of Commons whose members are elected by the people. There are ten provinces and three territories whose legislative authority is somewhat structured by the federal constitutional acts of 1867 and 1982 (Central Intelligence Agency, 2020; Estes et al., 2017).

Certain authors argue that while Islamophobia is direct and explicit in the United States, it is indirect and implicit in Canada (Bahdi & Kanji, 2018). Such a statement is not supported by the current research. As in the U.S., troubled race relations and associated violence have long been a part of the Canadian society (Parent & Ellis, 2014). In 2004 and 2005, Canada's minority communities, particularly its Muslim and Arab-Canadian communities, raised concerns about unequal treatment and discriminatory National Security policing measures. Muslims expressed their feelings of being marginalized, ostracized, or under suspicion for being terrorists or terrorist supporters. They were asked inappropriate religion-based questions and asked to remove their turbans or hijabs in public. They were denied requests for protection against law enforcement and security personnel for mishandling them or their Holy Book, the Qur'an (Hanniman, 2008).

On June 16, 2019, Quebec's National Assembly proposed Bill 21 and passed legislation that would ban the wearing of religious symbols like hijabs and turbans by certain public servants in positions of authority, including judges, teachers, and police officers, overriding their fundamental rights (Authier, 2019). This ban impacted Muslim women wearing the hijab and/or Muslims men wearing turbans who worked within educational institutions of the province of Quebec. A poll of 1212 Quebecers, conducted by Léger Marketing research firm and commissioned by the Association for Canadian Studies, found that anti-Muslim sentiments appeared to be the main motivation for those who supported a ban on religious symbols (Magder, 2019).

5.3.2 Political Parties

In the U.S, political parties are highly polarized in the sense that "there are substantial differences in political perspectives across a single ideological dimension. Liberals versus conservatives" (Campbell, 2018, p. 1). Political polarization was evident in the U.S. in the past, but the level of division and animosity has recently increased and deepened. This has caused political instability as represented by the storming of the Capitol Building on January 6, 2021 (NPR, 2021), the gridlock between political parties, and the negative sentiments among partisans toward the members of the opposing party (Layman, 2001; Pew Research Center, 2019). Notably, evangelical Protestants are the force behind an increasingly strong religious faction in the Republican Party (Todd, 2011). In political and public spheres, evidence has indicated that white evangelical and Republican identities are fused together (Lewis, 2019). In addressing the impact of increased political polarization on American society, Gallup (2019) indicated that partisans on both sides increasingly view institutions in the U.S. not as beneficial and necessary, but as part of an effort by the other side to gain advantage and to perpetuate its power and ideological positions.

Such political schisms have a negative impact on Muslim Americans. Particularly during the Donald Trump presidency (2017–2021), the Republican Party advocated Islamophobic and anti-Muslim sentiment. For example, Republican candidates in the primaries of the 2016 election were able to manipulate the stereotype of Islamophobia by framing Muslims as cultural enemies, outsiders, and others (Braunstein, 2017; Whitehead et al., 2018). Anti-Muslim discrimination was directly related to views that challenge fundamental democratic norms and values (Institute for Social Policy and Understanding, 2018).

Table 5.1 Views of Islam and Muslims by U.S. Political Parties (Democrats and Republicans)

Political Party	Islam encourages violence more than any other religion (%)	Muslim Americans are extremists (%)	The majority of Muslim Americans are anti-America (%)	Islam is not part of mainstream American society (%)	Islam and democracy are not compatible (%)
Democrats	26	22	17	37	30
Republicans	63	56	34	68	65

Source: Adapted with modification from Pew Research Center (2017) *U.S. Muslims concerned about their place in society*

Republican or conservative figures have made most of the offensive and negative comments about Islam and Muslims since 9/11 (Kalkan et al., 2009). According to the Pew Research Center (2017), Republicans and those who lean toward the GOP tend to hold much more negative views about Islam than do Democrats and those who lean toward the Democratic Party. For instance, Republicans were three times (63%) more likely than Democrats (26%) to state that Islam encourages violence more than any other religion. Comparably, 56% of Republicans and 22% of Democrats believed that Muslim Americans were extremists. Republicans (34%) were twice as likely as Democrats (17%) to view Muslim Americans as being anti-America. Additionally, two-thirds of Republicans (68%) said Islam was not part of mainstream American society, while fewer Democrats (37%) expressed this view. Republicans (65%) more than doubled Democrats (30%) in viewing Islam and democracy as incompatible (Pew Research Center, 2017) (Table 5.1).

In 2016, Muslim Americans expressed more positive views about Democrats' attitudes toward the Muslim community than about Republicans' attitudes. About 43% said the Democratic Party was friendly toward Muslim Americans, and an additional 35% said the party was neutral toward Muslims. Just 13% said the Democratic Party was unfriendly toward Muslims. However, about 59% of Muslim Americans stated that the Republican Party as a whole was unfriendly toward Muslim Americans, up from 48% who expressed this view in 2011. About 69% of Muslim women viewed the GOP as unfriendly toward Muslims compared with 49% of Muslim men who expressed this view. Wariness of the GOP was higher among U. S.-born Muslims than among immigrants (Pew Research Center, 2017).

About 66% of Muslim Americans identified with the Democratic Party. Only 13% of Muslim Americans identified with the Republican Party, while 20% say they preferred another party or are political independents and do not lean toward either major party. Moreover, attachment to the Democratic Party was strong among U.S.-born and foreign-born Muslims alike, scoring 67% and 66%, respectively. Only 21% of Muslims described themselves as ideological conservatives compared with 36% of the general American public. About 39% of Muslims described themselves as politically moderate as compared with 32% of general American population (Pew Research Center, 2017).

Although Canada is known for having more political parties than the U.S., the most dominant political parties are the Conservative Party of Canada and the Liberal

Party of Canada. There are deep divisions between them on public issues, particularly those that relate to Islamophobia and anti-Muslim racism. Canadian conservatives overwhelmingly share ideologies and values of the U. S. conservatives, particularly those related to the Republican Party (Marche, 2016).

Except for the Liberal Party of Canada and the New Democratic Party of Canada (Lansford, 2019), the Conservative Party of Canada as well as the People's Party of Canada are known for being on the right of the political spectrum advocating anti-Muslim, anti-immigration, anti-diversity, and anti multi-multiculturalism policies (Froese, 2019; People's Party of Canada, 2019). It is worth noting that the founding members of the People's Party of Canada included associates of the extreme far-right, Pegida Canada, neo-Nazi organizations, Soldiers of Odin, and anti-immigrant groups (Global News, 2019).

In December of 2016, the 42nd Canadian Parliament introduced Motion 103 (M-103) condemning Islamophobia and all forms of racism and religious discrimination. Initially, the motion was rejected by members of the Parliament from the Conservative Party of Canada who wanted to remove the word of *Islamophobia* from the text. A survey published by the Angus Reid Institute (2017) proposed that 42% of Canadians, not MPs, would vote against the motion, while just 29% would vote in favor of it, displaying a public split concerning anti-Muslim sentiments and discrimination in society. After three months of debate, however, the Motion was passed by a vote of 201–91 on March 23, 2017 (CBC News, 2017).

5.3.3 White Supremacists and Far-Right Organizations Targeting Muslims

Islamophobia in North America is expressed by zealous groups such as far-right extremists, followers of neo-Nazism, the Ku Klux Klan (K.K.K.), and white supremacists or white nationalists (el-Aswad, el-S. et al. 2020). The latter has claimed that they are superior to people of other races and should dominate them. Extreme white nationalism leads to fascism (Griffin, 1993; Stanley, 2020). A study conducted by the Muslim Public Affair Council (2012) pointed out that a non-Muslim extremist category consists mostly of violent right-wing extremists: specifically, Christian extremists, white nationalists, and anti-government militias. Moreover, the Study of Terrorism and Responses to Terrorism (START) stated that just "as many state-police agencies (62%) view Neo-Nazis as posing a serious threat to their own state's security as consider Islamic Jihadists to pose a serious threat" (Muslim Public Affair Council, 2012, p. 6).

Such white supremacists, supported by former president Trump and related far-right groups, have depicted Islam as a backward or false religion, and have worked to spread Islamophobia, undermining the diversity and multiculturalism of North America (Gorski, 2017). One of the far-right militia groups is the neo-fascist organization, the Proud Boys, founded by Vice Media co-founder Gavin McInnes in the midst of the U.S. 2016 election. The Proud Boys are known for their white supremacist pandering, premeditated anti-Muslim rhetoric and close ties with more publicly violent extremists (The Hill, 2020b). Far-right extremists and fascists "mask their destructive goals with the language of liberalism, or 'social justice'" (Stanley, 2020, p. 187). White supremacist groups are involved in many incidents of terrorist attacks and homicides in the U.S. (Gruenewald et al., 2013). The overwhelming presence of white men in "the far-right extremist movement has factored into some explanations of why extremist crimes occur" (Gruenewald, 2011, p. 190). In brief, the prevailing form of paranoid politics or Islamophobia has been exacerbated by American far-right and Zionist groups, both Christian and Jewish, whose dislike of Muslims has a long history (Davidson, 2011). In September 2020, FBI director, Christopher Wray, declared that racially motivated violent extremism, mostly from white supremacists, is behind the majority of domestic terrorism threats (The Hill, 2020a).

Race and whiteness are considered norms that have helped construct Canada as a white country in such a way that "Non-white and Indigenous people have been excluded from that norm. . . since the nation's inception" (Baldwin et al., 2011, p. 1). In Canada, rhetoric from far-right, white supremacist and extremist groups trickle down to street-level hate crimes. In 2017, there was a surge in attacks against Muslims as well as on mosques in Toronto (Abedi, 2020; Dickson, 2020). A Canadian woman, wearing a 'Make Canada Great Again' hat (with reference to Trump's slogan 'make America great again') was chanting 'Islam is evil'. She has been seen at multiple anti-Islam demonstrations (Khandaker & Krishnan, 2017).

5.3.4 Political Leadership

Political leaders have relied on anti-Muslim rhetoric to secure and mobilize voters (Fording & Schram, 2020; Jones, 2020; Stanley, 2020). In the U.S., elected officials and politicians such as Peter King and Michele Bachmann played a core role in reaching the public with misinformed narratives about Islam and Muslims. For example, Peter King, a former U.S. representative and a member of the Republican Party, falsely claimed that "80–85% of mosques in this country are controlled by Islamic fundamentalists" (Center for American Progress, 2011, p. 111). Additionally, there is a strong link between Islamophobia, the leadership of former President Trump, and Trump supporters (Blair, 2016; Hell & Steinmetz, 2017; Jones, 2017). Even before Trump, numerous political leaders were involved in the anti-Muslim and anti-Arab Islamophobia industry (Musaji, 2012). Douglas Todd (2011) stated that three out of four evangelicals voted for the presidential power of George W. Bush who led wars against Muslim-majority countries, Iraq and Afghanistan. By the same token, in the 2016 presidential election white Evangelicals represented 26% of the voters despite that their proportion of the population fell to 17% (Jones, 2017).

Nevertheless, several scholars have indicated that based on the strong role that Islamophobia was shown to play in fortifying support for Trump, and because Islam is often viewed as the antithesis of American identities, the expectation is that "Trump support, Christian nationalism, and Islamophobia" are "closely related" (Whitehead et al., 2018, p. 153). Citizens often follow indications from leaders who share their political predispositions (Kalkan et al., 2009). According to a survey conducted in 2018 by the Public Religion Research Institute (PRRI), 54% of Americans said that Trump's attitudes and behavior have encouraged white supremacist group (Jones, 2020).

Donald Trump, manipulating the issue of race in American politics and courting white supremacists, "embodies the hatreds and fears that have been part of America's politics since its founding" (Glaude, 2018, p. 42). Trump fueled generalized outgroup hostilities, including Muslims, to gain votes while instantaneously normalizing racism in American politics (Fording & Schram, 2020). Voting for Donald Trump in 2016 was for many Americans a Christian nationalist response to perceived threats to their identity (Whitehead et al., 2018). For example, approximately two thirds of white Christians favored Trump's travel ban, preventing people from some Muslim countries from entering the U.S. (Jones, 2020). Following the 2016 election, exit polls suggested that 81% of white voters who self-identified as evangelical cast their ballots for Trump (Lewis, 2019). According to the Baylor Religion Survey (2017, p. 8), there is a collection of values and attitudes from the core ethos of what might be called Trumpism, which is "a new form of nationalism which merges pro-Christian rhetoric with anti-Islam, anti-feminist, anti-globalist, and anti-government attitudes."

Islamophobia has been politically used by authoritarian leaders to deepen the fear that can lead voters to elect them. This fear is a useful driver used by politicians to mobilize voters during elections. For example, during the 2016 presidential election Trump said, "Islam hates us" (Schleifer, 2016). He also attacked Barak Obama as being covertly Muslim, a depiction refuted by Obama (Jones, 2020; Nimer, 2011; Stanley, 2020). The literature on authoritarianism suggests this is not just simple Islamophobia, but rather reflects a broader phenomenon wherein, according to conspiracy theories, authoritarians feel threatened by people they identify as outsiders (Gorski, 2017; Stanley, 2020; Taub, 2016).

Such a phenomenon of authoritarianism has intensified under Trump, causing political upheaval and instability as exhibited by the rise of the far-right, the unprecedented spread of Islamophobia, Muslims' anger in response to a travel ban, African Americans' protests for racial equality (Sanchez, 2020), and decline in the trust in the President (Trump), particularly since his failure to protect Americans against the COVID-19 during the pandemic which he called a hoax (New York Times, 2020; Stanley, 2020; Woodward, 2020).

During the first 2020 presidential debate (Sept. 29, 2020), Trump declined to explicitly condemn white supremacy; rather, he instructed the Proud Boys to *stand back and stand by*. The group celebrated Trump's comments. One social media account affiliated with the self-described *white chauvinist* organization added Trump's comments to the Proud Boys logo (The Hill, 2020b). Trump's supporters

Table 5.2 Americans' favorable views of the overall performance of former President Trump

Respondents	Muslim	Jewish	Catholic	Protestant	White Evangelical	Non-affiliated	General Public
Score	13%	31%	36%	41%	72%	17%	35%s

Source: Adapted with modification from the Institute for Social Policy and Understanding (2018)

have come to embrace such extreme policies including mass deportation of millions of people (Taub, 2016). It is worthy to note that not all Americans share Trump's bigotry. Two-thirds of Americans actually disapprove of politicians engaging in hate speech toward Muslims (Whitehead et al., 2018).

This political cataclysm has negatively impacted American Muslims. According to the Pew Research Center (2017), 68% of Muslim Americans stated that Trump made them feel worried, while 45% said he made them feel angry. Only 17% of Muslim Americans stated that Trump made them feel happy. Muslim women were especially likely to express skepticism of Trump's attitude toward Muslims. Fully 80% of Muslim women, compared with 68% of men, said that Trump was unfriendly toward Muslims (Pew Research Center, 2017).

A poll conducted by the Institute for Social Policy and Understanding (2018), examining the views of Americans toward Trump's performance, concluded that at 13%, American Muslims were the least likely group to report a favorable view of Donald Trump as President. Non-affiliated (17%) and Jewish (31%) sentiments were more positive than Muslims. Catholic views (36%) hovered right around the general public average (35%), and Protestants' views (41%) were slightly higher. However, White Evangelicals (72%) were the group most likely to approve of Trump's performance (Table 5.2).

Similar results related to Americans' views of the overall performance of Trump were revealed in 2019 by a survey conducted by the Institute for Social Policy and Understanding (2019). In less than two weeks before the 2020 presidential election (November 3), a poll conducted by Gallup (2020) revealed that 56% of U.S. voters said Donald Trump did not deserve reelection, while 43% he did.

In an interview with Zainab Salim, a politically oriented female activist living in Dearborn, she revealed that she had supported the Republican Party and voted for Trump in 2016, but ended this political affiliation. She said, "I thought that the travel ban against Muslims was a part of Trump's election campaign, not a serious plan. After I heard and watched the TV news about the racist rally of white supremacists and far-right groups in Charlottesville [in August 2017] in which a woman was killed and other people injured by a white supremacist's car, I changed my mind and affiliated myself with the Democratic Party. I could not believe that Trump, the President of our country, was giving signals supporting those criminals. Later, he [Trump] attacked Muslim congresswomen, showing a biased and failed leadership."

In Canada, Trump has had great impact on the right-wing. It is worth pointing out that conservative leaders in Canada have used discourses borrowed from Trump's campaign on anti-immigration, anti-refugee and anti-Muslims (Al-Solaylee, 2017) to fuel their discourse. Additionally, Quebec has shown a readiness as a province in

Canada "to take up the sort of right-wing populous rhetoric championed by Trump, particularly with respect to Islamophobia" (Perry & Scrivens, 2019, p. 159). Another example is Steve King, a U.S. Republican congressman from Iowa who has a history of making racist, anti-Muslim and anti-immigrant remarks. He has made comments in support of white nationalism and is connected to far-right figures around the world. In an October 2018 tweet, he publicly supported the Canadian anti-Muslim and far-right politician, Faith Goldy, who at the time was running for mayor of Toronto (Bridge, 2019; Perry & Scrivens, 2019).

In an interview with Ali Mugahid, a Canadian Muslim and car dealer living in Windsor, about his reaction to the 2020 U.S election, he said, "Most North Americans are not aware that there are politically active Muslims in the U.S. who played a significant role in the 2020 election, defeating Trump and his corrupt and Islamophobic circle."

5.4   Conclusion

This chapter has shown how North American's most influential right-wing think-tanks have used the fear of Islam to achieve economic and political goals by spreading Islamophobic ideologies as well as for sustaining an authoritarian political agenda for their benefit. Islamophobia has been economically and politically used by North American governments and authoritarian leaders to deepen the fear that can lead to dominate minority groups, including Muslims. The problem is that profiling by government officials has increased public suspicion of American Muslims, giving permission to private actors to think that they can handle security issues their own way.

Viewed within a market framework of supply and demand, Islamophobia in North America involves business tycoons and people of the far-right political spectrum, Christian evangelical extremists and white supremacists who depict Islam as a backward, inferior and false religion. Far-right extremist groups inspire hate, disgust, contempt and violence toward Muslims as well as toward those who disagree with them.

Financial and political support of the Islamophobia industry undermines the issues of diversity, equality, and equity among citizens of North America and promotes racist rhetoric and violence towards Muslims as well as other minority groups. Muslim minority groups, as well as other minority groups are finding support within their communities and forming organizations, (e.g. Black Lives Matter) and mobilizing efforts gain political and financial resources to combat racist attitudes in an effort to find representation in a democratic society.

References

Abedi, M. (2020, January 29). A look at Islamophobia in Canada, 3 years after the Quebec mosque shooting. *Global News*. Retrieved from https://globalnews.ca/news/6472549/muslim-canadians-islamophobia-quebec-city-shooting/

Al-Solaylee, K. (2017, April 14). Anti-Muslim hate has been in Canada – and our politics – long before the violence. *The Globe and Mail*. Retrieved from https://www.theglobeandmail.com/opinion/in-the-culture-of-hate-toward-muslims-dont-forget-the-made-in-canada-politicalcontributions/article33847973/

Angus Reid Institute. (2017, March 23). *M-103: If Canadians, not MPs, voted in the House, the motion condemning Islamophobia would be defeated*. Retrieved from http://angusreid.org/islamophobia-motion-103/

Authier, P. (2019, Jun 18). *Bill 21: Quebec passes secularism law after marathon session*. The Montreal gazette. Retrieved from https://montrealgazette.com/news/quebec/quebec-passes-secularism-law-after-marathon-session

Bahdi, R., & Kanji, A. (2018). What is islamophobia? *University of New Brunswick Law Journal, 69*, 325–363.

Baldwin, A., Cameron, L., & Kobayashi, A. (2011). Introduction: Where is the great white north? Spatializing history, historicizing whiteness. In A. Baldwin, L. Cameron, & A. Kobayashi (Eds.), *Rethinking the great white north: Race, nature, and the historical geographies of whiteness in Canada* (pp. 1–19). UBC Press.

Baylor Religion Survey. (2017). *American values, mental health, and using technology in the age of trump: Findings from the Baylor religion Survey, Wave 5*. Retrieved from https://www.baylorisr.org/wp-content/uploads/2019/09/BaylorISR_BRSw5-08242017-web-FINAL-1.pdf

Bazian, H. (2014). National entry-exit registration system: Arabs Muslims and Southeast Asians and post-9/11 "Security Measures.". *Islamophobia Studies Journal, 2*(1), 82–98.

Blair, K. L. (2016, October 10). *A 'basket of deplorables'? A new study finds that trump supporters are more likely to be Islamaphobic, racist, transphobic, and homophobic*. American politics and policy blog. Retrieved from: http://eprints.lse.ac.uk/68398/.

Braunstein, R. (2017). Muslims as outsiders, enemies, and others: The 2016 presidential election and the politics of religious exclusion. *American Journal of Cultural Sociology, 5*(3), 355–372. https://doi.org/10.1057/S41290-017-0042-X

Bridge. (2019, March 9). *Factsheet: Faith Goldy*. Retrieved from https://bridge.georgetown.edu/research/factsheet-faith-goldy/

Campbell, J. E. (2018). *Polarized: Making sense of a divided America*. Princeton University Press.

CBC News. (2017, March 23). *House of commons passes anti-islamophobia motion*. Retrieved from https://www.cbc.ca/news/politics/m-103-islamophobia-motion-vote-1.4038016

Center for American Progress. (2011, August 26). *Fear, Inc. The roots of the Islamophobia network in America*. Retrieved, 26 August, from https://www.americanprogress.org/issues/religion/reports/2011/08/26/10165/fear-inc/

Center for American Progress. (2015, February 11). *Fear, Inc. 2.0: The Islamophobia network's efforts to manufacture hate in America*. Retrieved from https://cdn.americanprogress.org/wp-content/uploads/2015/02/FearInc-report2.11.pdf?_ga=2.8220529.278273326.1603753559-1225250106.1603753559

Central Intelligence Agency. (2020). *The world fact book*. Central Intelligence Agency. Retrieved from https://www.cia.gov/library/publications/the-world-factbook/geos/us.html

Council on American Islamic Relations. (2013). *CAIR report: Islamophobia network funded with $119 million 2008 to 2011*. Retrieved from https://ca.cair.com/sandiego/updates/cair-report-islamophobia-network-funded-with-119-million-2008-to-2011/

Council on American-Islamic Relations. (2018). *U.S. Islamophobia Network: Islamophobic organizations*. Retrieved from http://www.islamophobia.org/islamophobic-organizations.html

Council on American-Islamic Relations & University of California, Berkeley Center for Race and Gender. (2016). *Confronting fear. Islamophobia and its impact in the United States*. retrieved from file:///Users/elaswad/Downloads/2013–2015%20Confronting%20Fear_%20Islamophobia %20and%20its%20Impact%20in%20the%20U.pdf.

Curtis, E. E. (2013). The black Muslim scare of the twentieth century: The history of state islamophobia and its post 9/11 variations. In C. W. Ernst (Ed.), *Islamophobia in America: The anatomy of intolerance* (pp. 75–106). Palgrave Macmillan.

Davidson, L. (2011). Islamophobia, the Israel lobby and American paranoia: Letter from America. *Holy Land studies: A multidisciplinary journal (Edinburgh University Press), 10*(1), 87–95.

Dickson, J. (2020, November 4). *Ottawa says measures meant to curb no-fly-list discrimination have come into force.* The Globe and Mail. Retrieved from https://www.theglobeandmail.com/ politics/article-ottawa-says-measures-meant-to-curb-no-fly-list-discrimination-have/

el-Aswad, el-S. (2013). Images of Muslims in Western scholarship and media after 9/11. *Digest of Middle East Studies, 22*(1), 39–56.

el-Aswad, el-S., Sirgy, M., Estes, R., & Rahtz, D. (2020, December 17). Global jihad and international media use. In *Oxford research encyclopedia of communication.* Oxford University Press. https://doi.org/10.1093/acrefore/9780190228613.013.1151

Estes, R. J., Land, K. C., Michalos, A. M., Phillips, R., & Sirgy, M. J. (2017). Well-being in Canada and the United States. In R. J. Estes & M. J. Sirgy (Eds.), *The pursuit of human Well-being: The untold global history* (pp. 257–299). Springer.

Fording, R. C., & Schram, S. F. (2020). *Hard white: The mainstreaming of racism in American politics.* Oxford University Press.

Froese, I. (2019, July 19). *People's Party board in a Winnipeg riding quits over concerns about racism.* CBC News. Retrieved from https://www.cbc.ca/news/canada/manitoba/people-party- canada-winnipeg-elmwood-transcona-resigns-quits-1.5215988

Gallup. (2019, December 5). *Polling matters: The impact of increased political polarization.* Retrieved from https://news.gallup.com/opinion/polling-matters/268982/impact-increased-polit ical-polarization.aspx

Gallup. (2020, October 22). *56% of U.S. voters say Trump did not deserve reelection.* Retrieved from https://news.gallup.com/poll/322340/voters-say-trump-not-deserve-reelection.aspx?utm_ source=alert&utm_medium=email&utm_content=morelink&utm_campaign=syndication

Glaude, E. S. (2018, September 06). Our racist soul: Don't let the loud bigots distract you. America's real problem with race cuts far deeper. *Time* (pp. 40–46). Retrieved, from http:// time.com/5388356/our-racist-soul/

Global News. (2019, March 23). *Tensions high as protestors clash at Toronto anti-Islam demon- stration.* Retrieved from https://globalnews.ca/video/5089698/tensions-high-as-protestors- clash-at-toronto-anti-islam-demonstration#autoplay

Gorski, P. (2017). Why evangelicals voted for trump: A critical cultural sociology. *American Journal of Cultural Sociology, 5*(3), 338–354. https://doi.org/10.1057/s41290-017-0043-9

Griffin, R. (1993). *The nature of fascism.* Routledge.

Gruenewald, J. (2011). A comparative examination of homicides perpetrated by far-right extrem- ists. *Homicide Studies, 15*(2), 177–203.

Gruenewald, J., Chermak, S., & Freilich, J. D. (2013). Far-right lone wolf homicides in the United States. *Studies in Conflict & Terrorism, 36*(12), 1005–1024.

Hanniman, W. (2008). Canadian Muslims, islamophobia and national security. *International Journal of Law, Crime and Justice, 36*, 271–286.

Hell, J., & Steinmetz, G. (2017). A period of 'wild and fierce fanaticism': Populism, theo-political militarism, and the crisis of US hegemony. *American Journal of Cultural Sociology, 5*, 373–391. https://doi.org/10.1057/s41290-017-0041-y

Horowitz, D. (2006). *The Professors: The 101 most dangerous academics in America.* Regnery Publishing.

Institute for Social Policy and Understanding. (2018). *American Muslim Poll (2018): Pride and prejudice featuring the first-ever national American Islamophobia Index.* Retrieved from https:// www.ispu.org/american-muslim-poll-2018-full-report/

Institute for Social Policy and Understanding. (2019). *Predicting and preventing Islamophobia.* Retrieved from https://www.ispu.org/american-muslim-poll-2019-predicting-and-preventing- islamophobia/

Jones, R. P. (2017). *The end of white Christian America*. Simon & Schuster Paperbacks.

Jones, R. P. (2020). *White too long: The legacy of white supremacy in American Christianity*. Simon & Schuste.

Kalkan, K. O., Layman, G. C., & Uslaner, E. M. (2009). 'Bands of others'? Attitudes toward Muslims in contemporary American society. *Journal of Politics, 71*(3), 847–862.

Kaplan, R. D. (1993). *The Arabists: The romance of an American elite*. Free Press.

Khandaker, T., & Krishnan, M. (2017). 'Islam is evil': Protesters clash at Toronto anti-M-103 rally. *Vice*. Retrieved from https://www.vice.com/en/article/ez8nja/protestors-clash-at-pro-islamophobia-anti-m-103-rally-in-toronto

Krueger, A. B. (2003, May 29). Economic scene; cash rewards and poverty alone do not explain terrorism. *New York Times*. Retrieved from https://www.nytimes.com/2003/05/29/business/economic-scene-cash-rewards-and-poverty-alone-do-not-explain-terrorism.html.   (Business section).

Krueger, A. B. (2007). *What makes a terrorist: Economics and the roots of terrorism*. Princeton University Press.

Kumar, D. (2012). *Islamophobia and the politics of empire: The cultural logic of empire*. Haymarket Books.

Lansford, T. (2019). *Political handbook of the world 2018–2019*. CQ Press, Sage Publication.

Layman, G. (2001). *The great divide: Religious and cultural conflict in American party politics*. Columbia University Press.

Lean, N. (2017). *The islamophobia industry: How the right manufactures fear of Muslims*. Pluto Press.

Levin, J. (1975). *The functions of prejudice*. Harper & Row.

Lewis, A. R. (2019, August 28). The inclusion-moderation thesis: The U.S. republican party and the Christian right. In *Oxford research encyclopedia of communication*. Oxford University Press. https://doi.org/10.1093/acrefore/9780190228637.013.665

Love, E. (2017). *Islamophobia and racism in America*. New York University Press.

Lowrie, A. L. (1995). The campaign against Islam and American foreign policy. *Middle East Policy, 4*(1/2), 210–219.

Magder, J. (2019, May 18). *A new poll shows support for bill 21 is built on anti-Islam sentiment*. The Montreal gazette. Retrieved from https://montrealgazette.com/news/local-news/a-new-poll-shows-support-for-bill-21-is-built-on-anti-islam-sentiment

Marche, S. (2016, November 1). *Canadian exceptionalism*. Open Canada.org. Retrieved from https://www.opencanada.org/features/canadian-exceptionalism/

Montréal Antifasciste. (2017, October 26). *Critical report on bill 62, adopted by the Québec National Assembly on October 18, 2017*. Retrieved from https://montreal-antifasciste.info/en/2017/10/26/critical-report-on-bill-62-adopted-by-the-quebec-national-assembly-on-october-18-2017/

Musaji, S. (2012, October 15). *A who's who of the anti-Muslim/anti-Arab/Islamophobia industry*. The American Muslim. Retrieved from http://theamericanmuslim.org/tam.php/features/articles/a_whos_who_of_the_anti-muslimanti-arabislamophobia_industry

Muslim Public Affair Council. (2012). *Policy report: Data on post-9/11 terrorism in the United States*. Retrieved from https://www.mpac.org/assets/docs/publications/MPAC-Post-911-Terrorism-Data.pdf

New York Times. (2020, September 17). *Trump scorns his own scientists over virus data*. Retrieved from https://www.nytimes.com/2020/09/16/us/politics/trump-cdc-covid-vaccine.html?campaign_id=9&emc=edit_nn_20200917&instance_id=22266&nl=the-morning&regi_id=134650621&section_index=2&section_name=three_more_big_stories&segment_id=38344&te=1&user_id=b2303d48cd3121f31bc49b51ed0df287

Nimer, M. (2011). Islamophobia and anti-Americanism: Measurements, dynamics, and consequences. In J. L. Esposito & I. Kalin (Eds.), *Islamophobia: The challenge of pluralism in the 21st century* (pp. 77–92). Oxford University Press.

NPR, (National Public Radio). (2021, January 15). *January 6: Inside the Capitol siege*. Retrieved from https://www.npr.org/2021/01/15/957362053/january-6-inside-the-capitol-siege

Parent, R. B., & Ellis, J. O. (2014). *Right-wing extremism in Canada. The Canadian network for research on terrorism, security, and society.* Retrieved from https://www.publicsafety.gc.ca/lbrr/archives/cnmcs-plcng/cn31894-eng.pdf

Patel, F. (2017, April 19). *The Islamophobic administration.* Brennan Center for justice. Retrieved from https://www.brennancenter.org/our-work/research-reports/islamophobic-administration

People's Party of Canada. (2019). *2019 Electoral platform: Canadian identity: Ending official multiculturalism and preserving Canadian values and culture.* Retrieved from https://www.peoplespartyofcanada.ca/canadian_identity_ending_official_multiculturalism_and_preserving_canadian_values_and_culture

Perry, B., & Scrivens, R. (2019). *Right-wing extremism in Canada.* Cham.

Pew Research Center. (2017, July 26), *U.S. Muslims concerned about their place in society, but continue to believe in the American Dream.* Retrieved from https://www.pewforum.org/2017/07/26/findings-from-pew-research-centers-2017-survey-of-us-muslims/

Pew Research Center. (2019, October 10). *Partisan antipathy: More intense, more personal.* Retrieved from https://www.pewresearch.org/politics/2019/10/10/partisan-antipathy-more-intense-more-personal/?utm_source=link_newsv9&utm_campaign=item_268982&utm_medium=copy

Russell, A., & Bell, S. (2019, September 23). *Former neo-Nazi, Pegida Canada official among People's Party of Canada signatories.* Global News. Retrieved from https://globalnews.ca/news/5929770/former-neo-nazi-pegida-canada-official-among-peoples-party-of-canada-signatories/

Sanchez, R. (2020, July 23). *Black lives matter protests across America continue nearly 2 months after George Floyd's death.* CNN. Retrieved from https://www.cnn.com/2020/07/23/us/black-lives-matter-protests-continue/index.html

Saylor, C. (2014). The U.S. islamophobia network: Its funding and impact. *Islamophobia Studies Journal, 2*(1), 99–118.

Schafer, J. A., Mullins, C. A., & Box, S. (2014). Awakenings: The emergence of white supremacist ideologies. *Deviant Behavior, 35*(3), 173–196.

Schleifer, T. (2016, March 10). *Donald Trump: 'I think Islam hates us.'* CNN. Retrieved from https://www.cnn.com/2016/03/09/politics/donald-trump-islam-hates-us/

Sirgy, M. J., Estes, R., el-Aswad, el-S., & Rahtz, D. (2019). *Combatting jihadist terrorism through nation-building: A quality-of-life perspective.* Springer.

Smith, S. J. (2020). Challenging islamophobia in Canada: Non-Muslim social workers as allies with the Muslim community. *Journal of Religion & Spirituality in Social Work: Social Thought, 39*(1), 27–46.

Southern Poverty Law Center. (2011, June 17). *The anti-Muslim inner circle.* Retrieved from https://www.splcenter.org/fighting-hate/intelligence-report/2011/anti-muslim-inner-circle

Stanley, J. (2020). *How fascism works: The politics of us and them.* Random House.

Stern, J. (2003). *Terror in the name of God: Why religious militants kill.* Harper Collins.

Taub, A. (2016, March 1). *The rise of American authoritarianism.* Vox. Retrieved from https://www.vox.com/2016/3/1/11127424/trump-authoritarianism

The Hill. (2020a, September 17). *Wray: Racially motivated violent extremism makes up most of FBI's domestic terrorism cases.* https://thehill.com/policy/national-security/516888-wray-says-racially-motivated-violent-extremism-makes-up-most-of-fbis

The Hill. (2020b, September 30). *Trump aides struggle to defend proud boys remarks at debate.* Retrieved from https://thehill.com/homenews/administration/518937-trump-aides-struggle-to-defend-proud-boys-remarks-at-debate?userid=463715

Todd, D. (2011, October 30). The state of evangelicalism: Canada differs from U.S. *Vancouver sun.* Retrieved from https://vancouversun.com/news/staff-blogs/the-state-of-evangelicalism-canada-different-from-u-s

Whitehead, A. L., Perry, S. L., & Baker, J. O. (2018). Make America Christian again: Christian nationalism and voting for Donald Trump in the 2016 presidential election. *Sociology of Religion, 79*(2), 147–171. https://doi.org/10.1093/socrel/srx070

Woodward, B. (2020). *Rage.* Simon & Schuster.

Chapter 6
Religious and Cultural Drivers of Islamophobia

6.1 Introduction

The relationship between Islamophobia and its religious and cultural drivers in North America merit scholarly attention. For the past two decades, the rising tide of Islamophobia in the religious cultures in North America has caused social and cultural mayhem (Powell, 2011). There continues to be growing hatred and enmity towards Muslim communities as identified by indicators of religious and cultural differences. Unfortunately, "countries that once imagined themselves as 'racial democracies' in which racially different people lived side by side... are now admitting the harsh reality of entrenched and historic racism" (Baldwin, 2017, pp. 9–10). Interestingly, Julian Weinberg (2010, p. 143) has argued that, "the percentages seeing the conflict as religious and cultural are higher in the West than they are in the Muslim East. When Western writers publish books entitled, 'Why Do they Hate Us?', perhaps we should also be questioning ourselves, 'Why Do Some of Us Hate them?'"

This chapter addresses important interrelated themes that include the place of religion in North America, the religious drivers of Islamophobia with a special focus on the extreme religiosity of evangelical Protestants, and the cultural drivers of Islamophobia mirrored in prejudice, intolerance and ignorance of Islam and Muslim cultures.

6.2 Place of Religion in North America

Religious trends in the United States may be different from those in the rest of the world. According to the Pew Research Center (2018), 53% of Americans, as compared with 27% of Canadians, said that religion plays an important role in their lives, while about 66% of Muslim Americans said that religion played

el-S. el-Aswad, *Countering Islamophobia in North America*, Human Well-Being Research and Policy Making, https://doi.org/10.1007/978-3-030-84673-2_6

important role. Sixty-eight percent of Christian Americans, compared with 39% of Canadians, reported religion to be important in their lives. Around 37% of Americans stated that churches and other houses of worship have too much influence on politics rather than too little (28%), while 34% said that the influence of religious groups on politics was about right. Almost half of Americans (49%) said that the Bible should influence U.S. laws; 28% favored it over the will of the people (Pew Research Center, 2020).

Researchers have argued that religion plays a political role in the United States and that almost all religious indicators are more feeble in western and central Europe than they are in the United States. They have stated that Europe lacks the massive presence of Evangelical Protestantism, which is a crucial part of the American scene (Berger et al., 2008). According to Gallup's 2020 estimate, Protestants constitute 45% of the American population, making them the largest religious group in the U.S. (Gallup, 2021). A survey, conducted in 2018 in Canada, found that 55% of Canadian adults reported to be Christian, including 29% who were Catholic and 18% who were Protestant. About 29% of Canadian Christians said religion was very important to them—higher than the share who expressed the same view in the UK, France and most other Western European countries (Pew Research Center, 2019a). Currently, Christian nationalism operates an independent ideology that influences political actions by calling forth a defense of narratives about America's distinctively Christian heritage and future (Whitehead et al., 2018).

According to the Pew Research Center (2018), Americans pray more often, attend weekly religious services, and attribute higher weight to faith in their lives than people in other Western countries, including Canada, Australia and most European states. About 55% of Americans said they pray daily, compared with 25% in Canada, 18% in Australia, 6% in Great Britain, and 22% in the average European country. Around 36% of Americans reported attending weekly worship services, compared with 20% of Canadians. Accordingly, about 59% of Muslim Americans said they pray daily and 43% reported attending weekly services (Pew Research Center, 2017).

Americans are similar to people in poorer, developing nations—including South Africa (52%), Bangladesh (57%) and Bolivia (56%) in the frequency of their daily prayer practices—than people in richer countries. Some sociologists have argued that there is a link between relatively high levels of income inequality in the U.S. and continued high levels of religiosity. These researchers posit that less-well-off people in the U.S. and other countries with high levels of income inequality may be more likely to seek comfort in religious faith because they experience financial and other insecurities. Younger Americans have not been found to be less religious than their elders, challenging the notion that older people are more religious (Pew Research Center, 2018).

Politically, the religious makeup of the United States' 116th Congress, which convened on January 3, 2019, was very different from that of the U.S. population in that it was overwhelmingly Christian. Christians made up 88.2% of the congressional representatives, while they constituted 71% of the public. Protestant members comprised 55% of the Congress and 48% of the public, while Catholic members comprised 30.5% of the Congress and 21% of the public (Pew Research Center, 2019b). Additionally, Protestants held majorities in both the House (54% including 136 Republicans and 97 Democrats) and the Senate (60% including 40 Republicans and 20 Democrats), while Catholics held 32.5% of the House (including 87 Democrats and 45 Republicans) and 22% of the Senate (including 12 Democrats and 10 Republicans). However, Catholics made up a larger share of the lower chamber than the upper chamber; there were 141 Catholics in the House (32%) and 22 in the Senate (22%). In the same 116th Congress, only two of the 252 Republicans did not identify as Christian, while 61 members of the 282 Democrats did not identify as Christian. About 35% of congressional Democrats were Catholic, compared with 25% of Republicans in Congress. There numbered three Muslim Democrats (0.6%) in the House including two Muslim women joining the House for the first time in 2019 (Pew Research Center, 2019b).

The 117th U.S. Congress, which convened on January 3, 2021, looked similar to the 116th Congress in that it was heavily Christian. Christians comprised about 88.1% of all congressional representatives, while they constituted 65% of the general public. Protestant members made up 55.4% of the Congress and 43% of the public, while Catholic members comprised 30% of the Congress and 20% of the public. However, fully 99% of the Republicans in Congress identified as Christians of whom 68% were Protestants. Democrats (43%) were less likely than Republicans (68%) to identify as Protestant. Conversely, Catholics made up a higher number of Democrats (34%) than Republicans (26%). Democrats held a slim majority in the House, and they narrowly controlled the Senate in January 20, 2021. The same three Muslim Democrats (0.6%) kept their seats in the 117th U.S. Congress (Pew Research Center, 2021).

The share of the population that belongs to faiths other than Christianity has grown much faster in Canada than in the United States. As of 2011, about 10% of Canadians self-identified as Muslim, Sikh, Hindu, Buddhist, Jewish, or adherents of other religions. By contrast, the share of U.S. adults who belong to smaller religious groups has increased over the last 30 years, and reached 6% in 2012 (Pew Research Center, 2013). The steady rise of non-Christian faiths is viewed by Christians as a threat that must be countered by, for example, the evangelization of Muslims. Tom Gibbons (2016, p. 6) stated, "in 1949 the Baptist preacher Billy Graham began mass rallies in the United States that continue to reach many nations across the world today through the Billy Graham Evangelistic Association (BGEA), founded in 1950." Several studies acknowledge the presence of a Christian norm within North America that undervalues the concerns of citizens from marginalized religions that include Muslims and other faith community members (Joshi, 2018).

According to the Social Progress Index (2020), the U.S. and Canada have interesting comparisons regarding indicators of "freedom of religion," "freedom of expression," and "access to justice" (Table 6.1). Both the U.S. and Canada scored within range of each other on "freedom of religion" and "access to justice" with the U.S. ranking higher globally in both categories. However, Canada outperformed the U.S. by ranking first globally in the category of "freedom of expression."

Table 6.1 Freedom of religion/expression and access to justice in Canada and the U.S. (2020)

Country	Freedom of religion		Freedom of expression		Access to justice	
	Score (4 = full Freedom)	Global rank (out of 163)	Score (1 = full Freedom)	Global rank (out of 163)	Score (1 = Justice accessed)	Global rank (out of 163)
Canada	3.71	45	0.98	1	0.90	37
U.S.	3.78	32	0.90	63	0.93	25

Source: Adapted with modification from Social Progress Index (2020)

6.3   Religious Driver of Islamophobia

Peter Berger (1999) pointed out that since the late twentieth century, people have been observing the desecularization of the world due to the rise of religious devotions. One of the religious drivers of Islamophobia in North America is the increase of Christian religiosity, particularly among white evangelicals. This section addresses this specific religious driver pertaining to the resurgence of Christian religiosity as reflected in white evangelical and Christian nationalism, with political impact on far-right and white supremacist groups. Despite North Americans' commitment to religious freedom and access to justice, religious minorities have been stigmatized, misunderstood, and deprived of justice (Braunstein, 2017).

6.3.1   Extreme Religiosity

The concept of religiosity includes doctrinal, experiential, ritualistic, ideological, communal, moral, and cultural components of personal involvement in religion (Sirgy et al., 2019). Regarding the doctrinal aspect, extremism often takes the form of hardened dogmatism and rigidity of thought. As Harvey Whitehouse (2004, p. 9) pointed out, "Cognitively costly aspects of religion are driven and sustained by powerful motivational systems... such systems are evidenced by all kinds of expressions of religious enthusiasm, ranging from evangelism and missionization to crusade and holy wars" (Whitehouse, 2004, p. 9). A poll conducted in 2019 found that 71% of Muslims and 82% of white Evangelicals were more likely than other faith groups and non-affiliated Americans to say religion was very important in their daily lives. However, white Evangelicals scored highest on the Islamophobia Index with 44% holding unfavorable opinions about Muslims, which is twice that of those holding favorable opinions (20%) (Institute for Social Policy and Understanding, 2019).

When addressing Christian religiosity, it has become evident that "white supremacy has become embedded in the DNA of American Christianity" (Jones, 2020, p. 3). Whitehead et al. (2018, p. 150) state, "historical and contemporary appeals to Christian nationalism are often quite explicitly evangelical, and consequently, imply the exclusion of other religious faiths or cultures." White supremacy and white privilege exist at the micro level of the person and the macro level of society and culture. At the national level, the "United States is where racism, white supremacy and white privilege run rampant" (Sullivan, 2019, p. 4).

Extreme religiosity and conservative theological beliefs, mostly of evangelical conviction, can give rise to fanaticism. Increased religiosity and intolerance in North America play a significant role in the incidence of Islamophobia (Sherrard, 2017). Paul Djupe and Brian Calfano (2012, p. 518) argued "that more religious Americans are less tolerant... In particular, fundamentalist Christians who regard the Bible as the literal word of God hold a set of beliefs that strongly influence their political beliefs... encouraging them to reject 'unbiblical' lifestyles."

Several researchers disclose that white Christians, particularly white evangelical Protestants, spread negative attitudes about racial, ethnic and religious minorities, including Muslims, in addition to instigating class-based anxieties, xenophobia and Islamophobia (Gorski, 2017; Jones, 2020). Many white evangelical Protestants see Islam and the Islamist movement as a war against Judeo-Christianity (Braunstein, 2017). Douglas Todd (2011) stated that evangelicals, or at least some of them, are the most antagonistic towards Muslims. These negative forms of Islamophobia "are empirically related to Christian nationalism... which is a proxy for evangelical Protestant affiliation, traditionalist religiosity, or political conservatism and affiliation with the Republican Party" (Whitehead et al., 2018, pp.164–165).

There is profound compatibility between white supremacist ideology and white Christian theology. White Christian Churches in the U.S. "have been responsible for constructing and sustaining to protect white supremacy" (Jones, 2020, p. 6). And, "Whatever the explicit public proclamations of white denominations and individual Christians, the public opinion data reveal that the historical legacy of white supremacy lives on in white Christianity today" (Jones, 2020, p. 10).

While not all white supremacists identify as Christian, Jones (2020, p. 80) revealed that these extremists embrace beliefs of cultural power of "the lost dominance of Christendom." And the extreme behavior of religiously unaffiliated white supremacists may be seen as a reactionary and secularized version of white Christian nationalism (Gorski, 2017; Jones, 2017, 2020). Muslims feel they are situated between the religiosity of militant white supremacists, affiliated with white evangelical Christians, and the extreme secularism of capitalist society. Muslims are accused of being reluctant to accommodate themselves to North American secular society as well as to the holding of ideas and beliefs that are different from mainstream conventions (Kalkan et al., 2009).

During the first half of the nineteenth century evangelism was the predominant religious force in American society, with "a commitment to evangelizing or 'spreading the Word'" (Layman, 2001, p. 4). Evangelicals, composing up to 35% of the U.S. population (Todd, 2011), have been active in proselytizing and evangelizing non-Christians. In the 1970s there was a call on all evangelicals to unite for the evangelization of the whole world, including Muslims. The 1978 North American Conference on Muslim Evangelization, convened in Colorado, was an example of this effort. The topics of this conference included:

"the failure of American Christian evangelization of Muslims, the need for a culturally relevant gospel for Muslims, and the urgency for further systemization of evangelical missionary work among Muslims" and "the greatest reason for the lack of Western success in evangelizing Muslims was...that Christian missionaries had so often assumed that 'Islamic cultures are totally evil'" (Kidd, 2009, p. 123).

Steven Fink (2014, p. 27) pointed out that "American Christian Zionism is a subsection of American evangelical Christianity" which emphasizes persistent support for the nation of Israel by distorting the image of Muslims, including Palestinians (Mearsheimer & Walt, 2008; Sherrard, 2017). Brooke Sherrard (2017, pp. 8–9) wrote, "Christian Zionists often operate with some of the same old tropes of Islam as a despotic and devilish tradition that will be swept away before the end of time as have existed throughout the history of American Protestantism." For Evangelicals there is a strong correlation "between Islam and the Anti-Christ... Further, their understanding of end-times scripture leads to a strong pro-Israel bias, to the point where they will either 'support Israel or be counted as God's enemy'" (Johnston, 2016, p. 170). David L. Johnston (2016) argued that the vast majority of American evangelicals support the pro-Zionist camp, and hence the Christian Right's alliance with the spreaders of hateful and rigid anti-Islamic discourse like Pamela Geller, David Horowitz, Daniel Pipes, Steve Emerson, and Glenn Beck, among others.

The number of Christian Zionists in 2009 was probably in the range of 50–60 million, demonstrating a significant Christian Zionist presence in the United States, and therefore a large number of Americans "are regularly exposed to anti-Islamic discourse" (Fink, 2014, p. 27). Fink argued that American Christian Zionist leaders connect Islam with violence threatening the security and survival not only of the U. S, but also the entire world (Fink, 2014). John Bunzl (2004, p. 9) stated, "Evangelical Christian support for right-wing Israeli agenda has been strengthened, especially after 9/11, to a large extent by dubious attractiveness of these developments, which seem in the eyes of the Evangelical Christians to corroborate their pro-Israel and anti-Islamic attitudes." Most of the post-9/11 literature draws sharper boundaries between Islam and Christianity and asserts that Islam is an essentially violent religion (Cimino, 2005; Walker, 2019).

Within the Islamophobic context, the following indicators display general patterns of how American Christian groups view Muslim Americans as being violent, extremist, anti-America, undemocratic, and not part of American mainstream (Pew Research Center, 2017). White evangelical Protestants tend to express more reservations about Muslims and Islam than do those in other Christian groups. Table 6.2 shows that 63% of white evangelicals said, 'Islam encourages violence more than any other religion'; 'Muslim Americans are extremists' (51%); 'the majority of Muslim Americans are anti-America' (38%); 'Islam is not part of mainstream American society' (67%); and 'Islam and democracy are not compatible' (72%). However, roughly half or fewer of those in other major Christian groups expressed these views.

White evangelical Protestants "view Muslims negatively because of their traditionalist religious orientations and their strong support for Israel and an aggressive

Table 6.2 Christian groups' views of Islam and Muslims in the U.S.

Christian Groups	Islam encourages violence more than any other religion (%)	Muslim Americans are extremists (%)	The majority of Muslim Americans are anti-America (%)	Islam is not part of mainstream American society (%)	Islam and democracy are not compatible (%)
Catholic	41	33	25	55	43
Protestant	51	43	32	56	55
White evangelical	63	51	38	67	72
White mainline	47	40	26	51	54
Black Protestant	n/a	32	28	39	47

Source: Adopted with modification from Pew Research Center (2017): *U.S. Muslims concerned about their place in society*

posture toward Islamic extremism" (Kalkan et al., 2009, p. 4). Meanwhile, Robert Jones developed a Racism Index focusing on general perceptions of race and racism. He stated that attending church more frequently does not make white congregants less racist. Conversely, "there is a positive relationship between holding racist attitudes and white Christian identity among both frequent (weekly or more) and infrequent (seldom or never) church attenders" (Jones, 2020, p. 184). The Racism Index confirmed the general pattern that white Christians are more likely than white religiously unaffiliated Americans to register higher scores. This is to say that "white evangelical Protestants have the highest median score (0.78) on the Racism Index" (Jones, 2020, p. 170). The median scores of white Catholics (0.72) and white mainline Protestants (0.69) were very close, compared with the median scores of the general population (0.57), white religiously unaffiliated Americans (0.42) and Black Protestants (0.24). There is no significant relationship between white religiously unaffiliated identity and holding racist attitudes. The Racism Index revealed that the more racist attitudes a person holds, the more likely he or she is to identify as a white Christian and vice versa (Jones, 2020).

In 2018, the ISPU developed an Islamophobia Index examining views of Christian, Jewish, Muslim, and religiously non-affiliated groups measuring the following indicators: 1- Most Muslims living in the United States are more prone to violence than other people. 2- Most Muslims living in the United States discriminate against women. 3- Most Muslims living in the U.S. are hostile to the United States. 4- Most Muslims living in the United States are less civilized than other people. 5- Most Muslims living in the United States are partially responsible for acts of violence carried out by other Muslims (Institute for Social Policy and Understanding, 2018) (Table 6.3).

Table 6.3 shows that the indicators of the Islamophobia Index survey revealed that the religiously unaffiliated group (14%) and Muslims (17%) expressed the lowest levels of Islamophobia, while white evangelicals (40%) and Protestants

Table 6.3 Islamophobia Index of religiously affiliated and unaffiliated groups in the U.S.

Most Muslims living in the U.S. (net % agree shown)	Muslim	Jewish	Catholic	Protestant	White Evangelical	Non-affiliated	General Public
Are more prone to violence	18%	25%	12%	13%	23%	8%	13%
Discriminate against women	12%	23%	29%	30%	36%	18%	26%
Are hostile to the United States	12%	13%	9%	14%	23%	8%	12%
Are less civilized than other people	8%	6%	4%	6%	10%	1%	6%
Are partially responsible for acts of violence carried out by other Muslims	10%	16%	11%	12%	14%	8%	12%
Index (0 min–100 max)	17%	22%	22%	31%	40%	14%	24%

Source: Adopted with modification from the Institute for Social Policy and Understanding (2018)

(31%) expressed the highest levels of Islamophobia. The higher scores on the Islamophobia Index are associated with support for discriminatory policies toward Muslims, such as the Muslim travel ban, the surveillance of American mosques, and the acceptance for targeting civilians (Institute for Social Policy and Understanding, 2018, 2019). In brief, North American evangelicals have been at the forefront of the widespread attempts to demonize Muslims (Bendroth, 2017; Todd, 2011).

While evangelicals make up to 10% of the Canadian population and are often less fundamentalist than their militant American counterparts, the evangelical Fellowship of Canada oversees and exercises power over more than 160 different evangelical denominations and organizations (Coren, 2017; Todd, 2011).

It might be insightful to make a comparison between militant Evangelical Protestants and militant Islamist jihadists (el-Aswad, el-S. et al., 2020). Both evangelical Protestants and militant Islamists use religion to rationalize their political ideologies, seeking power over the other. They divide the world into good and evil, based, respectively, on those supporting or opposing each of them. They also spread hate rhetoric and condemn each other. Both of them believe that violence against one's enemies is a sign of bravery and commitment supported by God. Finally, both are involved in the apocalyptic fight against the Antichrist, despite their ideological differences.

6.4 Cultural Drivers of Islamophobia

There are attitudes, policies, and practices that are destructive to cultures and consequently to the groups and individuals within the culture (Tajfel, 1982). The extreme examples of this orientation are programs, agencies, and/or institutions that participate in cultural dehumanization of minority groups. The effects of Islamophobia on North American Muslims' well-being and their everyday experiences of belonging, health and safety are detrimental. Religion becomes the focus of prejudice in the sense that "it is the pivot of the cultural tradition of a group" (Allport, 1979, p. 446). With reference to North America, white evangelical culture serves as a cultural code that helps white Americans form symbolic boundaries that exclude non-white racial minorities (Edgell, 2016). Recent studies show how religious commitment shapes cultural membership in North American life (Stewart et al., 2017). Cultures dominated by extreme religious outlook and biased ideology generate an unhealthy social environment. Racism and prejudice have negative impact on people's mental and physical health (Paradies, 2006; Sirgy, 2020). The cultural drivers significant to the production of Islamophobia in North America include prejudice against Muslim and ignorance of their religion.

6.4.1 Prejudice

Prejudice is defined as *"thinking ill of others without sufficient warrant"* (Allport, 1979, p. 7, italics original). Prejudice, an aspect of affect or feeling toward a group, is characteristically negative and conjuring of stereotypic images or views (Allport, 1979; Baldwin, 2017). Prejudice is a form of social rejection, leading to, and caused by stigma, "an attribute that is deeply discrediting" (Goffman, 1963, p. 3). In this context, Islamophobia is defined as "a rejection of Islam, Muslim groups and Muslim individuals on the basis of prejudice and stereotypes. It may have emotional, cognitive, evaluative as well as action-oriented elements" (Stolz, 2005, p. 548). Cultural and ethnic prejudice "is an antipathy based upon a faulty and inflexible generalization... It may be directed toward a group as a whole, or toward an individual because he is a member of that group" (Allport, 1979, p. 9). Incidents of culture-based prejudices include, for example, police brutality based on racial group, social or class divisions, or anti-Islamic bullying (Baldwin, 2017).

As mentioned in Chap. 2, there are three types of minorities in North America: religious minorities (e.g., non-Christian) racial minorities (e.g., non-white), and cultural minorities (e.g., different from North American mainstream culture). Therefore, Muslims in North America fall within "other" cultural, religious and racial minorities as there are Arab Muslims, Asian Muslims, Black Muslims and White Muslims, being targets of Islamophobia. This unique positioning necessitates a focus on the cultural implications of discrimination against Muslims as "cultural others" in

North America, despite the increase of pluralism and multiculturalism (Kalkan et al., 2009).

The "essentialization or classification of the other implies executing physical, psychological and symbolic violence upon them" (el-Aswad, el-S., 2021). The category of cultural others implies a form of discrimination and exclusion based in the conjecture that Muslims are unable to assimilate into civic life in North America. Cultural others are cultural minority groups viewed based on behaviors or values that the majority people find unacceptable (Costarelli & Gerłowska, 2015; el-Aswad, el-S., 2003, 2004, 2005, 2013b; Stewart et al., 2017). To reiterate, Muslims appear to be unique among minority groups in that attitudes toward them are associated with evaluations of cultural minority groups, ethnic groups, and racial minorities. There is a limited, "but significant, correlation between the cultural factor and the racial and religious factor—attitudes toward them may be distinct, but they are positively related" (Kalkan et al., 2009, p. 5).

In North America "religion and race intersect to form a strong white evangelical subculture that fosters attitudes about social and political issues, including race and racial inequality" (Edgell & Tranby, 2007, p. 267). Religious conservatism may lead to an even greater intolerance of cultural diversity (Fredrickson, 1981). While efforts to purify the Christian nation rely on an ethno-religious vision of American nationhood, a considerate civic logic is also at work in efforts to frame religious minorities, including Muslims, as uncivil threats to American values and norms (Braunstein, 2017). Several cultural factors that trigger discriminatory attitudes against Muslims in North America include religious conservatism, authoritarianism, patriotism, fear, and ignorance of Islam.

As aforementioned (Chap. 5), authoritarian elites and political leaders expect full conformity from all people, including minorities (Baldwin, 2017). However, from an authoritarian point of view, Muslims' cultural orientations, behaviors and attitudes do not conform fully to the ideological orientations of authoritarian elites. Such a cultural conflict drives authoritarians to discriminate against Muslims. As far as patriotism is linked to strong inclination to ingroups and insofar as Muslims are depicted as hostile to the United States, patriotic people in North America are likely to embrace discrimination against Muslims (Kalkan et al., 2009). The Islamophobia industry renders Muslims alleged foes as conceived fear and threat increase suspicion of perceived enemies (Gottschalk & Greenberg, 2008). In brief, cultural-racial discrimination is a durable and dynamic stratifying element in North America (Goodman et al., 2012).

Discrimination against Muslims in the U.S. escalated from 58% in 2009, to 59% in 2014, and to 69% in 2017, particularly during the presidency of Donald Trump. Research study found that there was a strong correlation between former President Trump's tweets on Islam-related topics and the number of anti-Muslim hate crimes after his campaign start (Müller & Schwarz, 2018; Walker, 2019). For comparison purposes, Table 6.4 shows that in 2017, 69% of Muslims faced a great deal of discrimination, exceeding discrimination against blacks (59%), Hispanics (56%), and gays and lesbians (58%) (Pew Research Center, 2017).

Table 6.4 Discrimination against minorities in the U.S. (2009–2017)

Minority/Year	2009 (%)	2014 (%)	2017 (%)
Muslims	58	59	69
Blacks	49	54	58
Hispanics	52	50	56
Gays & lesbians	64	65	58

Source: Adopted with modification from Pew Research Center (2017): *U.S. Muslims concerned about their place in society*

Table 6.5 Religious groups experiencing racial/religious discrimination (2012)

Religious groups	Percentage of discrimination (%)
Muslims	48
Jews	21
Catholics	20
Protestants	18

Source: adapted with modification from Gallup (2013). *Islamophobia: Understanding anti-Muslim sentiment in the west*

Table 6.6 Muslims less likely to experience racism from other Muslims than from general public

	Never experienced discrimination from own ethnic/faith group (%)	Never experienced discrimination from outside ethnic/faith group (%)
Arab Muslim	73	35
Asian Muslim	65	34
Black Muslim	67	44
White Muslim	69	57

Source: Adapted with modification from Institute for Social Policy and Understanding (2017)

According to Gallup (2013), 48% of Muslims were more likely than Americans of other major religious groups to say they, personally, had experienced racial or religious discrimination in 2012. In other words, Muslim Americans were more than twice as likely as American Jews (21%), Catholics (20%), and Protestants (18%) to say they experienced such discrimination (Gallup, 2013) (Table 6.5).

About 64% of those whose appearance was identifiably Muslim said they had experienced a sort of discrimination, compared with 39% among Muslims who said they did not have a distinctively Muslim appearance but reported an experience of discrimination (Pew Research Center, 2017).

In a poll conducted by the Institute for Social Policy and Understanding (2017), a Muslim person was asked if he/she experienced discrimination by another member of his/her faith community because of his/her race in the past. The same Muslim person was asked if he/she experienced discrimination by someone from outside his/her faith community because of his/her race in the past. Table 6.6 shows that the majority of non-white Muslims have experienced some race-based discrimination in the past from outside their faith community. A minority of Muslims of all ethnic backgrounds also reported experiencing racism from other Muslims in the past.

In the U.S. a higher proportion of Muslims (61%), more than any other faith group (or the unaffiliated groups), reported experiencing religious discrimination. Muslim women (75%) also reported experiencing more racial discrimination than women in the general public (40%), whereas Muslim women and those in the general public were on par in terms of gender discrimination. For Muslim women, however, racial (75%) and religious (69%) discrimination occurred more often than gender discrimination (51%).

Discrimination and intolerance lead to violence and hate crimes. In Texas, there were five reported attacks and assaults against Arab and Muslim institutions in 2017, including the vandalizing of an Islamic cemetery, which is a felony. The most recent hate crime statistics from the FBI show that anti-Arab and anti-Muslim assaults are the worst on record. Hate crimes were up 91% for the first six-months of 2017 compared with the same period in 2016. This hatred can be tragic and deadly as when two non-Muslim men were stabbed to death for coming to the defense of a veiled Muslim woman who was being harassed on a Portland, Oregon train (Arab–American Anti-Discrimination Committee, 2018).

In Canada, networks of discrimination, hate and violence, targeting Muslims, have had more than one hundred years to develop from white supremacy into a complex series of groups inclusive of Nazism. They have had strong ties with the American leadership of the KKK and other racist hate groups. These groups have recently augmented despite the disagreement of the majority of Canadians with their beliefs and actions (Kinsella, 1994). In June 2021, in London, Ontario, a man ran over a Muslim family, killing 4 persons and injuring a 9-year-old boy, with his truck because of their religion. Police said the terrorist attack was planned (NPR, 2021).

Prejudice against Muslim women is evidenced in Canada where 49% of Canadians said a woman wearing a *hijab* or *niqab* (a veil that covers the entire face except the eyes) in a public zone should be prohibited from visiting government offices. Only 29% of Canadians said such behavior should be discouraged but tolerated (Angus Reid Institute, 2017). Within a comparative analysis, 47% of Canadians would ban Muslim head scarfs in public, compared with just 30% of Americans. Likewise, 51% of Canadians liked the idea of monitoring what happens in mosques, compared with 46% of Americans (Geddes, 2017).

6.4.2 Ignorance

The deep ignorance about Islam and Muslims is one of the key drivers of Islamophobia. The "grave ignorance about Muslims and their stereotypical images in scholarship and press the world over is responsible for the emerging conflict between the West and Muslims as represented in Samuel Huntington's theory (1996) of the clash of civilizations" (el-Aswad, el-S., 2013a, p. 44), depicted by Edward Said (2001) as a clash of ignorance. In 1961, Paul Findley, a Republican

Table 6.7 Americans' views indicating that the majority of American Muslims are Arab

Response	Total (%)	Dem. (%)	Rep. (%)	Ind. (%)	Generations young old		White (%)	Non-White (%)
					18–29 (%)	65+ (%)		
Agree	30	25	40	25	36	27	30	30
Disagree	33	56	32	30	23	26	34	30

Source: Adapted with modification from Arab American Institute (2014)

Presbyterian Christian, became a member of the U.S. House of Representatives, and later wrote, "I had no idea what the words Islam and Muslims meant. . .At the same time, most of my colleagues on Capitol Hill shared similar levels of ignorance and disinterest about the Muslim world" (Findley, 2001, pp. 8–9).

Charles Mills distinguished between what he called white ignorance, a cognitive phenomenon contingent on race or racialized causality, from the general pattern of ignorance in which race is not a factor. He uses the term "ignorance" to mean both "false belief and the absence of true belief" (Mills, 2007, p. 16). White ignorance, linked to white supremacy, upholds the Racial Contract, which is "a contract between those categorized as white *over* nonwhites, who are thus the objects rather than the subjects of the agreement" (Mills, 1997, p. 12, emphasis in original). This "Racial Contract establishes a racial polity, a racial state, a racial juridical system where the status white and nonwhite is clearly demarcated, whether by law or custom" (Mills, 1997, pp. 13–14). The Racial Contract implies a system of group-based social hierarchy, embracing groups at the top and bottom (Mills, 1997; Harris, 1993). For instance, the "'mainstream' groups in American society—whites, Protestants, perhaps Catholics. . .—should associate groups like Muslims that fall outside of the mainstream with other minority groups" (Kalkan et al., 2009, p. 2). Hostility "toward Muslims as a racial outgroup is much more widespread among white racial extremists and that Muslims now occupy a place that is similar to those of black and Latinx immigrants within the extremist community" (Fording & Schram, 2020, p. 63).

White ignorance is not confined to whites; it is also shared by nonwhites due to the power relations and the patterns of ideological hegemony involved. However, whites tend not to see themselves in racial terms. White ignorance is not uniform across the white population as there are other factors such as "class, gender, nationality, religion and so forth, and these factors will modify. . .the bodies of belief and cognitive patterns of the subpopulation concerned" (Mills, 2007, p. 23).

The problem of ignorance is that a large number of Americans, particularly Republicans, have said inaccurately that the majority of American Muslims are Arab, and the majority of Arab Americans are Muslim as represented in Tables 6.7 and 6.8.

Of Americans who said they have no personal prejudice toward Muslims, 29% said they have no knowledge at all about Islam (Gallup, 2013). Even among Americans who reported no personal prejudice toward Muslims, more than

Table 6.8 Americans' views indicating that the majority of Arab Americans are Muslim

| Response | Total (%) | Dem. (%) | Rep. (%) | Ind. (%) | Generations young old | | White (%) | Non-White (%) |
					18–29 (%)	65+ (%)		
Agree	44	41	50	42	43	47	44	43
Disagree	24	21	28	22	25	23	25	20

Source: Adapted with modification from Arab American Institute (2014)

one-third (36%) said they have an unfavorable opinion about Islam. And those indicating they have a great deal of prejudice toward Muslims are the most unknowledgeable about and unfavorable toward Islam (91% unfavorable). That one-third of those with no reported prejudice have an unfavorable opinion of Islam is alarming because it indicates that those who embrace no reported prejudice for the people maintain negative views about the religion (Gallup, 2013). According to the Institute for Social Policy and Understanding (2019), three in four Jews, about half of the U.S. general public, but only about one in three white Evangelicals know an American who is Muslim. The core point here is whether Americans hold prejudice against Muslims or not, the majority of them show ignorance about Islam, leading to fear or Islamophobia.

The Arab American Institute (2014) found that favorable attitudes of Americans toward Muslims declined from 35% in 2010 to 27% in 2014 and toward Arabs from 43% in 2010 to 32% in 2014. A direct consequence of this disturbing discriminatory trend is that 42% of Americans support the use of profiling by law enforcement against both Muslim and Arab Americans (Arab American Institute, 2014).

Additionally, Republicans and Democrats showed a deep divide on the issue of discrimination as related to whether or not profiling of Muslim Americans by law enforcement is justified. A majority of Democrats (54%) did not find profiling justifiable, while a majority of Republicans (59%) did. This divide continues between older and younger Americans, and White and Non-White respondents (Table 6.9).

The actions of Terry Jones, an American anti-Islamic pastor, further exemplifies how ignorance facilitates the spread of Islamophobia worldwide. After he burned a Qur'an, on March 20, 2010, he called for an *International Burn a Koran Day*. Jones organized anti-Muslim protests and sermons in different cities inside and outside the U.S. He was also an active player in the national controversy and opposition to the construction of Park 51 (otherwise known as the Ground Zero mosque) in New York City (Goldman, 2010), which was seen as a violation of Muslims' right to freedom of religion.

Although Canada endeavors to maintain a multicultural, liberal-democratic society, anti-Muslim sentiment continues to flourish due to the view of Islam by a non-Muslim population as being incompatible with democracy, revealing a form of ignorance about Islam. Because Muslims have religious and cultural backgrounds unfamiliar to most other Canadians, they face questions about their commitment to

Table 6.9 Americans' views regarding profiling Muslim Americans by law enforcement

Response	Total (%)	Democrats (%)	Republicans (%)	Independent (%)	Generations young old		White (%)	Non-White (%)
					18–29 (%)	65+ (%)		
Agree	42	32	59	38	32	53	47	29
Disagree	40	54	25	37	54	34	34	57

Source: Adapted with modification from Arab American Institute (2014)

becoming part of Canadian society (Environics Institute, 2016). In 2015, 44% of Canadians viewed Muslims negatively, while 15% viewed them positively. Conversely, 44% of Canadians viewed Protestants positively, while 8% viewed them negatively (Angus Reid Institute, 2015). In 2016, over 35% of Canadian Muslims, compared with 21% of non-Muslims, reported "having experienced discrimination in the past five years" due to mainstream people's misunderstanding of Islam, which is above the levels of discrimination experienced by the population-at-large (Environics Institute, 2016, p. 3).

Several scholars have argued that the dominant Canadian culture is rooted in race, and founded on white and Eurocentric colonial beliefs. Moreover, race and racism are imbedded in North American institutions and in everyday lives (Goodman et al., 2012). Racial discrimination here is more about culture than about biology (Mills, 1997). In Canada, Christians, particularly white evangelicals, believe that whites are the true chosen people that should be protected from religious and cultural others (Parent & Ellis, 2014). Accordingly, as is the case in the U.S., fear of Islam and militant Muslims forms a cultural drive of Islamophobia in Canada.

6.5 Conclusion

This chapter has shown that the increase of Christian religiosity, particularly among white evangelicals, constitutes one of the most critical drivers of Islamophobia in North America. The white supremacist hatred of Muslims is a disrupting force that fuels the socio-cultural web and economy of both America and Canada.

Cultural drivers that are significant in the production of Islamophobia in North America include ignorance of Islam and discrimination against Muslims. Despite North Americans' commitment to religious freedom and freedom of expression, religious minorities have become increasingly stigmatized, excluded, and deprived of justice especially since the events of 9/11 and the Presidency of Donald Trump.

In North America, Muslims feel they are situated between the religiosity of militant white evangelical Christians, affiliated with white supremacists, and the extreme secularism of a capitalist society. Muslims are accused of being incapable of accommodating themselves to North American secular society. However, there is little evidence to support this all-inclusive claim especially within well-established Muslim American communities. Religious and political authoritarians in North America underscore conformity and convention and this translates into intolerance for groups such as Muslims who are viewed and promoted as outside of the mainstream.

Muslims have been viewed by the North American mainstream as constituting religious, cultural and racial minorities, making them distinct from other minority groups. However, North American discrimination against Muslims represent self-serving and ignorant cultural-religious attitudes that substantiate the perceived decadence and self–aggrandizement of such racially oriented cultures that attack Muslims in the name of freedom of speech.

Material presented in this chapter display that North America has gone against its claimed standards of civilization, including freedom, democracy and support of human rights, when it stigmatizes Muslim Americans and their religion, Islam. Advocates of the Islamophobia industry deprive Muslims of the promise for their religious freedoms and human rights. Religious drivers, represented in extreme religiosity, and cultural drivers, displayed in discrimination against Muslims and ignorance of Islam, result in negative consequences for both the Muslim minority and mainstream, democratic society.

References

Allport, G. W. (1979). *The nature of prejudice*. Addison-Wesley Publisher.

Angus Reid Institute. (2015, March 26). *Religion and faith in Canada today: Strong belief, ambivalence and rejection define our views*. Retrieved from http://angusreid.org/faith-in-canada/

Angus Reid Institute. (2017, March 23). *M-103: If Canadians, not MPs, voted in the House, the motion condemning Islamophobia would be defeated*. Retrieved from http://angusreid.org/islamophobia-motion-103/

Arab American Institute. (2014, July 29). *American attitudes toward Arabs and Muslims*. Retrieved from https://b.3cdn.net/aai/3e05a493869e6b44b0_76m6iyjon.pdf

Arab–American Anti-Discrimination Committee. (2018, February 13). *Anti-Sharia legislation, Islamophobia rises under Trump*. Retrieved from https://www.adc.org/anti-sharia-legislation-islamophobia-rises-under-trump-2/

Baldwin, J. (2017, January 25). Culture, prejudice, racism, and discrimination. In *Oxford research encyclopedia of communication* (pp. 1–26). Oxford University Press. https://doi.org/10.1093/acrefore/9780190228613.013.164

Bendroth, M. (2017, February 27). Christian fundamentalism in America. In *Oxford research encyclopedia of religion*. Oxford University Press. https://doi.org/10.1093/acrefore/9780199340378.013.419

Berger, P. L. (1999). The desecularization of the world: A global overview. In P. L. Berger (Ed.), *The desecularization of the world: Resurgent religion and world politics* (pp. 1–18). W.B. Eerdmans.

Berger, P., Davie, G., & Fokas, E. (2008). *Religious America, secular Europe?* Ashgate Publishing Company.

Braunstein, R. (2017). Muslims as outsiders, enemies, and others: The 2016 presidential election and the politics of religious exclusion. *American Journal of Cultural Sociology, 5*(3), 355–372. https://doi.org/10.1057/S41290-017-0042-X

Bunzl, J. (2004). Introduction: In God's name? In J. Bunzl (Ed.), *Islam, Judaism, and political tole of religions in the Middle East* (pp. 1–16). Florida University Pres.

Cimino, R. (2005). No god in common: American evangelical discourse on Islam after 9/11. *Review of Religious Research, 47*(2), 162–174.

Coren, M. (2017, December 27). How powerful is the religious right in Canada? *Maclean's*. Retrieved from https://www.macleans.ca/opinion/how-powerful-is-the-religious-right-in-canada/

Costarelli, S., & Gerłowska, J. (2015). Ambivalence, prejudice and negative behavioural tendencies towards out-groups: The moderating role of attitude basis. *Cognition and Emotion, 29*, 852–866.

Djupe, P. A., & Calfano, B. R. (2012). American Muslim investment in civil society political discussion, disagreement and tolerance. *Political Research Quarterly, 65*(3), 516–528.

Edgell, P. (2016, December 15). *Seeing the white in Christian America*. The Society Pages. https://thesocietypages.org/specials/seeing-the-white-in-christian-america/.

Edgell, P., & Tranby, E. (2007). Religious influences on understandings of racial inequality in the United States. *Social Problems, 54*(2), 263–288.

el-Aswad, el-S. (2003). Sanctified cosmology: Maintaining Muslim identity with globalism. *Journal of Social Affairs, 24*(80), 65–94.

el-Aswad, el-S. (2004). Review of Islam, Judaism, and the political role of religions in the Middle East. *Digest of Middle East Studies, 13*(2), 53–55.

el-Aswad, el-S. (2005). Review of Islam in urban America: Sunni Muslims in Chicago. *Digest of Middle East Studies, 14*(1), 78–81.

el-Aswad, el-S. (2013a). Images of Muslims in Western scholarship and media after 9/11. *Digest of Middle East Studies, 22*(1), 39–56.

el-Aswad, el-S. (2013b). Muslim Americans. In C. E. Cortés (Ed.), *Multicultural America: A multimedia encyclopaedia* (pp. 1525–1530). Sage.

el-Aswad, el-S. (2021). Oriental images and ethics: British empire and the Arab gulf (1727-1971): A perspective from historical anthropology. *Anthropos, 116*(2), in press.

el-Aswad, el-S., Sirgy, M., Estes, R., & Rahtz, D. (2020, December 17). Global jihad and international media use. In *Oxford research encyclopedia of communication* (pp. 1–29). Oxford University Press. https://doi.org/10.1093/acrefore/9780190228613.013.1151

Environics Institute. (2016). *Survey of Muslims in Canada 2016*. https://nsiip.ca/wp-content/uploads/survey_of_muslims_in_canada_2016_final_report.pdf

Findley, P. (2001). *Silent no more: Confronting America's false images of Islam*. Amana Publications.

Fink, S. (2014). Fear under construction: Islamophobia within American Christian Zionism. *Islamophobia Studies Journal, 2*(1), 26–43.

Fording, R. C., & Schram, S. F. (2020). *Hard white: The mainstreaming of racism in American politics*. Oxford University Press.

Fredrickson, G. M. (1981). *White supremacy: A comparative study in American and south African history*. Oxford University Press.

Gallup. (2013, September 21). *Islamophobia: Understanding anti-Muslim sentiment in the West*. Retrieved from http://www.gallup.com/poll/157082/islamophobia-understanding-anti-muslim-sentimentwest.aspx

Gallup. (2021, May 28). *Americans' religion and their sympathies in the Middle East*. Retrieved from https://news.gallup.com/opinion/polling-matters/350435/americans-religion-sympathies-middle-east.aspx?utm_source=alert&utm_medium=email&utm_content=morelink&utm_campaign=syndication

Geddes, J. (2017, February 9). On one issue, Canadians are a lot less tolerant than Americans. *Maclean's*. Retrieved from https://www.macleans.ca/politics/ottawa/on-one-issue-canadians-are-a-lot-less-tolerant-than-americans/

Gibbons, T. (2016, October 26). Christianity as public religion in the post-secular 21st century. In *Oxford research encyclopedia of communication* (pp. 1–16). Oxford University Press. https://doi.org/10.1093/acrefore/9780190228613.013.115

Goffman, E. (1963). *Stigma: Notes on the management of spoiled identity*. Prentice Hall.

Goldman, R. (2010, September 7). *Who is Pastor Terry Jones: Pastor behind 'burn a Koran day'*. ABC news. Retrieved from https://abcnews.go.com/US/terry-jones-pastor-burn-koran-day/story?id=11575665

Goodman, A. H., Moses, Y. H., & Jones, J. L. (2012). *Race: Are we so different?* Wiley-Blackwell.

Gorski, P. (2017). Why evangelicals voted for trump: A critical cultural sociology. *American Journal of Cultural Sociology, 5*(3), 338–354. https://doi.org/10.1057/s41290-017-0043-9

Gottschalk, P., & Greenberg, G. (2008). *Islamophobia: Making Muslims the enemy*. Rowman & Littlefield Publishers.

Harris, C. I. (1993). Whiteness as property. *Harvard Law Review, 106*(8), 1707–1791.

Huntington, S. (1996). *The clash of civilizations and the remaking of the world order.* Simon & Schuster.

Institute for Social Policy and Understanding. (2017). *American Muslim poll 2017: Muslims at the crossroads.* Retrieved from https://www.ispu.org/american-muslim-poll-2017/

Institute for Social Policy and Understanding. (2018). *American Muslim poll 2018: Pride and prejudice featuring the first-ever national American Islamophobia Index.* Retrieved from https://www.ispu.org/american-muslim-poll-2018-full-report/

Institute for Social Policy and Understanding. (2019). *American Muslim poll 2019: Predicting and preventing Islamophobia.* Retrieved from https://www.ispu.org/american-muslim-poll-2019-predicting-and-preventing-islamophobia/#4t

Johnston, D. L. (2016). American evangelical islamophobia: A history of continuity with a hope for change. *Journal of Ecumenical Studies, 51*(2), 224–235. https://doi.org/10.1353/ecu.2016.0018

Jones, R. P. (2017). *The end of white Christian America.* Simon & Schuster.

Jones, R. P. (2020). *White too long: The legacy of white supremacy in American Christianity.* Simon & Schuste.

Joshi, K. Y. (2018, May 24). Race and religion in U.S. public life. In *Oxford research encyclopedia of religion.* Oxford University Press. https://doi.org/10.1093/acrefore/9780199340378.013.460

Kalkan, K. O., Layman, G. C., & Uslaner, E. M. (2009). 'Bands of others'? Attitudes toward Muslims in contemporary American society. *Journal of Politics, 71*(3), 847–862.

Kidd, T. S. (2009). *American Christians and Islam: Evangelical culture and Muslims from the colonial period to the age of terrorism.* Princeton University Press.

Kinsella, W. (1994). *Web of hate: Inside Canada's far right network.* Harper Collins.

Layman, G. (2001). *The great divide: Religious and cultural conflict in American party politics.* Columbia University Press.

Mearsheimer, J. M., & Walt, S. M. (2008). *The Israel lobby and U.S. foreign policy.* Farrar, Straus and Giroux.

Mills, C. (1997). *The racial contract.* Cornell University Press.

Mills, C. (2007). White ignorance. In S. Sullivan & N. Tuana (Eds.), *Race and epistemologies of ignorance* (pp. 13–38). State University of New York Press.

Müller, K., & Schwarz, C. (2018). *Making America hate again? Twitter and hate crime under Trump.* SSRN Electronic Journal. Retrieved from https://papers.ssrn.com/sol3/papers.cfm?abstract_id=3149103

NPR (National Public Radio). (2021, June 8). *A man ran over a Muslim family with his truck because of their religion.* Retrieved from https://www.npr.org/2021/06/08/1004304899/man-ran-over-muslim-family-truck-canada-london-afzal

Paradies, Y. (2006). A systematic review of empirical research on self-reported racism and health. *International Journal of Epidemiology, 35*(4), 888–901.

Parent, R. B., & Ellis, J. O. (2014). Right-wing extremism in Canada. *The Canadian network for research on terrorism, security, and society (TSAS).* Retrieved from https://www.publicsafety.gc.ca/lbrr/archives/cnmcs-plcng/cn31894-eng.pdf

Pew Research Center. (2013, June 27). *Canada's changing religious landscape.* https://www.pewforum.org/2013/06/27/canadas-changing-religious-landscape/

Pew Research Center. (2017, July 26), *U.S. Muslims concerned about their place in society, but continue to believe in the American dream.* Retrieved from https://www.pewforum.org/2017/07/26/findings-from-pew-research-centers-2017-survey-of-us-muslims/

Pew Research Center. (2018, June 13). The age gap in religion around the world. Retrieved from https://www.pewforum.org/2018/06/13/the-age-gap-in-religion-around-the-world/

Pew Research Center. (2019a, July 1). *5 facts about religion in Canada.* Retrieved from https://www.pewresearch.org/fact-tank/2019/07/01/5-facts-about-religion-in-canada/

Pew Research Center. (2019b, January 3). *Faith on the Hill: The religious composition of the 116th Congress.* Retrieved from https://www.pewforum.org/2019/01/03/faith-on-the-hill-116/

Pew Research Center. (2020, July 15). *Half of Americans say Bible should influence U.S. laws; 28% favor it over the will of the people.* Retrieved from https://www.pewresearch.org/fact-tank/2020/

07/16/8-facts-about-religion-and-government-in-the-united-states/ft_20-07-16_churchstate_
bible420px/

Pew Research Center. (2021, January 4). *Faith on the Hill: The religious composition of the 117th
Congress*. Retrieved from https://www.pewforum.org/2021/01/04/faith-on-the-hill-2021/

Powell, K. A. (2011). Framing Islam: An analysis of US media coverage of terrorism since 9/11.
Communication Studies, 62(1), 90–112.

Said, E. W. (2001, October 4). *The clash of ignorance*. The Nation. Retrieved from http://www.
thenation.com/article/clash-ignorance

Sherrard, B. (2017, December 19). Islam and the Middle East in the American imagination. In
Oxford research encyclopedia of communication (pp. 1–14). Oxford University Press. https://
doi.org/10.1093/acrefore/9780199340378.013.508

Sirgy, M. J. (2020). *Positive balance: A theory of Well-being and positive mental health*. Springer
Nature.

Sirgy, M. J., Estes, R., el-Aswad, el-S., & Rahtz, D. (2019). *Combatting jihadist terrorism through
nation-building: A quality-of-life perspective*. Springer.

Social Progress Index. (2020). *Social progress imperatives*. Retrieved from https://www.
socialprogress.org

Stewart, E., Edgell, P., & Delehanty, J. (2017). The politics of religious prejudice and tolerance for
cultural others. *Sociological Quarterly, 59*(1), 17–39. https://doi.org/10.1080/00380253.2017.
1383144

Stolz, J. (2005). Explaining islamophobia: A test of four theories based on the case of a Swiss city.
Swiss Journal of Sociology, 31(3), 547–566.

Sullivan, S. (2019). *White privilege*. Polity.

Tajfel, H. (1982). Social psychology of intergroup relations. *Annual Review of Psychology, 33*(1),
1–39.

Todd, D. (2011, October 30). The state of evangelicalism: Canada differs from U.S. *Vancouver sun*.
Retrieved from https://vancouversun.com/news/staff-blogs/the-state-of-evangelicalism-canada-
different-from-u-s

Walker, N. C. (2019, August 28). *Political contempt and religion. Oxford research encyclopedia of
politics*. Oxford University Press. https://doi.org/10.1093/acrefore/9780190228637.013.1156

Weinberg, J. (2010). New Gallup report: Muslim-west discourse. *Arches Quarterly, 4*(7), 142–146.

Whitehead, A. L., Perry, S. L., & Baker, J. O. (2018). Make America Christian again: Christian
nationalism and voting for Donald Trump in the 2016 presidential election. *Sociology of
Religion, 79*(2), 147–171. https://doi.org/10.1093/socrel/srx070

Whitehouse, H. (2004). *Modes of religiosity: A cognitive theory of religious transmission*. Rowman
and Littlefield Publishers, Inc.

Chapter 7
Media Drivers of Islamophobia

7.1 Introduction

Muslims "in most of the Western media, especially since the events of September 11, 2001, are stereotypically and uncritically depicted as fundamentalist, intolerant, violent, terroristic, and as the threatening 'Other'" (el-Aswad, el-S., 2012, p. 6). Media plays a powerful role in the creation and maintenance of Islamophobic images impacting the way majority group members perceive and treat Muslims. Moreover, media is an influential driver in communicating distorted messages and stereotypes about Muslims to the public (Ahmed & Matthes, 2017; Karim, 2003; el-Aswad, el-S., 2014).

What most non-Muslims know about Islam and Muslims comes from one of two sources: the mass media and online networks which frame Muslims through the lens of terrorism and violence; and an ideologically oriented Islamophobia network, operated mostly by right-wing bloggers, advocates, authors, and politicians who make a living demonizing Muslims (Green, 2019). Furthermore, digital technologies and social media platforms such as Facebook, Twitter, and Instagram enable secrecy, anonymity and partial participation, extenuating the social, legal, and political implications and consequences of actions involving bigotry and hate (Waltman & Mattheis, 2017). In brief, media representations of Muslims impact the attitudes of North Americans toward Muslims (Said, 1997).

The core objective of Islamophobic media is to work diligently to keep the fear of terrorism and Islamophobia alive. Although Jack Shaheen stated (2001, 2017) that since 1918, more than 1200 American films, and hundreds of television programs have created negative images of Muslims, the 'war on terror' "marked an intensification of existing Islamophobia in the media" (Perry & Poynting, 2006, p. 5).

This chapter aims to investigate the underlying media drivers of Islamophobia in North America by focusing on how Islam and Muslims in North America are viewed through three core media drivers: mediated ideology of far-right conservatism, bias and misrepresentations of Islam and Muslims, and mediated politicization of Islamophobia.

7.2 Mediated Ideology of Far-Right Conservatism

Access to "a mediated public sphere and communications technology, new and print media, has given rise to a quintessential shift in information seeking behavior and is rapidly transforming the production, distribution, and consumption of knowledge and information in many parts of the world" (el-Aswad, el-S., 2021, pp. 164–165). Moreover, people, including media professionals, can be socially and politically pro and con certain extreme ideologies, resulting in media bias.

Media anchors and journalists are unlikely to use frames that reference concepts unknown within those journalists' culture or subculture. They might have certain ideologies, beliefs and preconceptions about the causes and consequences of problems, and those ideologies and beliefs can influence how they frame the news (Moy et al., 2016, p. 9). In other words, ideological differences in media source preferences may bring about distinct audience orientations for many media channels (Pew Research Center, 2014). And "[d]ifferences in expression carry ideological distinctions" (Fowler, 2007, p. 4).

In the U.S., research published by the Pew Research Center (2014), investigated the relationship between media platforms and mainstream ideologies by examining 36 news outlets. The study focused on five ideological groups, namely consistent liberals, mostly liberals, mixed liberals-conservatives, mostly conservatives and consistent conservatives. The research stated that despite that some mainstream American media outlets such as CNN (Cable News Network), ABC News (American Broadcasting Company) and Fox News, are recognized by at least 90% of respondents, they are viewed differently based on people's ideological views.

It is interesting to recognize that those with the most consistent ideological views on the left (liberals) and right (conservatives) have information streams that are very distinct from those of individuals with more mixed political views as well as from each other. Within the context of political polarization, those with both farther left and farther right ideological views have a greater impact on the political process than do those with more mixed ideological views (Pew Research Center, 2014).

The study further found that 47% of conservatives focused on a single news source, specifically Fox News as their main source for news. Other far-right media sources included Breitbart News, the National Review, the Washington Times, and the radio shows of Sean Hannity, Rush Limbaugh and Glenn Beck (Gramlich, 2020). However, fully 88% of conservatives said they trusted Fox News, while they distrusted 24 of the 36 news sources measured in the survey, including mainstream sources, such as CNN, MSNBC, the New York Times, the Washington Post, USA Today, NPR and Yahoo News (Pew Research Center, 2014).

According to the Public Religion Research Institute (2011), Americans who said they most trusted Fox News held negative views about Islam and American

Table 7.1 Major media outlets and mainstream ideologies in North America

Country	Conservative/right	Liberal/Left	Mixed
USA	Fox News	CNN	Local TV
	Rush Limbaugh	MSNBC	Google News
	Glenn Beck	NPR	Yahoo News
	Sean Hannity	New York Times	
		Washington Post	
Canada	National Post	Toronto star	Globe and mail
	Toronto sun	Maclean's magazine	CBC
	The rebel		

Source: compiled by the author from multiple sources

Muslims. Conservative and far-right media outlets have adopted an anti-Islam ideology and conspiracy theory that negatively affect Muslims in North America. It is to be noted that about 87% of those who tune in to Fox News identified their race and ethnicity as non-Hispanic white (Gramlich, 2020).

By contrast, those with liberal views relied on a greater range of news outlets and expressed more trust than distrust of 28 of the 36 news outlets, including, for instance, CNN, MSNBC, NPR, and the New York Times. About 81% of liberals distrusted Fox News, and 75% distrusted the Rush Limbaugh Show. For those who reported a mix of ideological views, their main news sources included CNN, local TV, and Fox News, along with Yahoo News and Google News, which aggregate stories from a wide assortment of outlets (Benkler et al., 2017) (Table 7.1).

Bypassing traditional mass media outlets, people are increasingly getting news from social media which are becoming major spheres for competing politicians (Dixon, 2017; Enli, 2017; Waltman & Mattheis, 2017). In the U.S., 47% of conservatives are twice as likely as the conventional Facebook user (23%) to view political opinions on Facebook that are in alignment with their right-wing ideology. Conversely, liberals are exposed to a broader range of views with about 32% of them viewing posts in accordance with their ideological positions (Pew Research Center, 2014). It is to be noted that, in 2014, 92% of Republicans were more conservative than the median Democrat, while 94% of Democrats were more liberal than the median Republican (Pew Research Center, 2014). The majority of Republicans are known for their unfavorable attitudes toward Islam. (Smith & Haberman, 2010).

Facebook is among the regular social media sources for news in North America (Face Book, 2018). In a recent survey, Facebook ranked first in 2020, with 36% of Americans accessing news regularly. YouTube followed with 23% of the adult population and Twitter with 15% of the adult population obtaining their news from these sites (Pew Research Center, 2021). It is worth noting that based on a sample of more than 100 million tweets, a study found that "Trump's anti-Muslim tweets are widely shared by his followers, who produce further xenophobic content in response, such as messages containing the hashtags '#StopIslam' and '#BanIslam'" (Müller & Schwarz, 2018, p. 4).

New media and online websites that attack Islam and Muslims virtually have increased. And a number of ideologically-driven blogs and websites have become important information centers for the far-right. Some of these websites include, for example, the Jihad Watch, Stop the Islamization of America, the Gateway Pundit, the Daily Stormer, and the Three Percenters, among others, that participate, though differently, in attacking and dehumanizing Muslims (Marwick & Lewis, 2017). Activities on the internet and such websites have promoted and encouraged anti-Muslim sentiment enticing followers to carry out violent and terrorist actions targeting Muslims and their institutions (Coleman, 2017). For example, more than 60 anti-mosque incidents were carried out across the U.S in 2008 (American Civil Liberties Union, 2020).

In Canada, there is also competition between conservative and less-conservative outlets. For instance, the National Post, known for being conservative, competes directly with the Globe and Mail (Potter, 2014), an outlet with a large circulation that holds a centrist political position (Bothwell, 2017; Granatstein & Anderako, 2015; Potter, 2014). It worth noting that a great deal of mass media in Canada tend to be conservative (Vipond, 2011, p.12). Left or liberal audiences, however, depend on leading liberal news outlets including, for instance, the Toronto Star and Maclean's magazine. Those who have a mix of ideological views, rely on the Canadian Broadcasting Corporation (CBC) as well as the Globe and Mail (Table 7.1).

7.3 Media Bias and Misrepresentations of Islam and Muslims

Generally, there are various drivers of media bias and prejudice. For example, media corporations may have a strong bias for one political party or policy issue and may influence their media outlets to reflect that bias. In addition, individual newscasters and journalists may favor one side of an issue and reflect that bias, consciously or unconsciously, in the way they cover news stories. This driver relates to the ethnic blame discourse in North America in the sense that ethnic and racial minorities are responsible for their own problems (Dixon et al., 2019). Also, characterizing stereotypes makes processing and attending to media messages appealing and easier for audience members. Within the framework of market supply and demand, since stereotypes appeal to and are easily processed by wide-ranging audiences, the misrepresentation of racial and ethnic groups enables good revenue and profits. Media coverage of Islamophobia can be exceptionally profitable. Another driver relates to the fact that a majority of media anchors and commentators in North America are white leading to high potential for biased reporting on minority groups (Dixon et al., 2019; Snyder & Ballentine, 1996; Tattrie, 2019a, 2019b).

Literature review shows that several studies have focused on the media bias and misrepresentations of Islam, Muslims and Arabs in the West (Ahmed and Matthes 2017; Belt 2016; Ciftci, 2012; el-Aswad, el-S., 2013; el-Aswad, el-S. et al., 2020;

Farouqui, 2009; Kanji, 2018; Karim, 2003; Poole & Richardson, 2006; Richardson, 2004). Several mainstream media commentators, journalists, Islamophobes, right-wing bloggers, authors, and academics have been involved in creating and spreading false narratives of the moral system of Islam and the stereotypically adverse attributes of Muslims (Brown, 2006). As opposed to rumors and mistakes, fake news "are intentionally and verifiably false" (Allcott & Gentzkow, 2017, p. 231). Fake news, a critical tool of information warfare, has been employed to incite violence between ethnic groups (Hills, 2019). Fake news not only spreads faster than the truth, but also reaches more people than the truth (Jasny, 2018). And repeating false information makes it more believable. Even when false information is debunked, it may continue to shape people's attitudes (Marwick & Lewis, 2017).

There is worldwide concern over false information as it influences people's political, economic, social and health well-being. It is worth noting that new media and social technologies, which facilitate rapid information sharing and extensive information flows, "can enable the spread of misinformation" (Vosoughi et al., 2018, p. 1146). Studies have shown that 80% of the news coverage of Muslims is false and extremely negative, portraying Islam, individual Muslims and Muslim organizations as roots of hostility and violence (Abdelaziz, 2018). Several media outlets have fabricated images of Muslims including, for example, bearded terrorists, mad religious imams, cartoon bombs involving Muslims in turbans, veiled and dangerous Muslim women, airplane hijackings, skyscraper terrorism, and suicide bombers (Russel, 2013; Springer et al., 2009; Wiktorowicz, 2005). Moreover, when a mosque burns, U.S. media outlets do not cover the event as when a church or synagogue burns (Shaheen, 2017). In addition, Alex Jones and his team at Infowars have been on the attack spreading false information and lies about Islam and Muslims (Media Matters, 2018).

The subsequent paragraphs focus on the drivers of media bias attacking Muslims in the U.S. and Canada.

7.3.1 The U.S.

Anti-Muslim media bias has impacted both Muslims and non-Muslims. Media coverage has remarkable social and psychological impact on the well-being of Muslim communities. Although media outlets plan to reach the public, the main drive behind their attack of Muslim is to serve conservative Republicans or provide media supply to right-wing groups. A poll conducted by the Pew Research Center (2017) shows that 53% of the U.S. general public think coverage of Islam and Muslims by American news organizations is generally unfair, compared with 39% who think the media of Islam and Muslims is fair. However, 60% of American Muslims think coverage of Islam and Muslims by American news organizations is generally unfair, compared to 27% who think that coverage of Islam and Muslims by the U.S. media is fair (Pew Research Center, 2017) (Table 7.2).

Table 7.2 Americans' views of the U.S. media coverage of Islam and Muslims

U.S. media coverage of Islam and Muslims is generally...	U.S. Muslims (%)	U.S. general public (%)
Fair	27	39
Unfair	60	53
Other/do not know	13	8
Total	100	100

Source: Adopted with modification from Pew Research Center (2017)

Table 7.3 Americans' views of Islam as part of mainstream society

Do American people see Islam as part of mainstream society?	U.S. Muslims (%)	U.S. general public (%)
Yes	29	43
No	62	50
Other/do not know	9	7
Total	100	100

Source: Adopted with modification from Pew Research Center (2017)

Influenced by biased media, American people do not see Islam as part of mainstream American society, despite the growing number of Muslim communities and agencies throughout the U.S. These views are largely echoed by U.S. adults 50% of which say they do not see Islam as part of mainstream society, as compared with 43% who say that Islam is part of mainstream society. On the other hand, 62% of American Muslims say they do not see Islam as part of mainstream society, as compared with 29% who say that Islam is part of mainstream society (Table 7.3). These negative media portrayals of Muslims as well as Trump's attitudes and policies toward Muslims, epitomized in several media outlets, are the most critical problems facing the Muslim community in the U.S. (Pew Research Center, 2017).

Islamophobes and anti-Muslim media outlets in North America use fake facts, represented, for example in Frank Gaffney's blog (2012), to claim that Muslims have been engaged in a stealth or civilizational jihad to infiltrate the U.S. legal system and other public institutions and bring America under Islamic law (Isaacs, 2018). More mainstream American media, such as Fox News, view Islam negatively and necessarily anti-democratic (el-Aswad, el-S., 2013; Farouqui, 2009). The vast majority of North American media, radio, television programs, online posts, and articles make a direct link between Islam and violence, terrorism, irrationality, backwardness and dishonesty. In other words, the terms Islam and Muslim in media are linked to extremism, Islamic war, Islamic terror, and militant jihadists, as if they belonged together inextricably and naturally (el-Aswad, el-S., 2013; The Guardian, 2005).

The New York Times was the focus of the 416 Labs report. In 2015, the report investigated news headlines in the New York Times newspaper. It detected significant bias against Islam and Muslims who were depicted in terms of militancy and terrorism. According to the report, Islam was portrayed negatively in 57% of the New York Times headlines, compared with cancer, alcohol and cocaine, which were negatively evaluated respectively at 34%, 44% and 47%. The latter terms, however, were often associated with health risks, disease, poverty or drug related violence (Arshad et al., 2015).

The Media has rarely distinguished between the religion of Islam and the political-religious affairs that occur in most Islamic countries, including global and non-state terrorist or jihadist groups such as al-Qa'ida, ISIS and IS (Da'ish) or the Islamic State of Iraq and the Levant (ISIL) (el-Aswad, el-S. et al., 2020). One study pointed out that in the 14 years since the 9/11 terror attacks, nearly twice as many people have been killed in the United States by white supremacists and anti-government radicals than by Muslim jihadists (Washington Times, 2015). White supremacists and extreme right-wing paramilitaries stormed the U.S. Capitol on January 6, 2021, in an unprecedented episode of turmoil and domestic terrorism in American history (Snyder, 2021). In his book, *Hateland* (2019), Daryl Johnson stated that in the U.S., there has been continuous processes of radicalization of Americans, particularly those associated with far-right and white supremacy organizations, generating unparalleled cases of violence and crimes against Muslims.

Within this unhealthy and toxic environment, anti-Muslim media provide baseless anti-Islam propaganda (Kalsnes, 2018). Even Americans express suspicion and skeptical views about media representations. For example, Americans perceive news organizations as lacking in transparency with respect to the work they do and the inner workings of their companies. Not only do many Americans see news outlets as opaque in how they produce their stories and choose their sources but a large majority (72%) have said news organizations do an insufficient job explaining to the public where their information comes from (Pew Research Center, 2020).

Additionally, 69% of Americans think news organizations generally try to cover up mistakes and misinformation when they do occur. There are different reasons for why Americans think these mistakes highlight the distrust that significant portions of the public feel. For instance, 55% of Americans think that mistakes and misinformation in news narratives are due to careless reporting, while 44% think the mistakes or misinformation are driven by a desire to mislead the public. In a nutshell, Americans think that trust and truth in the media have declined (Pew Research Center, 2020).

Another survey poll indicated that 64% of Americans said social media has a mostly negative effect on the way things are going in the U.S. There are again different reasons behind this perception of the negative effect of social media: 28% of Americans think that it is due to the spread of misinformation and fake news, while 16% of Americans think it is due to explicit messages of hate, harassment, and extremism. About 11% of Americans think this negative effect is caused by a lack of critical thinking skills among many users, facilitating concern that people who use these sites either believe everything they see or read, or are unsure about what to believe (Auxier, 2020).

Media Matter (2017) reported that immediately after former President Donald Trump initiated the first iteration of a travel ban targeting Muslims, prime-time television hosted a group of 176 experts (of whom 14 were Muslims) to discuss the ban, despite the fact that the ban principally targeted several Muslim-majority countries. The fourteen Muslim guests were invited by Fox News (five Muslims), CNN (seven Muslims) and MSNBC (two Muslims). Fox News' Bill O'Reilly, while speaking to two non-Muslim guests, stated that he did not care if any Muslims were alienated by the United States due to the ban (Media Matter, 2017).

7.3.2 Canada

In Canada, a recent Abacus Data poll conducted from January 15–18, 2021 showed overwhelming concern for online hate and racism among Canadians. The poll indicated that 93% of Canadians think online hate and racism is a problem; 20% of Canadians have experienced online hate, harassment, or violence, including 40% of 18–29 year-olds, and 29% of racialized Canadians (Abacus Data, 2021; Farber & Balgord, 2021).

Another research (Kanji, 2018) investigated the phenomenon of negative and biased media framing of Muslims in Canadian national news media, including the Globe and Mail, the National Post, and CBC. The research compared representations of ideological violence committed by Muslim versus non-Muslim perpetrators, specifically white supremacists and right-wing extremists. Major findings of the research indicated that acts of Muslim violence received 1.5 times more coverage on average, than non-Muslim crimes, while obstructed Muslim plots received five times more coverage. Muslim incidents were depicted not as crimes, but as terrorist acts and associated with other occurrences of violence. Here, the depiction of terrorism is critical as terrorism is viewed by Canadian political leaders and judiciary as posing an existential threat to Canada that is consequently used to justify a pre-emptive and punitive response by law enforcement. In this particular context, Muslim perpetrators were categorized by their religious and ethno-racial identities (Kanji, 2018). However, there were exceptional cases where some media outlets, such as the Toronto Star, offered relatively balanced or unbiased coverage of Islam and Muslims (Perry & Poynting, 2006; Poynting & Perry, 2007).

7.4 Mediated Politicization of Islamophobia

Islamophobia has become an ideological construction "upon which governmental policies and social practices are framed" (Sheehi, 2011, p. 31). The underlying political ideologies of politicians and media professionals have played critical roles in spreading Islamophobia at national and international levels. Internationally, social and political forces that advocate wars against several Muslim countries (Afghanistan, Iraq, Syria and Libya, for example) have used and disseminated concepts of terrorists and extreme jihadists via the media to justify for their aggressive actions (el-Aswad, el-S. et al., 2020). Western media has repeatedly stressed the reality of terrorist acts, bomb blasts, flag burning, and the misconduct of Muslims, especially imams or men of religious learning accused of politically mobilizing Muslim people (el-Aswad, el-S., 2013). Nationally, several government and non-government media outlets, in both Canada and the U.S, have played a principal role in the creation of fabricated images of Muslims for ideological and political gains. These media drivers have contributed to the rapid spread of Islamophobia in North America. Politically oriented organizations and media platforms, using fear and anger to spread negative messages about Muslims, have moved from the fringes of public discourse into the mainstream media (Bail, 2012).

The following subsection address, in detail how the media politicize Islamophobia in the U.S and Canada.

7.4.1   The U.S.

In the U.S., the media have dealt with Islamophobia as an ideological phenomenon fulfilling and promoting political and economic goals, both nationally and internationally. Islamophobia is used as a powerful political construction that sustains an American Empire (Kumar, 2012; Sheehi, 2011). The deep-seated negative perceptions of Islam in the U.S. affect discourses and actions of Muslims who have become subject to the web of racism (el-Aswad, el-S., 2013). As Doris Graber (2003) maintained, when politicians control the media, they proliferate their ideologies and are able to dominate people and society. For politicians and pundits, the media is "a political institution that plays an important role in politics along with many other institutions" (Graber, 2003, p. 140). However, politicians have implemented a political strategy of labeling news sources that do not support their ideologies as unreliable or fake news, whereas sources that support their positions are labeled reliable and true (Vosoughi et al., 2018).

Using media as a *power ideology* is one of the major drivers of cultural, religious and political domination of minorities in America. Islamophobia here is understood not only as a fear of the 'other,' but also as a political campaign and a main focal point of political action that is tied to American power and discursive processes that subject Muslim minorities to the power of the state (Tutt, 2013). Anti-Muslim hatred and racism are utilized as tools, effectively normalizing dangerous rhetoric and moving Islamophobia from the realm of harassment to possibly fully politicized and institutionalized legislations (Islamophobia Studies Center, 2020).

Many diverse ideologies, particularly those of conservatives, evangelicals, far-right extremists, and white supremacists, have used various media to induce racist rhetoric and actions in America, including instances of racial animosity, anti-Muslim racism, and anti-government views. American far-right communities "may feel that by manipulating media outlets, they gain some status and a measure of control over an entrenched and powerful institution, which many of them distrust and dislike" (Warwick & Lewis, 2017, p. 31).

The politicization of Islamophobia is reflected in the phenomenon that several Christians, particularly evangelical groups in the U.S. tend to "associate Christianity with nationalistic, right-wing causes" (Ward, 2008, p. 170), acting contrary to biblical teaching, in the process of defending themselves against outsiders. Literature shows the impact of religiously oriented media on audience political views (Djupe & Calfano, 2019; Lewis, 2019). For instance, a video clip, posted by Fox News 2 Detroit, Michigan (2019), featured an anti-Muslim event organized by the Bloom-field Hills Baptist Church, during which a pastor called himself a 'proud Islamophobe' and claimed that Muslims and Islam constituted a threat to the U.S. and the entire world (Fox News 2 Detroit, 2019). On the 700 Club, a Christian Broadcasting Network, televangelist Pat Robertson on recorded video hosted the Republican activist, Michele Bachmann who appeared and warned about media whitewash on Muslim terrorism. Robertson described Muslims as people who want to destroy Western civilization. He claimed that Muslims wanted to bring people back to the Arabia of the seventh and eighth centuries (Tashman, 2012). On NBC, in November 2001, evangelical minister Franklin Graham called Islam a very evil and wicked religion signaling at least some American evangelical Christians' negative views of Islam (Sherrard, 2017).

For evangelicals, the main source of information is the Christian media. According to a survey conducted in 2005, "more than 90 percent of evangelicals consume some form of evangelical media—radio, television, websites, magazine—each month" (Pasha, 2016, p. 228). However, evangelical media, "owned and operated primarily by white Anglo-Saxon" (Schultze & Woods, 2008, p. 284), have expressed fear and suspicion about Islam (Fortner 2009; Bruner, 2008). Yet, it is quite odd to hear evangelicals claim that Islamophobia is a political tool designed and used by Muslims to silence Christians and distract them from danger-ous movements in the Muslim world (Milstein, 2019).

The electronic Church, through radio, television and the Internet, has kept the evangelical informed about the war with Islam going beyond the domestic issues of Muslim Americans (Trammell, 2016) to take a global-apocalyptic tune. Evangelicals believe that before the Messiah returns, the Temple in Jerusalem must be rebuilt on its original site. However, Al-Aqsa Mosque, one the most sacred places of Islam, currently sits on the Temple Mount. Therefore, "Islam is literary a tool of Satan's fanatical but ultimately doomed determination to prevent of the Second Coming and the establishment of Christ millennial rule on earth" (Trammell, 2016, p. 235). The evangelical author and television host Hal Lindsey wrote, "Islam represents the single greatest threat to the continued survival of the planet" (Trammell, 2016, p. 236).

Personalities, particularly of the political and religious elites contribute to the major narrative for constructing and perpetuating media stereotypes, including dehumanizing Islamophobic ideology. Elites play a major role in the "discursive reproduction processes of the system of racism" as the folk follow their elites' ideologies (Van Dijk, 1997, p. 32). Specifically, presidents and other political elites have used media and political-religious rhetoric throughout American history to varying extents, though how they used them changed during the Trump era to be much more exclusive, rather than inclusive, when compared with the language of past presidents (Djupe & Calfano, 2019; Reilly, 2018; Uberti, 2016).

Islamophobic political ideology is also reflected in the speech of media professionals, such as Fox News' hosts Tucker Carlson and Judge Jeanine Pirro, who have a history of attacking Islam and Muslims. Carlson, shown in a video clip released by Fox News (2019), accused Ilhan Omar, a Muslim congresswoman from Minnesota, of being an anti-American politician. By the same token, Judge Pirro, shown in a YouTube published by the Washington Post (2019), questioned the patriotism of Ilhan Omar and asked whether the Somali-American's Islamic religious beliefs stood in opposition to the U.S. constitution (Stelter, 2020, p. 242). Pirro pressed down on one of the Fox News' favorite fear themes: Shari'a law. And she demonized Omar even more than her colleagues had.

Additionally, Marjorie Taylor Greene, a far-right Congresswoman from Georgia, filmed herself visiting the U.S. Capitol, shown in a video clip (Media Matters, 2020), where she accused Ilhan Omar and U.S. Representative Rashida Tlaib of Michigan of supporting Shari'a Islamic law and of not being legitimate congresswomen because they were sworn into office using a Qur'an instead of a Bible. She wanted them to re-take their oaths of office on a Bible (Media Matters, 2020; Southern Poverty Law Center, 2019).

The previous statement indicates how media has been able to create another source of Islamophobia related to the fear that Muslim Americans aspire to impose the Islamic law (Shari'a law) on American people, including non-Muslims, threatening the social fabric of American society (Elliot, 2011). Far-right extremists associated with QAnon, Trump's supporters, are known among conspiracy-oriented groups for issuing alerts that Shari'a law will be enforced on the U.S. (Fraser, 2020).

7.4.2   Canada

In Canada, negative media portrayals of Islam, together with discriminatory policies and practices at the level of the state, "create an enabling environment that signals the legitimacy of public hostility toward Muslim communities" (Perry & Poynting, 2006, pp.1–2). Such discriminatory practices conducted by the media and the state, have reinforced a racist and Islamophobic ideology. Use of online and social media platforms has reduced the geographical distance between members in such a way that hate groups, including anti-Muslim racists, are currently able to reach wider audiences (Waltman & Mattheis, 2017).

White supremacist and far-right violence have been documented as forming the most threatening factor in Canada (Henry & Tator, 2006; Perry & Scrivens, 2019; Schafer et al., 2014). A study about the white nationalist website, Stormfront, found that Islamophobic sentiments were more prominent among Canadian subscribers than Americans in the United States (Schafer et al., 2014). Another study revealed that between 1994 and 2004, 64.7% of Canadian national television news reports included evangelicals from Canada, while 32.7% featured evangelicals from the United States (Haskell, 2007).

The anti-Muslim movement in Canada is a network of groups and individuals, active online and offline, who share the fear that western cultures are threatened by an Islamic takeover. Anti-Muslim groups view Islam as a political ideology (Plante, 2015). The Canadian Defence League is an example of one of these anti-Muslim groups that has spread hateful anti-Muslim messages on their Facebook page (Davey et al., 2020). Anti-Muslim hate speech has moved from being a phenomenon to a social disease. Certain Canadian politicians, aided by a few media outlets inflaming Islamophobia, have used the Muslim community in a politically hot game in hopes of gaining more votes during election periods (Canadian Muslim Forum, 2016).

In Canada, politically oriented conservatives claimed that Islam "is intolerant and hateful of anything different from itself" (Marine, 2017, p. 325). They also stated, "mainstream Islam is the culture of enemy" (Marine, 2017, p. 331). Islamophobes attack not only Canadian Muslims, but also any institution or person who shows fair attitudes toward them. For example, Islamophobes, using media, Internet and online networks, smeared Justin Trudeau for his support of minorities, including Muslims (Lim, 2019).

These examples have highlighted how extensive anti-Muslim activity is represented in various forms of media, cyberspace and online social networks. It is worthy to note the irrational fear, explicitly among Islamophobes, of the mere thought of the implementation of Shari'a law in Canada (Selby & Korteweg, 2012), despite the fact that Canadian Muslims do not seek to displace Canadian law with Shari'a law (Noor Cultural Center, 2018).

7.5 Conclusion

This chapter has addressed media outlets that propagate anti-Muslim racism, shedding light on the underlying media drivers that has resulted in the rapid expansion of Islamophobia in North America. Print media, social media platforms, Internet memes, websites, cyber forums, political podcasts, online chats, and videos, among other media channels and digital communication technologies, have become effective tools for spreading Islamophobia in North America. While Islamophobia is one of other types of racism, it has developed its exceptional feature as being linked to the irrational fear of Islam.

This study has focused on three core media drivers of Islamophobia: 1-mediated ideologies of far-right conservatism, 2-media bias and misrepresentations of Muslims, and 3-mediated politicization of Islamophobia. These drivers have negatively impacted the attitudes of North Americans toward Muslim communities. The problem of media outlets is that they deal with Muslims as if they were forming a monolithic and homogenous community. Muslims in North American media are stereotypically and uncritically depicted as fundamentalist, fanatics, violent, terroristic, and as the threatening 'Other.' Muslim symbols and attire, headscarves, veils (*hijabs*), beards, turbans, prayers, and mosques are recurrent topics of media misrepresentations.

These systemic misrepresentations not only breed hate, fear and suspicion which distance Muslims from the rest of the North American mainstream, but also cause cultural polarization in which Muslims are depicted as aliens. Media have contributed to increasing levels of Islamophobia by normalizing voices of racism, prejudice and hatred, in the name of augmenting public discourses.

Although this study tackles media outlets influenced by two ideological groups, specifically conservatives (right-wing) and liberals (left-wing), it concludes that far-right conservatives are the foremost drivers of Islamophobia in North America, driven by economic-political and ideological gains. Islamophobia also relates to various drivers of media bias ranging from the manufacture of fake news and the dispersion of propaganda ideology to the dehumanization of minorities. The media's stereotypes and biased depictions of Muslims as being violent might cause social volatility and political instability, leading to animosity and conflict between Muslims and non-Muslims, as well as conservatives and liberals.

This chapter has provided documented material confirming that most North American media outlets are biased in their depiction of Islam and Muslims. Other media outlets that are not associated with the far-right wing, such as CNN and the New York Times among others, have also produced unfavorable coverage of Muslims, though not on as immense a magnitude as that of the far-right media. This might be explained by the fact that most media reporters tend to present Islam and Muslims in a way that corresponds to their own ideologies and to the values of the societies to which they belong.

Mediated politicization of Islamophobia is another critical media driver. This has been clearly evident in the political far-right extremist camps of both the U.S. and Canada, mobilizing the public against Muslim minorities via different media outlets. Negative media portrayals affect the overall well-being of Muslims and their perception of themselves.

Media has played a decisive part in creating radicalized antagonists, generating chaos in North American countries. The problem is not confined to those who confront Muslim Americans, but it extends to include both majorities and minorities within the entire society. Radicalization has intensified to embrace far-right extremists and white supremacists who, in their insurrection and attack on the U.S. Capitol/Congress (on January 6, 2021), represented a real threat to democracy and civil rights.

References

Abacus Data. (2021, January). *Online hate and racism. Canadian race relations foundation.* Retrieved from https://www.crrf-fcrr.ca/images/CRRF_OnlineHate_Racism_Jan2021_FINAL.pdf

Abdelaziz, A. (2018, July 3). *Coverage of American Muslims is bigoted and inaccurate.* HuffPost. Retrieved from https://www.huffingtonpost.com/entry/muslim-coverage-bigoted-inaccurate_us_5b3be3cee4b09e4a8b284a59

Ahmed, S., & Matthes, J. (2017). Media representation of Muslims and Islam from 2000 to 2015: A meta-analysis. *The International Communication Gazette, 79*, 219–244.

Allcott, H., & Gentzkow, M. (2017). Social media and fake news in the 2016 election. *Journal of Economic Perspectives, 31*(2), 211–236.

American Civil Liberties Union. (2020). *Nationwide anti-mosque activity*. Retrieved from https://www.aclu.org/issues/national-security/discriminatory-profiling/nationwide-anti-mosque-activity?redirect=map-nationwide-anti-mosque-activity

Arshad, O., Setlur, V., & Siddiqui, U. (2015). Are Muslims collectively responsible? A sentiment analysis of the New York Times. *416Labs* (pp. 1–29). Retrieved from https://static1.squarespace.com/static/558067a3e4b0cb2f81614c38/t/564d7b91e4b082df3a4e291e/1505087319147/416LABS_NYT_and_Islam.pdf

Auxier, B. (2020, October 15). 64% of Americans say social media have a mostly negative effect on the way things are going in the U.S. today. *Pew research Center*. Retrieved from https://www.pewresearch.org/fact-tank/2020/10/15/64-of-americans-say-social-media-have-a-mostly-negative-effect-on-the-way-things-are-going-in-the-u-s-today/

Bail, C. A. (2012). The fringe effect: Civil society organizations and the evolution of media discourse about Islam since the September 11th attacks. *American Sociological Review, 77*(6), 855–879. https://doi.org/10.1177/0003122412465743

Belt, D. D. (2016). Anti-Islam discourse in the United States in the decade after 9/11: The role of social conservatives and cultural politics. *Journal of Ecumenical Studies, 51*(2), 210–223.

Benkler, Y., Faris, R., Roberts, H., & Zuckerman, E. (2017, March 13). Study: Breitbart-led right-wing media ecosystem altered broader media agenda. *Columbia Journalism Review*. Retrieved from https://www.cjr.org/analysis/breitbart-media-trump-harvard-study.php

Bothwell, R. (2017, November 8). *Toronto Star. The Canadian Encyclopedia*. Retrieved from https://www.thecanadianencyclopedia.ca/en/article/toronto-star

Brown, M. D. (2006). Comparative analysis of mainstream discourses, media narratives and representations of Islam in Britain and France prior to 9/11. *Journal of Muslim Minority Affairs, 26*(3), 297–312.

Bruner, K. (2008). Thinking outside the tribal TV box. In Q. J. Schultze & R. H. Woods (Eds.), *Understanding evangelical media: The changing face of Christian communication* (pp. 47–57). IVP Academic.

Canadian Muslim Forum. (2016, October). *Islamophobia is now a Canadian concern*. Retrieved from https://www.fmc-cmf.ca/islamophobia-is-now-a-canadian-concern/

Ciftci, S. (2012). Islamophobia and threat perceptions: Explaining anti-Muslim sentiment in the west. *Journal of Muslim Minority Affairs, 32*(3), 293–309.

Coleman, N. (2017, August 7). *On average, 9 mosques have been targeted every month this year*. CNN. Retrieved, from https://www.cnn.com/2017/03/20/us/mosques-targeted-2017-trnd/index.html

Davey, J., Hart, M., & Guerin, C. (2020). *An online environmental scan of right-wing extremism in Canada: Interim report*. Institute for Strategic Dialogue. Retrieved from https://www.isdglobal.org/wp-content/uploads/2020/06/An-Online-Environmental-Scan-of-Right-wing-Extremism-in-Canada-ISD.pdf

Dixon, T. L. (2017). How the internet and social media accelerate racial stereotyping and social division: The socially mediated stereotyping model. In R. A. Lind (Ed.), *Race and gender in electronic media: Challenges and opportunities* (pp. 161–178). Routledge.

Dixon, T. L., Weeks, K. R., & Smith, M. A. (2019, May 23). Media constructions of culture, race, and ethnicity. *Oxford Research Encyclopedia of Communication*. Oxford Press. Retrieved from https://doi.org/10.1093/acrefore/9780190228613.013.502.

Djupe, P. A., & Calfano, B. R. (2019, August 28). *Communication dynamics in religion and politics. Oxford research encyclopedia of politics*. Oxford University Press. https://doi.org/10.1093/acrefore/9780190228637.013.682

el-Aswad, el-S. (2012). *Muslim worldviews and everyday lives*. AltaMira Press.

el-Aswad, el-S. (2013). Images of Muslims in Western scholarship and media after 9/11. *Digest of Middle East Studies, 22*(1), 39–56.

el-Aswad, el-S. (2014). Communication. In K. Harvey (Ed.), *Encyclopedia of social media and politics* (Vol. 1, pp. 304–308). SAGE.

el-Aswad, el-S. (2021). Rethinking knowledge and power hierarchy in the Muslim world. In A. Fromherz & N. Samin (Eds.), *Knowledge, authority and change in Islamic societies: Studies in honor of Dale F. Eickelman* (pp. 157–171). Leiden.

el-Aswad, el-S., Sirgy, M., Estes, R., & Rahtz, D. (2020, December 17). *Global jihad and international media use. Oxford research encyclopedia of communication.* Oxford University Press. https://doi.org/10.1093/acrefore/9780190228613.013.1151

Elliot, A. (2011, July 30). *The man behind the anti-Shariah movement.* The New York Times. Retrieved from http://www.nytimes.com/2011/07/31/us/31shariah.html?_r=2&hp

Enli, G. (2017). Twitter as arena for the authentic outsider: Exploring the social media campaigns of trump and Clinton in the 2016 US presidential election. *European Journal of Communication, 32*(1), 50–61.

Face Book: Politikal Memes. (2018, November 20). *Imam admits Justin Trudeau will allow sharia law in Canada if re-elected.* Retrieved from https://www.facebook.com/politikalmemes/videos/2170991046496582/

Farber, B., & Balgord, E. (2021, January 25). *Overwhelming Canadian support for new consequences/regulations around online hate and racism.* Canadian Race Relations Foundation. Retrieved from https://www.antihate.ca/support_new_regulations_consequences_online_hate_racism_policy?utm_campaign=jan_27&utm_medium=email&utm_source=antihate

Farouqui, A. (2009). *Muslims and media images: News versus views.* Oxford University Press.

Fortner, R. S. (2009). Internationalizing evangelical media. In Q. J. Schultze & R. H. Woods (Eds.), *Understanding evangelical media: The changing face of Christian communication* (pp. 239–251). IVP Academic.

Fowler, R. (2007). *Language in the news: Discourse and ideology in the press.* Routledge.

Fox News. (2019, July 10). *Tucker: Rep. Ilhan Omar attacks the country that took her family in.* Retrieved from https://video.foxnews.com/v/6057198316001#sp=show-clips

Fox News 2 Detroit. (2019, September 5). *'Proud Islamophobe' pastor hosts anti-Muslim event on 9/11 at Bloomfield Hills church.* Retrieved from https://www.fox2detroit.com/news/proud-islamophobe-pastor-hosts-anti-muslim-event-on-9-11-at-bloomfield-hills-church

Fraser, S. (2020, October 15). *The United States of paranoia: From the Salem witch hunt to conspirator-in-chief Donald Trump.* TomDispatch: A regular antidote to the mainstream media. Retrieved from https://tomdispatch.com/steve-fraser-was-american-history-a-conspiracy/

Gaffney, F. (2012, April 23). *Losing the Jihadists' war on America.* Middle East and Terrorism. Retrieved from https://israelagainstterror.blogspot.com/2012/04/losing-jihadists-war-on-america.html

Graber, D. (2003). The media and democracy: Beyond myths and stereotypes. *Annual Review of Political Science, 6*, 139–160. https://doi.org/10.1146/annurev.polisci.6.121901.085707

Gramlich, J. (2020, April 8). *5 facts about fox News.* Pew Research Center. Retrieved from https://www.pewresearch.org/fact-tank/2020/04/08/five-facts-about-fox-news/

Granatstein, J. I., & Anderako, M. (2015). *Maclean's. The Canadian encyclopedia.* Retrieved from https://www.thecanadianencyclopedia.ca/en/article/macleans

Green, T. (2019, April 26). *Islamophobia. Oxford research encyclopedia of religion.* Oxford University Press. https://doi.org/10.1093/acrefore/9780199340378.013.685

Haskell, D. M. (2007). News media influence on nonevangelical coders' perceptions of evangelical Christians: A case study. *Journal of Media and Religion, 6*(3), 153–179.

Henry, F., & Tator, C. (2006). *The colour of democracy: Racism in Canadian society.* Thomson Nelson.

Hills, T. T. (2019). The dark side of information proliferation. *Perspectives on Psychological Science, 14*(3), 323–330.

Isaacs, A. (2018, July 31). *American Islamophobia's fake facts: Their 'proof' is not what they say.* TomDispatch: A regular antidote to the mainstream media. Retrieved from https://tomdispatch. com/arnold-isaacs-the-con-game-of-america-s-anti-muslims/#more

Islamophobia Studies Center. (2020, August 18). *Islamophobia on the 2020 Campaign Trail.* Retrieved from https://iphobiacenter.org/2020-campaign-trail/

Jasny, B. R. (2018). Lies spread faster than the truth. *Science, 359*(6380), 1114–1115. https://doi. org/10.1126/science.359.6380.1114-h

Johnson, D. (2019). *Hateland: A long, hard look at America's extremist heart.* Prometheus Books.

Kalsnes, B. (2018, September 26). Fake News. *Oxford research encyclopedia of communication.* New York: Oxford Press. Retrieved from https://doi.org/10.1093/acrefore/9780190228613.013. 809.

Kanji, A. (2018). Framing Muslims in the "war on terror": Representations of ideological violence by Muslim versus non-Muslim perpetrators in Canadian national news media. *Religion, 9*(9), 274–300. https://doi.org/10.3390/rel9090274

Karim, H. (2003). *Islamic peril: Media and global violence.* Black Rose Books.

Kumar, D. (2012). *Islamophobia and the politics of empire.* Haymarket Books.

Lewis, A. R. (2019). *The inclusion-moderation thesis: The U.S. republican party and the Christian right.* Oxford research encyclopedia of politics & religion. Retrieved from https://doi.org/10. 1093/acrefore/9780190228637.013.665

Lim, J. (2019, July 15). *Trudeau criticizes racist Trump remarks attacking four congresswomen.* Ipolitics. Retrieved from https://ipolitics.ca/2019/07/15/trudeau-criticizes-racist-trump-remarks-attacking-four-congresswomen/

Marine, S. (2017). Stephen Harper and the radicalization of Canadian foreign policy. In J. P. Lewis & J. Everitt (Eds.), *The blueprint: Conservative parties and their impact on Canadian politics* (pp. 314–342). University of Toronto Press.

Marwick, A., & Lewis, R. (2017, May 15). *Media manipulation and disinformation online.* Data & Society Research Institute. Retrieved from https://datasociety.net/library/media-manipulation-and-disinfo-online/

Media Matters. (2018, August 20). *Alex Jones: I am Islamophobic.* Retrieved, 20 August, from https://www.mediamatters.org/video/2018/08/20/alex-jones-i-am-islamophobic/221030

Media Matters. (2020, August 18). *Marjorie Taylor Greene visited the capitol and tried to get reps. Ilhan Omar and Rashida Tlaib to retake their oaths on the Bible.* Politico. Retrieved from https://www.mediamatters.org/congress/marjorie-taylor-greene-visited-capitol-and-tried-get-reps-ilhan-omar-and-rashida-tlaib

Milstein, A. (2019, May 31). *Islamophobia – The 21st-century weapon to silence our freedom of speech?* CBN News: The Christian Perspective. Retrieved from https://www1.cbn.com/ cbnnews/israel/2019/may/islamophobia-ndash-the-21st-century-weapon-to-silence-our-freedom-of-speech

Moy, P., Tewksbury, D., & Rinke, A. M. (2016). Agenda-setting, priming, and framing. In K. B. Jensen & R. T. Craig (Eds.), *The international encyclopedia of communication theory and philosophy* (pp. 1–13). John Wiley & Sons.

Müller, K., & Schwarz, C. (2018). *From hashtag to hate crime: Twitter and anti-minority sentiment.* SSRN electronic journal. Retrieved from https://ssrn.com/abstract=3149103

Noor Cultural Center. (2018). *Islamophobia in Canada: Myths and facts.* Retrieved from https:// noorculturalcentre.ca/wp-content/uploads/2018/03/Islamophobia-Myths-and-Facts-1.pdf

Pasha, S. (2016). American apocalypse: Portrayal of Islam and Judaism in the post-9/11 electric church. In M. Ward (Ed.), *The electronic church in the digital age: Cultural impacts of evangelical mass media (How evangelical media engage American culture)* (Vol. 2, pp. 227–252). Praeger, ABC-CLIO, LLC.

Perry, B., & Poynting, S. (2006). Inspiring islamophobia: Media and state targeting of Muslims in Canada since 9/11. *Paper presented at TASA conference*, University of Western Australia & Murdoch University, 4–7 December. Retrieved from https://web.archive.org/web/ 20180417175416/https://tasa.org.au/wp-content/uploads/2015/02/PerryPoynting.pdf

Perry, B., & Scrivens, R. (2019). *Right-wing extremism in Canada*. Palgrave.

Pew Research Center (2014, June 12). *Political polarization in the American public*. Retrieved from https://www.pewresearch.org/politics/2014/06/12/section-1-growing-ideological-consistency/

Pew Research Center. (2017, July 26), *U.S. Muslims concerned about their place in society, but continue to believe in the American Dream*. Retrieved from https://www.pewforum.org/2017/07/26/findings-from-pew-research-centers-2017-survey-of-us-muslims/

Pew Research Center. (2020, August 31). *Americans see skepticism of news media as healthy, say public trust in the institution can improve*. Retrieved from https://www.journalism.org/2020/08/31/americans-see-skepticism-of-news-media-as-healthy-say-public-trust-in-the-institution-can-improve/?utm_source=Pew+Research+Center&utm_campaign=0f3ef94846-Weekly_2020_09_05&utm_medium=email&utm_term=0_3e953b9b70-0f3ef94846-400057377

Pew Research Center. (2021, January 12). *News use across social media platforms in 2020*. Retrieved from https://www.journalism.org/2021/01/12/news-use-across-social-media-platforms-in-2020/

Plante, C. (2015, October 1). *Québec Solidaire motion condemning 'islamophobia' passes unanimously in National Assembly: Québec Solidaire wants Quebecers to tone down the rhetoric when it comes to Islam*. Montreal gazette. Retrieved from https://montrealgazette.com/news/quebec/quebec-solidaire-calls-for-calm-as-use-of-term-islamophobia-debated

Poole, E., & Richardson, J. E. (2006). *Muslims and the news media*. I. B. Tauris.

Potter, J. (2014, July 3). *The National Post*. The Canadian Encyclopedia. Retrieved from https://thecanadianencyclopedia.ca/en/article/the-national-post

Poynting, S., & Perry, B. (2007). Climates of hate: Media and state inspired victimisation of Muslims in Canada and Australia since 9/11. *Current Issues in Criminal Justice, 19*(2), 151–171.

Public Religion Research Institute. (2011, September 6), *What does it mean to be American?* Retrieved from https://www.prri.org/spotlight/what-does-it-mean-to-be-american/

Reilly, R. (2018, February 15). *A Federal appeals court just said Trump's tweets show he's an anti-Muslim bigot*. HuffPost. Retrieved from https://www.huffingtonpost.com/entry/trump-anti-muslim-travel-ban_us_5a85c085e4b0774f31d3307c

Richardson, J. E. (2004). *(Mis)representing Islam: The racism and rhetoric of British broadsheet newspapers*. John Benjamins.

Russel, W. F. (2013). *Islam: A threat to civilization*. First Edition Design Pub..

Said, E. W. (1997). *Covering Islam: How the media and the experts determine how we see the rest of the world*. Vintage Books.

Schafer, J. A., Mullins, C. A., & Box, S. (2014). Awakenings: The emergence of white supremacist ideologies. *Deviant Behavior, 35*(3), 173–196.

Schultze, Q. J., & Woods, R. H. (2008). Conclusion: Being self- critical about evangelical media. In Q. J. Schultze & R. H. Woods (Eds.), *Understanding evangelical media: The changing face of Christian communication* (pp. 282–287). IVP Academic.

Selby, J. A., & Korteweg, A. C. (2012). Introduction: Situating the sharia debate in Ontario. In A. C. Korteweg & J. A. Selby (Eds.), *Debating sharia: Islam, gender politics, and family law arbitration* (p. 12). University of Toronto Press.

Shaheen, J. G. (2001). *Reel bad Arabs: How Hollywood vilifies a people*. Olive Branch Press.

Shaheen, J. G. (2017). Introduction. In N. Lean (Ed.), *The islamophobia industry: How the right manufactures fear of Muslims by Nathan lean* (pp. xix–xxiii). Pluto Press.

Sheehi, S. (2011). *Islamophobia: The ideological campaign against Muslims*. Clarity Press.

Sherrard, B. (2017, December 19). Islam and the Middle East in the American imagination. In *Oxford research encyclopedia of communication*. Oxford University Press. https://doi.org/10.1093/acrefore/9780199340378.013.508

Smith, B., & Haberman, M. (2010, August 15). *GOP takes harsher stance toward Islam*. Politico. Retrieved from http://www.politico.com/news/stories/0810/41076.html

Snyder, T. (2021, January 9). *The American abyss: A historian of fascism and political atrocity on trump, the mob and what comes next*. New York time magazine. Retrieved from https://www.nytimes.com/2021/01/09/magazine/trump-coup.html

Snyder, J., & Ballentine, K. (1996). Nationalism and the marketplace of ideas. *International Security* 21(2), 5–40. Retrieved from https://doi.org/10.2307/2539069

Southern Poverty Law Center. (2019, August 16). *Marjorie Taylor Greene: How an outspoken MAGA fan built a following in a world of extremists.* Retrieved from https://www.splcenter.org/hatewatch/2019/08/16/marjorie-taylor-greene-how-outspoken-maga-fan-built-following-world-extremists

Springer, D. R., Regens, J. L., & Edger, D. N. (2009). *Islamic radicalism and global Jihad.* George Town University Press.

Stelter, B. (2020). *Hoax: Donald Trump, fox News, and the dangerous distortion of truth.* One Signal Publishers/Atria.

Tashman, B. (2012, April 16). *Pat Robertson and Michele Bachmann warn about media whitewash on terrorism.* Right Wing Watch. Retrieved, from http://www.rightwingwatch.org/content/pat-robertson-and-michele-bachmann-warn-about-media-whitewash-terrorism

Tattrie, J. (2019a, June 11). Fake news (a.k.a. disinformation) in Canada. *Canadian encyclopedia.* Retrieved from https://www.thecanadianencyclopedia.ca/en/article/fake-news-in-canada

Tattrie, J. (2019b, October 23). *Media bias in Canada.* Canadian Encyclopedia. Retrieved from https://www.thecanadianencyclopedia.ca/en/article/media-bias-in-canada

The Guardian. (2005, November 14). *Media has anti-Muslim bias, claims report.* Retrieved from https://www.theguardian.com/media/2005/nov/14/pressandpublishing.raceintheuk

Trammell, J. Y. (2016). Jesus? There is an app for that! Tablet media in the 'new' electronic church. In M. Ward (Ed.), *The electronic church in the digital age: Cultural impacts of evangelical mass media (How evangelical media shape evangelical culture)* (Vol. 1, pp. 219–238). Praeger, ABC-CLIO, LLC.

Tutt, D. (2013, June 25). *How should we combat islamophobia?* Huffpost. Retrieved from: https://www.huffingtonpost.com/daniel-tutt/how-should-we-combat-islamophobia_b_3149768.html

Uberti, D. (2016, December 15). The real history of fake news. Columbia Journalism Review. Retrieved from https://www.cjr.org/special_report/fake_news_history.php

Van Dijk, T. A. (1997). Political discourse and racism: Describing others in Western parliaments. In S. H. Riggins (Ed.), *The language and politics of exclusion: Others in discourse* (pp. 3–64). Sage.

Vipond, M. (2011). *The mass media in Canada.* James Lorimer Publishers.

Vosoughi, S., Roy, D., & Aral, S. (2018). The spread of true and false news online. *Science, 359* (6380), 1146–1151. https://doi.org/10.1126/science.aap9559. Retrieved from https://science.sciencemag.org/content/359/6380/1146

Waltman, M. S., & Mattheis, A. A. (2017, September 26). *Understanding hate speech. Oxford research encyclopedia of communication.* Oxford University Press. https://doi.org/10.1093/acrefore/9780190228613.013.422

Ward, A. (2008). Faith-based theme parks and museums: Multidimensional media. In Q. J. Schultze & R. H. Woods (Eds.), *Understanding evangelical media: The changing face of Christian communication* (pp. 161–172). IVP Academic.

Warwick, A., & Lewis, R. (2017, May 15). Media manipulation and disinformation online. *Data & Society.* Retrieved from https://datasociety.net/library/media-manipulation-and-disinfo-online/

Washington Post. (2019, March 12). *Jeanine Pirro's history of controversial comments on Islam.* Retrieved from https://www.youtube.com/watch?v=yCHdow7wvSw&ab_channel=WashingtonPost

Washington Times. (2015), June 24. *Majority of fatal attacks on U.S. soil carried out by white supremacists, not terrorists.* Retrieved from https://www.washingtontimes.com/news/2015/jun/24/majority-of-fatal-attacks-on-us-soil-carried-out-b/

Wiktorowicz, Q. (2005). *Radical Islam rising: Muslim extremism in the west.* Rowman & Littlefield.

Part IV
Policies to Combat Islamophobia

Chapter 8
Policies Confronting Biased Media

8.1 Introduction

This study contributes to the scholarship of public policies dealing with both the countering of biased media and the combating of Islamophobia. The previous chapter has examined the role of biased media outlets and social media networks in propagating and spreading stereotypes and misrepresentations of Islam and Muslims. This chapter, viewing biased media and Islamophobia as two sides of the same coin, aims at examining the efforts made by governments and NGOs or advocacy organizations to counter media bias and Islamophobia in North America. It is efficacious, however, to focus on the holistic picture that explains media's quality-of-life intervention policies and plans to reduce Islamophobia.

As false representations trigger strong reactions to refute and resist them (Vosoughi et al., 2012), this study proposes that misrepresentations about Islam and Muslims demand strong reactions to counter them. A plan to offset negative representations can be implemented by the adoption of counter—and more accurate—representations that seek to highlight negative depictions.

Several scholars point out that frequent exposures to biased media depictions tend to cause the viewers to accept such depictions as being proper reflections of reality (Gerbner et al., 1980). However, counter-discriminations deploring misrepresentations of a group enable individuals to make substantial evaluation of misleading media depictions (Power et al., 1996). Being aware of stereotypical information about Muslims increases the perceived credibility of Muslims and discredits biased media reports.

Public policy, affecting a portion of the public, indicates the process through which a government acts to improve people's quality of life or deals with the needs of its citizens through plans and actions defined by the law or its constitution (el-Aswad, el-S., 2019; Hersch, 2016). For public and social policy advocates, Islamophobia necessitates policies to counter all forms of injustice and discrimination directed at Muslims. This research provides recommendations for policymakers, political leaders, media reporters and viewers, Muslim and non-Muslim.

This chapter focuses on three core themes: approaches to combat biased media, countering biased media of conservative and far-right extremists, and combatting Islamophobia and hate activities on biased social Media.

8.2 Approaches to Combat Biased Media

Media play a large role in the fabrication of false images of Muslims (el-Aswad, el-S., 2013; el-Aswad, el-S. et al., 2020). Theoretically, there are two approaches that can work together to combat media bias and anti-Muslim racism. One approach proposes that policies advocating guidance and restrictions on biased media are the appropriate solutions, while the other approach prefers an open marketplace of ideas, where no expression is restricted (Walker, 2018). This chapter attempts to employ these approaches to better understand the intricate problem of combating biased media and the related Islamophobia industry.

It is hard to conceive of a media outlet that is completely unbiased or completely biased. For example, in the U.S., 64% of Republicans, 65% of Democrats, and 64% of Independents expressed their concern about the biases in others' news sources, rather than the one with which they identify (Gallup, 2020). To discern bias, it is more appropriate to compare media outlets to one another, establish a baseline of what is possible or realistic, and compare the content and relative extent to which media content is biased (Brinson, 2009; Garz, 2014).

While there are myriad different approaches within the media dealing with Islamophobia, there are two primary, opposing and competing paradigms that can be summarized as *war* and *peace* media approaches. As opposed to war media, spreading bias and conflict information as well as focusing on elite and bureaucratic sources, peace media promotes the contextualization of conflict narratives and seeks to supply opportunities for audiences to galvanize their empathic abilities through the humanization of actors in conflict narratives (Lynch, 2008). A study centering on countering Islamophobic media representations reveals that lower levels of Islamophobia are associated with reporting patterns that are consonant with a "peace journalism" approach, while higher levels of Islamophobia are associated with reporting patterns that are in the line with "war/violence journalism" (Anderson, 2015 p. 256). It is important to not minimize the victims' experiences by indicating that digitally mediated injury is less harmful than physical harm. The veracity of the emotional, social, and professional effect of digitally mediated harm should be taken into account (Phillips, 2018).

A society's economic, political and cultural well-being is advanced by numerous and independent media, while excessive media concentration may endanger the public's access to essential information or viewpoints (Baker, 2013; Stucke & Grunes, 2009). The concept of a marketplace of ideas refers to a domain in which intangible values compete for acceptance. The most favorable results can be better attained by free trade in ideas and the best assessment of truth is the power of the thought that gets accepted in the competitive market. In other words, truth prevails in the widest possible dissemination of information from diverse and opposed sources (Stucke & Grunes, 2009). It is to be noted that the marketplace of ideas is important to democracy, in the sense that democracy thrives when there is an unconstrained flow of information (Stucke, 2008; Stucke & Grunes, 2009). Within this theoretical scope, an unbiased and "competitive media, for example, (1) informs policy makers of the unintended social effects of their policies, (2) provides a voice to pressure the government for change, and (3) serves as a catalyst for institutional change to promote competition policy" (Stucke, 2008 p.1021), facilitating equality and better quality of life.

The problem here is that Islamophobes have used extended media means to compete for acceptability, spreading their hateful ideas to a large audience. More-over, this unhealthy presentation by Islamophobic media needs to be challenged and reformed. The best response to Islamophobic media is through debate that lets different ideas challenge it freely. Jake Lynch (2014 p. 6) states, "Good journalism… works against journalism itself, or at least against journalism-as-usual… It challenges accepted notions of 'us' and 'them'." Concerning the impor-tant role played by media in society, any reliable reform or competition policy must involve advancing a competitive market place of ideas with cost-effective measures to combat Islamophobic media (Stucke, 2008). It is essential to observe that, "Increased competition in the news market… can lead to lower bias…This finding was consistent with several other studies that show how competition among alter-native sources of media reduces bias" (Stucke & Grunes, 2009 p.120). Reforms in media could result in significant outcomes in terms of developed confrontation and contestation of dominant discourses that misrepresent Muslims and Islam, not merely in North American media networks but worldwide.

There is a more recent problem pertaining to the use of social media, the Internet, and interactive computer services such as Facebook, Twitter and YouTube among others, that have been granted immunity by Section 230 of the Communications Decency Act (CDA) of 1996 (U.S. Code, 2021; U.S. Department of Justice, 2020). Section 230 of the CDA gives interactive computer services and other interactive media ample immunity from liability for user-generated content posted on their sites. The U.S. policy objectives of Section 230 are "(1) to promote the continued development of the Internet and other interactive computer services and other interactive media; (2) to preserve the vibrant and competitive free market that presently exists for the Internet and other interactive computer services, unfettered by Federal or State regulation" (U.S. Code, 2021 p.1). It interesting to note that traditional media companies have expanded their Internet holdings, or sought to collaborate with well-known Internet platforms (Stucke & Grunes, 2009).

The purpose of granting immunity to platforms is to encourage them to take an active role in removing offensive content, as well as to avoid free speech problems of security censorship, implying the protection of free speech for platform users. Courts have grappled with how to locate online platforms within First Amendment doctrine, protecting freedom of speech, religion and the press. And scholars have debated how to constrain or control these platforms (Klonick, 2018). The "combination of significant technological changes since 1996 and the expansive interpretation that courts have given Section 230, however, has left online platforms both immune for a wide array of illicit activity on their services and free to moderate content with little transparency or accountability" (U.S. Department of Justice, 2020, p.1). Prior to the Internet, the publisher was the most critical constraint on the effect and power of speech. However, the "internet ended the speaker's reliance on the publisher by allowing the speaker to reach his or her audience directly" (Klonick, 2018 p. 1603). The main issue here relates to whether the First Amendment constrains the government's ability to regulate media platforms or, rather, supports such an effort (Stucke & Grunes, 2009).

8.3 Countering Biased Media of Conservative and Far-right Extremists

This section aims to enable and help researchers and policymakers understand how right-wing extremists have manipulated the media. The following subsections discuss how the U.S and Canada counter biased media of far-right extremists.

8.3.1 The U.S.

Bias is the ideological distortion of information, and that problem is built into the U.S.'s current system (Center for American Progress, 2005). Previous chapters have addressed the spread of Islamophobia in North America through misinformation campaigns orchestrated by right-wing media organizations and conservative Christian fundamentalist groups, among others. The far-right media are accused of bias against Islam and Muslims. Many far-right extremists share broader views of conservatism, expressed, for example, in their portrayal of immigrants, including Muslims, as geopolitical threats (Center for American Progress, 2020). Such extremist members are hidden behind the guise of conservatism to disseminate racist beliefs and hate ideologies, including Islamophobia, Christian nationalism, white supremacy, and anti-Semitism (Ryan, 2021). From a legal perspective, based on the U.S. Hate Crime Statistics Act, hate crimes are viewed to be criminal violations that manifest evidence of prejudice based on race, religion, sexual orientation, or ethnicity (Osterbur, 2020).

Far-right media organizations augment and disseminate Islamophobic views to wide audiences. Among the far-right media associates in the U.S. are the Fox News channel, the National Review magazine and its website, the Washington Times newspaper and website, and the Christian Broadcasting Network and website. Those in charge of these media networks often view themselves as unbiased, but their attitude, policy, and practice reflect their biased media. They invite and encourage Islamophobes to spread xenophobic and prejudiced views, claiming that what they do is based on freedom of expression (Center for American Progress, 2011). The American Center for Law and Justice, the conservative legal foundation founded by Pat Robertson and Jay Sekulow, has claimed that Muslims are compelled by their religion to fight America and other countries (Right Wing Watch, 2011).

The flow of information and exercise of freedom of expression cannot be used as an excuse for violating human rights or attacking religious beliefs. Article 20 of the International Covenant on Civil and Political Rights (United Nations, 1966) states that any propaganda for war and any advocacy of national, racial or religious hatred that constitutes incitement to discrimination, hostility or violence shall be prohibited by law. In the opinion of the Human Rights Committee, such prohibitions are fully compatible with the right to freedom of expression (United Nations, 2014).

It is interesting to note that on January 20, 2021, on his first day in office, U.S. President Joseph Biden, issued a proclamation ending and revoking the discriminatory travel ban that prevented Muslims from certain countries entry into the U.S. (The White House, 2021a). Another executive order was made to advance racial equity and support for historically underserved communities through the federal government. The policy of the administration confirms that the Federal Government should pursue a comprehensive approach to advancing equity for all, including people of color and others who have been historically disadvantaged, marginalized, and adversely affected by persistent poverty and inequality (The White House, 2021b).

Concerning policies countering media bias, religious discrimination and Islamophobic hate, a state's national action plan, while guaranteeing freedom of expression, in accordance with international law, should:

- Execute rigorous research and examination of Islamophobic discourses of right-wing extremists posted and displayed on media outlets;
- Initiate programs that aim to eradicate religious-racial discrimination disseminated by biased media;
- Establish mechanisms to ensure that media outlets assist in the promotion of religious tolerance;
- Train media producers and journalists to act objectively in providing unbiased information;
- Encourage members of media organizations to envision creative ways of combating Islamophobic media;
- Allocate federal resources to advance fairness and opportunity to invest sufficiently and equally in underserved communities;
- Combat bigotry in the biased media by holding anchors and producers accountable;
- Support international strategies to combat criminal right-wing extremist media content;
- Arrange virtual discussion groups about Islamic culture with participation of renowned Muslim scholars and anti-Islamophobia organizations;

- Invite diverse faith groups to engage in media and online interfaith dialogues (United Nations, 2014).

As to the approach of a marketplace of ideas in which media networks compete with each other, it is interesting to note that there are independent and competitive media outlets that counter biased media and hate issues. In the U.S., these competitive anti-Islamophobia media and organizations include, for example, Media Matters for America, the Center for American Progress, Arab–American Anti-Discrimination Committee, Muslim Advocates, Right Wing Watch, the Southern Poverty Law Center, and TomDispatch. However, this study does not claim that these organizations and media outlets are representative of the complex nature of anti-Islamophobia networks in the U.S. Yet, by examining the diverse views offered by these media and related organizations, the study aspires to achieve a better understanding of the rising phenomenon of countering Islamophobia in the U.S.

Media Matters (2019), criticizing the claims of Fox News and other right-wing media outlets that Muslims are a threat to the U.S., stated that right-wing extremism in America is an actual threat, and that conservative media downplaying the problem makes it worse. It also stated that white extremists pose an even greater terrorist threat than Muslims. According to the Anti-Defamation League, right-wing extremists were responsible for 73.3% of the murders committed between 2009 and 2018, compared to 3.2% for left-wing extremists and 23.4% for Islamist extremists (Media Matters, 2019). In addition, right-wing media have been criticized for its interference in Muslim legal affairs, attacking Muslims advocates for urging American Muslims to have attorneys when speaking to law enforcement (Media Matters, 2017). Such legal advice is standard guidance given by many legal rights advocacy groups, including the American Bar Association (Media Matters, 2011).

It is interesting to observe that *TomDispatch: A regular antidote to the mainstream media* (founded by Tom Engelhardt), has published several anti-Islamophobia articles criticizing and refuting Islamophobes and media organizations behind the propaganda that slams Muslims as being a threat to Western democracy. For example, Arnold Isaacs (2018a, 2018b) has criticized such Islamophobes as Brigitte Gabriel, John Bolton, Fred Fleitz, and John Guandolo. He criticized Gabriel, head of the organization of ACT for America, which is one of the most vocal anti-Muslim organizations in the U.S., for her contradictory statement that Muslims who believe in the teachings of the Qur'an, cannot be a loyal citizen to the United States (Isaacs, 2018b).

The Southern Poverty Law Center, a public policy research and advocacy organization, has provided critical reports concerning far-right extremists, disinformation media and conspiracy theories. It published several articles that countered Islamophobia and hate bigotry, including, for instance, *the anti-Muslim inner circle* (2011), *ten ways to fight hate: A community response guide* (2017), *hate crimes, explained* (2018), and *hate map* (2020). The following is a summary of the policies and recommendations offered by the Southern Poverty Law Center (2017) for fighting bias media and countering Islamophobia:

- Consider hate news a wake-up call that reveals tension in the community. Attack the problem.
- Take Islamophobic-hate crimes seriously and report on them prominently.
- Urge editorial writers, columnists, and hate experts to take a stand against hate.
- Remind editors that it is not fair to focus on small number of radical Muslims as representing all-inclusive Muslims worldwide.
- Do not debate Islamophobes and hate group members on conflict-driven talk shows. Your presence lends them legitimacy and publicity.
- Select a person from your group to be the main contact for the media. Invite the press to public events you hold.
- Perform a nuanced and thoughtful coverage. Propose human-interest narratives, such as the impact of Islamophobia on individuals.
- Don't allow hate groups to masquerade as white-pride civic groups or heritage organizations. On their media, they vilify certain groups of people, typically people of color, Jews, and Muslims.
- Sponsor a forum or other community media event tied to issues of combating Islamophobia and hate.

The Arab–American Anti-Discrimination Committee (2018) condemned Trump's administration for dehumanizing Muslims by the infamous Muslim ban that contributed to the increase in anti-Muslim racism and led 18 state legislatures in 2017 to introduce bills to ban Shari'a. Similarly, Muslim Advocates (2020) issued a response to news reports about right-wing Islomophobes who, driven by conspiracy theories, attacked Muslim Congresswomen claiming that they should go back to their Muslim countries as they hate America and support Shri'a, designed to impact the American legal system. However, there is no reliable evidence that Shari'a infiltrates the American legal system as conspiracy theorists claim (Isaacs, 2018a, 2018b). Such biased and antagonistic attitudes of the right-wing media toward Islam and Muslims cannot repudiate the exceptional contribution of Islamic civilization to humanity (el-Aswad, el-S., 2019).

Civil society and the public at large have a significant role to play in fighting religiously motivated hate rhetoric of media. Local and national leaders, scholars, lawmakers and stakeholders play a noteworthy role in combatting Islamophobic media of far-right extremists. The following example shows an exceptional case in which Islamophobia and biased media have been successfully combatted.

This case relates to an Islamophobic and anti-Muslim 9/11 anniversary event organized by the Bloomfield Hills Baptist Church in Michigan, covered by several local and national media outlets. The Bloomfield Hills Baptist Church had planned to host a two-day event (Sept. 11 and 12, 2019) entitled, "*9/11 Forgotten? Is Michigan Surrendering to Islam?*" that was canceled due to wide-scale confrontation and criticism from state and congressional political leaders, lawmakers and Christian scholars, who denounced the anti-Islamic orientation of the event (Beachum, 2019; Detroit Metro Times, 2019; Detroit Free Press, 2019a). In an interview conducted by Fox 2 News (2019) in Detroit, Donald McKay, pastor of the Baptist church, said he was proud to describe himself as an Islamophobe.

Without providing any evidence for his argument, McKay argued that Islam is a growing threat not merely to the U.S., but also to the entire world. Scholars of religious studies have stated that the event, grounded in a lack of biblical understanding, was ruled by the politics of fear and not the politics of Jesus (Beachum, 2019).

The contested event was scheduled to host speakers Shahram Hadian, a pastor (and Iranian born Muslim), and Jim Simpson, an extremist blogger. In response, the event was condemned by those who opposed the content for planning to present such topics as *How the interfaith movement is sabotaging America and the church*, and *How Islam is destroying America from within* (Detroit Free Press, 2019b). Despite the cancellation of the event, the event's flyer is still posted online (Faithconnector Event Flyer, 2019).

Michigan lawmakers publicly denounced this Islamophobic event. On September 4, 2019, State Representatives Abdullah Hammoud (D-Dearborn), and Mari Manoogian (D-Birmingham), issued a joint statement stating that the anti-Muslim event was an attempt to assign blame for 9/11 to the entire Muslim community. The statement urged Bloomfield Hills Baptist Church to reconsider hosting these events and instead seek opportunities to foster a positive dialogue within the community (Hammoud & Manoogian, 2019). On September 5, 2019, Congressman Andy Levin (MI-09) and Congresswoman Debbie Dingell (MI-12) issued a joint statement imploring the Bloomfield Baptist Church to forgo the anti-Muslim event and any future act of hatred (Levin & Dingell, 2019).

The important lesson learned here is that condemnation and cancellation of this anti-Muslim event was an orchestrated effort to expose and combat Islamophobia by people from diverse faith groups, including Jewish (Andy Levin), Christian (Mari Manoogian and Debbie Dingell) (Baptist News, 2019), and Muslim (Abdullah Hammoud), (Arab American News, 2017), among others.

Another example to support the combating of Islamophobic media is the open letter signed by more than 500 elected officials from across the U.S. posted online (Open Letter, 2016). According to People for the American Way (2016), this letter marked the start of a coordinated campaign in cities across the U.S. to counter the increasing number of attacks on immigrants and Muslims.

8.3.2   Canada

As is the case in the U.S., right wing extremism in Canada incorporates a wide range of activities, drawing on a shared ideology. According to a recent poll, 78% of Canadians are concerned about the spread of hate speech online, while 74% are concerned about the rise of right-wing extremism and terrorism (Canadian Race Relations Foundation, 2021).

In Canada, there is profound tension between the belief that the media represent the basis of a liberal democratic society, and the actual role of some media outlets as drivers of discriminatory discourse and advocates of a dominant white and economic-political elite. In short, biases are rooted in the culture of media organizations since those biases appear to be invisible to journalists and editors who are predominantly white (Henry & Tator, 2015). This problem, however, highlights the need for a multi-stakeholder response to right wing extremism, in which the government, law enforcement, tech platforms and civil society play a role (Davey et al., 2020).

In 2019, the Government of Canada initiated a program entitled *Building a Foundation for Change: Canada's Anti-Racism Strategy 2019–2022* according to which all Canadians benefit from equitable access to and participation in economic, socio-cultural, and political spheres. The program has planned to invest $30 million in community-based projects that aim to address racism and discrimination, in addition to $5 million for supporting community-led digital and civic literacy programming directed toward combating media disinformation. Another $6.2 million is to be used to increase reliable data and evidence regarding racism and discrimination. The program urges Canadians to refrain from broadcasting media stories, news items or imagery that may incite hatred or contempt of others, based on ethnic differences, skin color or religion (Government of Canada, 2019a).

In addition to government policies combating Islamophobic media, competitive media and grassroots' intervention play a decisive role in countering the misinformation targeting Muslims. The following two examples highlight two incidents in which rallies of anti-Muslim groups, particularly those belonging to the Worldwide Coalition Against Islam, were met by either counter-protests from anti-Islamophobia advocates or by rejection from local authorities.

The Worldwide Coalition Against Islam (WCAI) is a Calgary based right-wing extremist band, known as an anti-Islamic group (Payne, 2017) that has been associated with hosting rallies against Muslims across Canada. In August 2017, the WCAI organized an anti-Muslim rally that took place outside the Vancouver City Hall. In protest, this rally was met by thousands of counter demonstrators who condemned the hateful messages conveyed at the rally by the WCAI (Azpiri & Dooley, 2017).

The other example pertains to a rally also proposed by the WCAI to be held on August 11, 2018, commemorating the eve of the Unite the Right rally in Charlottesville (Virginia, U.S.) that was organized by far-right groups and white supremacists in the U.S. However, due to a negative response from the media, general population, and officials of Calgary city who denied issuing permits for the rally, the planned event by the WCAI was postponed and cancelled (Csillag, 2018; D'sa & Floody, 2018).

8.4   Combatting Islamophobia and Hate Activities on Biased Social Media

The transition of media from print, television and radio to digital and electronic communications has caused profound revolutions in the traditional media industry. Today consumers or audiences can access news and entertainment from personal digital audio and video devices. They can also create news and participate in the news discourse through citizen publishing, blogging, YouTube and other electronic communication developments (Stucke & Grunes, 2009). Online and social media platforms enable the collapsing of geographical distance between peoples in such a way that Islamophobic-hate groups have reached wider audiences (Waltman & Mattheis, 2017).

The following subsections highlight the role of government and non-government agencies of the U.S. and Canada in countering biased social media.

8.4.1   The U.S.

According to a Pew Research Center survey of U.S. adults conducted in July 2020, 64% of Americans say social media have a negative effect on the way things are going in the U.S. In addition, 86% of Americans say they get news from a smartphone, computer or tablet, compared with 40% from television, 16% from radio, and 10% from print publications (Auxier, 2020; Shearer, 2021). And, out of eleven social media sites used as regular sources of news, Facebook is ranked at the top with 36% of Americans using it regularly, followed by YouTube (23%), and Twitter (15%) (Shearer & Mitchell, 2021). The Internet offers endless lists of less institutionalized, more citizen-based, or alternative channels providing sociopolitical information (Boomgaarden & Schmitt-Beck, 2019).

The problem is that far-right, white supremacist and other organizations engaging in Islamophobic media are using online platforms to recruit supporters, raise funds, and regularize racism and religious prejudice. Cyber racism on the Internet has increased and Islamophobic discourse online has turned some social media a place of hostility, fear and intimidation for Muslims (Center for American Progress, 2018). In September 2019, the United Nations' Committee on the Elimination of Racial Discrimination expressed its concern about "the rise in hate speech, especially against ethnic-religious groups and foreigners of the Muslim faith, incitement to racial hatred and the propagation of ideas of racial superiority and involving racist stereotypes... in the media and on the Internet and social media" (United Nations, 2019 p. 3).

Tackling media bias and misinformation requires addressing several challenging issues, including fake accounts, deceptive behavior, and harmful content. The policies controlling misinformation and hate speech of several of the worldwide digital and social media platforms have developed substantially since 2016. For example, social media companies, including Facebook, Microsoft, Twitter, YouTube, Instagram, Snapchat, Dailymotion and TikTok, among other companies have agreed with and committed to the European Commission's "Code of conduct on countering illegal hate speech online," including Islamophobia. The outcome of such policies has been the removal of 72% of illegal hate speech content in 2019 compared with 28% in 2016 (European Commission, 2020 p. 2). In addition, per the request of the U.S. Congress, media platforms have made progress in eliminating certain hateful and misleading information. For instance, between October and December, 2020, Facebook disabled more than 1.3 billion (80% of) fake accounts, removed over 100 networks of coordinated forged behavior, and banned over 250 white supremacist groups and 890 militarized social movements. Also, Facebook has tripled the size of its teams working in safety and security since 2016 to over 35,000 people (Rosen, 2021). Another example of the consequences of using online platforms in a biased manner is the case of Laura Loomer, a high-profile, self-called proud Islamophobe, who described Islam as a cancer on humanity (Elfrink, 2020). Loomer's online accounts were banned from Twitter, Facebook and Instagram in 2018 over derogatory posts that violated their policies against hateful conduct that included inflammatory comments about Islam and Muslims, particularly targeting Congresswoman Ilhan Omar's Muslim faith (Givetash, 2018).

However, while Facebook's policies were applied globally, content moderators, conversely, were influenced by their own cultural inclinations and biases (Klonick, 2018). On March 25, 2021, lawmakers and members of the U.S. Congress questioned chief executives of media platforms, particularly Facebook, Google and Twitter about their handling of misinformation and online extremism that are still extensively rampant on the platforms (Fung, 2021).

At the heart of the policy issue conflict is the aforementioned Section 230 of the CDA of 1996 that grants media platforms legal immunity for much of the content posted by their users. From a legal point of view, Section 230 provides immunity to online platforms from civil liability based on third-party content as well as immunity for removal of bias and harmful content in certain circumstances (Code, 2021). Consequently, Islamophobia, related hateful activities, and unlawful, biased and dangerous content have disseminated online in unprecedented fashion.

To address this problem, the U.S. Department of Justice (2020) has provided a set of proposals and policies applicable to social media and online platforms. The following is a summary of those policies:

1. Incentivize online platforms to address illicit content. It makes little sense to immunize from civil liability an online platform that facilitates activity that would violate federal criminal law.
2. Clarify federal government civil enforcement capabilities. This policy aims to increase the ability of the government to protect citizens from illicit online activities.
3. Promote competition. This policy confirms that federal antitrust claims, promoting competition for the benefit of consumers, are not covered by the immunity stated in Section 230. It makes little sense to enable large online platforms

(particularly monopolistic ones) to invoke Section 230, where liability is based on harm to competition, not on third-party speech.

4. The benefits of immunity do not outweigh the costs when it comes to enabling serious offenses and harms, such as terrorism-related offenses.

5. Protect citizens from illicit and harmful content and activity online by addressing specific concerns over harmful content and activity where there is limited speech value.

6. Media platforms should address clearly illegal activity and material on their services.

7. An Internet platform must respect public safety by ensuring its ability to identify unlawful content. The provider must maintain the ability to assist government authorities to obtain content (i.e., evidence) in a comprehensible and usable format pursuant to court authorization (or any other lawful basis).

8. Civil and criminal enforcement efforts against cyberstalking are encouraged. Cyberstalking includes a course of conduct or series of actions by the perpetrator that places the victim in reasonable fear of death or serious bodily injury. Prohibited acts include repeated, unwanted, intrusive, and frightening communications from the perpetrator by phone, e-mail, or other forms of communications, as well as harassment and threats communicated through the Internet or social media sites and applications.

9. Carve out cyberstalking from Section 230 immunity, so that victims can seek civil recourse where platforms fail to exercise due care to prevent such illicit and harmful behavior.

10. Transparency reporting requirements: Large media platforms should regularly disclose data on the enforcement of their content moderation policies. Such disclosure would serve the following important objectives.

    (a) It would enable members of the public to identify best practices related to restricting harmful content.

    (b) Scholars, policymakers, and other platforms could use such information to improve content moderation practices and better protect against the range of unlawful material that appears online.

    (c) Enforcement data may help to alleviate suspicion of platforms if complaints of bias reflect that there are many anecdotal examples that individuals can refer to as evidence of bias.

    (d) Enforcement data may help inform consumer choices or policy solutions if they reveal that claims of bias are well-founded.

The United Nations' Committee on the Elimination of Racial Discrimination (United Nations, 2019 p. 3) evokes its general recommendation, No. 35 (2013), on combating racist hate speech and recommends that the State party take firm measures to combat hate speech, by:

(a) Condemning all expressions of racist hate speech, including by political and public figures, and firmly combating them, in particular by monitoring the media and social networks to identify persons or groups of persons expressing racist hate speech, and by investigating such acts, prosecuting those responsible and, if convicted, punishing them appropriately;

(b) Amending the Act on the media to abolish the requirement that violations be both serious and repeated in order for penalties to be imposed, so as to allow for more effective prosecution and punishment of all incidents of hate speech;

(c) Promoting understanding and tolerance between minorities, immigrants, refugees and the local population (United Nations, 2019 p. 3).

As representing one of the civil advocacy organizations, the Center for American Progress (2018) recommends policies for social media corporations to adopt and implement in order to address Islamophobia and hateful activities on their platforms. These policies are as follows:

- Users should not use social media services to engage in hateful activities or use these services to facilitate hateful activities, whether online or offline.
- Internet companies must have in place an enforcement strategy that recognizes the scope of the problem and reflects a commitment to continuously diminish hateful activities within their services.
- Users and outside organizations should have the ability to flag hateful activities on an Internet company's services, but responsibility for removing hateful activities from services should sit directly with the Internet company.
- Internet companies should let users who flag what they believe to be hateful activities know what actions the internet company has taken and why, including if the internet company has chosen to take no action. When media outlets do not respond positively, their advertisers should be boycotted.
- Consult civil and human rights organizations with experience in detecting hateful activities to assist Internet companies in identifying hateful activities.
- Internet companies should combine technology solutions and human actors to remove Islamophobic-hateful activities.
- Government actors should not be allowed to use Internet companies' flagging tools to attempt to remove content they find objectionable.
- Internet companies should be transparent with the actions that they are taking, why they are doing so, and who is affected (Center for American Progress, 2018 p. 4–10).

8.4.2 Canada

In Canada, 6660 accounts, channels, and pages associated with right-wing extremists have been identified. Notably, "Islam was the most commonly discussed religion, accounting for 60.5% of all discussion of religious communities, followed by Judaism (21.1%) and Christianity (18.3%)" (Davey et al., 2020 p. 28). Highly prolific extremist users of Twitter were engaged in anti-Muslim conversation, and spikes in activity often contained anti-Muslim conversation. Similarly, on Facebook, Muslims have been the most widely discussed minority community, and the most common target of posts containing explicit hate speech (Davey et al., 2020). The dissemination of misinformation, particularly in the form of false news distributed through social media platforms, can be exploited by organizations and individual actors to spread fear and invoke hatred (Canadian Center for Identity-based Conflict, 2019).

On May 9, 2019, the National Council of Canadian Muslims (NCCM) presented before the House of Commons Standing Committee on Justice and Human Rights on the perils of online hate and what must be done to counter it. The NCCM recommended that government take action in three key ways to combat online hate:

1. Reform the outdated Canadian Human Rights Act (CHRA) by opening the Act for legislative review. This will ensure that the CHRA meets the modern-day challenges of online hate and hate speech. This recommendation urges the government to address the rise of online hate and Islamophobia in balance with the rights of Canadians to engage in legitimate critique necessary for the full functioning of a democratic society. This recommendation is timely as the last extensive review of the CHRA was made in 2000, before social media platforms such as Facebook and Twitter had opened their doors.
2. A parliamentary study into how social media companies can be regulated to better protect Canadians and reduce online hate, while ensuring that free speech rights are protected. This policy is needed as around 84% of Canadians use Facebook, and a majority of Canadians get their news through social media that host hate activities, biased information, and fake news. Therefore, the study recommends that the government create a new regulatory system that would include some form of penalizing social media platforms for not removing unlawful material.
3. Federal funding to help NGOs, civil society organizations and industry run digital literacy programs to counter online hate through education and prevention efforts (National Council of Canadian Muslims, 2019).

As is the case with the U.S., efforts to address the problem of biased media, Islamophobia, and misinformation must be balanced against the right to freedom of expression (Ahmad, 2019) safeguarded by the Canadian Charter of Rights and Freedoms, particularly Subsection 2(b), which proposes that everyone has the fundamental freedom of thought, belief, opinion and expression, including freedom of the press and other media of communication (Government of Canada, 2019b). However, fundamental rights, including freedom of expression, are subject to section 1, which allows "reasonable" limits to be placed on those rights (Government of Canada, 2019b; Walker, 2018). The Supreme Court of Canada has declared that the harm instigated by online hate propaganda is not in keeping with the objectives of freedom of expression or the values of equality and multiculturalism expressed in the Canadian Charter of Rights and Freedoms (Walker, 2018).

The provincial and federal laws in Canada that pertain to defamation are examples of restrictions of free of speech. Canadian courts have made it clear that reasonable limits can be placed on people's freedom of expression in order to deal with hate issues. To be more specific, "Among the laws that have restricted freedom of expression are those referred to as anti-hate laws, for their purpose to restrict the

Table 8.1 Support/oppose of strong actions executed by the Canadian government to combat hate and racism online

Strong actions executed by the federal government	Support %	Oppose %
Strengthen laws to hold perpetrators accountable for what they say, share and do online	79	20
Create an independent oversight body to ensure large social platforms and media companies are following Canadian laws	73	25
Require social media companies to remove users who repeatedly share racist or hateful content	72	26
Strengthen laws to hold social media companies accountable for what appear in their platform	71	28
Require social media companies to remove racist or hateful content within 24 or 48 hours of it being posted, or face a fine	70	29

Source: Adapted with modification from the Canadian Anti-Hate Network (2021)

publication and public expression of messages intended to incite hatred towards members of particular groups. In other words, they prohibit hate propaganda" (Walker, 2018 p. 1).

A poll on online hate, conducted between March 1 and 5, 2021 by the Ekos Research suggested that 73% of Canadians consider online hate speech and racism as a problem in Canada, However, between 70% and 79% of the respondents strongly supported the federal government to introduce robust measures to combat hateful and racist content and behavior online.

Table 8.1 shows that 79% of Canadians are most supportive of the government's measure of strengthening laws to hold perpetrators accountable for their online speech and behavior. 73% of Canadians support the measure of creating an independent oversight body to make sure that large media companies follow the law, while 72% support the measure that requires social media companies to remove users who share racist or hateful content on their platforms. One of the most noteworthy findings is that 71% of the respondents support the measure of strengthening laws to hold social media companies accountable for what appears on their platforms. Finally, 70% of Canadians support the measure that requires social media companies to remove racist or hateful content within 24 or 48 hours of it being posted, or face fines. On all measures, both Liberals and New Democrats are more likely to support government intervention to stop hate and racism, while Conservatives are less likely (Canadian Race Relations Foundation, 2021).

8.5   Conclusion

The deep-seated negative depictions of Islam in the western and North American media affect discourses and actions of Muslims who have become subject to the web of racism that includes Islamophobia, hate crimes, media stereotypes, and dehumanizing ideology. These false media depictions of Muslims have not only aggravated sociopolitical problems and well-being difficulties among the Muslim minorities, but have also generated serious questions concerning civil and human rights of all minority groups in North America. However, this chapter has shown that biased media and anti-Muslim racism in North America have been challenged, resisted, and countered by policies and competitive media, endorsed by government and non-government agencies.

This chapter has investigated two policy approaches dealing with combating biased media and anti-Muslim racism. One approach suggests that policies providing guidelines and restrictions on biased media and online platforms are the proper remedy, while the other approach recommends an open marketplace of ideas, allowing full freedom of expression (Walker, 2018). These two approaches, however, have generated a sort of predicament of how to initiate and implement policies that combat media bias, religious discrimination and Islamophobic hate, while warranting freedom of expression, in accordance with international law.

There are differences between the U.S. and Canada in dealing with policy issues pertaining to biased media and Islamophobic hate. The U.S. provides immunity to media and online platforms, guaranteeing the protection of the free speech of platform users, but it also encourages platforms to take an active role in removing unlawful content, avoiding free speech drawbacks of collateral censorship. In Canada, however, two recent different surveys conducted by Abacus Data (January 2021) and the Canadian Anti-Hate Network (March 2021) show that the majority of Canadians endorse governmental regulations and consequences for both the perpetrators and social media platforms. In other words, anti-hate laws are among the laws that have restricted freedom of expression in Canada (Walker, 2018).

Both anti-biased media and anti-Islamophobia are crucial themes for scholars, political leaders, policymakers, and advocacy organizations. Addressing the policies that counter biased media and anti-Muslim racism is challenging as they express different official and non-official policies. This statement is substantiated by the fact that this chapter has focused on four types of policies: 1-International policies proposed by the United Nations, 2-national policies of the governments of both the U.S and Canada, 3-policies of anti-Islamophobic media organizations and 4-response of grassroots to formal and informal policies.

Countering biased media is more than attacking certain negative articles or posts generated by Islamophobes; rather, the thrust is on the extreme, conservative and radical ideology behind corrupt media. This chapter has tackled the underlying ideologies and contentions of certain misleading media and online platforms that manufacture and spread Islamophobic propaganda portraying Muslims and Islam as threatening elements to western and North American democracy.

Through applying the approach of a marketplace of ideas in which media networks compete each other, several Muslim and non-Muslim agents have been involved in countering biased media and opposing the negative images of Muslims. In their efforts to contest of media misrepresentations of Muslims and to provide significant insights to Islam and Muslims, advocates and media activists from both Muslim and non-Muslim backgrounds have established mediated organizations equipped with cyber communication and online facilities. Despite these on-going efforts, anti-Islamophobia organizations need to focus more on updating and using state of the art media technologies to be able to strengthen their virtual communications as well as to spread their messages to large audiences. They should also increase their funds and financial resources to be able to manage high quality and wider media outlets.

This study highlights the role played by local and national leaders, scholars, lawmakers, policymakers and stakeholders in countering Islamophobic media of far-right extremists. The collaboration of leaders of various faith groups (Christian, Jews and Muslims) has been another key element in confronting biased Islamophobic media.

References

Abacus Data. (2021, January 25). Detailed results: Online hate and racism. *Canadian Race Relations Foundation*. Retrieved from https://www.crrf-fcrr.ca/images/CRRF_OnlineHate_Racism_Jan2021_FINAL.pdf

Ahmad, T. (2019, September). Government responses to disinformation on social media platforms: Canada. *Library of Congress*. Retrieved from https://www.loc.gov/law/help/social-media-disinformation/canada.php

Anderson, L. (2015). Countering Islamophobic media representations: The potential role of peace journalism. *Global Media and Communication, 11*(3), 255–270. https://doi.org/10.1177/1742766515606293

Arab American News. (2017, June 30). *A day with Dearborn Rep. Abdullah Hammoud: A young Arab American strives for a more welcoming Michigan.* Retrieved from https://www.arabamericannews.com/2017/06/30/a-day-with-dearborn-rep-abdullah-hammoud-a-young-arab-american-strives-for-a-more-welcoming-michigan/

Arab–American Anti-Discrimination Committee (ADC). (2018, February 13). *Anti-Sharia legislation, Islamophobia rises under Trump.* Retrieved from https://www.adc.org/anti-sharia-legislation-islamophobia-rises-under-trump-3/

Auxier, B. (2020, October 15). 64% of Americans say social media have a mostly negative effect on the way things are going in the U.S. today. *Pew Research Center*. Retrieved from https://www.pewresearch.org/fact-tank/2020/10/15/64-of-americans-say-social-media-have-a-mostly-negative-effect-on-the-way-things-are-going-in-the-u-s-today/

Azpiri, J., & Dooley, B. (2017, August 20). Thousands protest against anti-Islam, anti-Immigration rally at Vancouver city hall. *Global News*. Retrieved from https://globalnews.ca/news/3682727/vancouver-anti-islam-anti-immigration-rally-and-counter-protest-planned-for-saturday/

Baker, C. E. (2013). *Media concentration and democracy: Why ownership matters.* Cambridge University Press.

Baptist News. (2019, September 11). *Under pressure, Baptist church drops plans for anti-Muslim program on 9/11.* Retrieved from https://baptistnews.com/article/under-pressure-baptist-church-drops-plans-for-anti-muslim-program-on-9-11/#.YFKtP5NKi8q

Beachum, L. (2019, September 10). Baptist church cancels 9/11 anti-Islam event after backlash from legislators, Christian scholars. *Washington Post*. Retrieved from https://www.washingtonpost.com/religion/2019/09/11/religion-scholars-baptist-church-your-anti-islam-event-isnt-very-christian/

Boomgaarden, H. G., & Schmitt-Beck, R. (2019). The media and political behavior. In *Oxford research encyclopedia of politics*. Oxford University Press. https://doi.org/10.1093/acrefore/9780190228637.013.621

Brinson, P. (2009, March 26). Reformulating news media bias: A new theoretical and methodological approach. *Study Mode Research*. Retrieved from https://www.studymode.com/essays/Media-Bias-198169.html

Canadian Anti-Hate Network. (2021, March 22). *Results: Poll online hate-conducted by the Canadian Anti-Hate Network and Ekos Research*. Retrieved from https://www.antihate.ca/results_poll_on_online_hate

Canadian Center for Identity-based Conflict. (2019, October 1). *Weaponized misinformation a.k.a #FakeNews*. Retrieved from https://vtsm.org/wp-content/uploads/2019/10/Fake-News-BN-CCIBC.pdf

Canadian Race Relations Foundation. (2021). *Online hate and racism: Canadian experiences and opinions on what to do about it*. Retrieved from https://www.crrf-fcrr.ca/images/CRRF_OnlineHate_Racism_Jan2021_FINAL.pdf

Center for American Progress. (2005, June 15). *On media bias*. Retrieved from https://www.americanprogress.org/issues/general/news/2005/06/15/1514/on-media-bias/

Center for American Progress. (2011, August 26). *Fear, Inc. The roots of the Islamophobia network in America*. Retrieved from https://www.americanprogress.org/issues/religion/reports/2011/08/26/10165/fear-inc/

Center for American Progress. (2018, October 24). *Recommended Internet company corporate policies and terms of service to reduce hateful activities*. Retrieved from https://cdn.americanprogress.org/content/uploads/2018/10/24111621/ModelInternetCompanies-appendix.pdf?_ga=2.133241933.2115433179.1616706657-630514323.1616706657

Center for American Progress (2020, January 31). *Expansion of Trump's illegal Muslim ban demonstrates policy guided by personal prejudice*. Retrieved from https://www.americanprogress.org/drumbeats/expansion-trumps-illegal-muslim-ban-demonstrates-policy-guided-personal-prejudice/

Csillag, R. (2018, August 9). Nationalist rally planned in Toronto on the anniversary of Charlottesville attack. *Canadian Jewish News*. Retrieved October 22, 2018, from http://www.cjnews.com/news/canada/nationalist-rally-planned-in-toronto-on-the-anniversary-of-the-charlottesville-attack

D'Sa, P., & Floody, C. (2018, August 9). Anti-Islam group postpones rally at Nathan Phillips Square. *Toronto Star*. Retrieved from https://www.thestar.com/news/gta/2018/08/09/anti-islam-group-postpones-rally-at-nathan-phillips-square.html

Davey, J., Hart, M., & Guerin, C. (2020). An online environmental scan of right-wing extremism in Canada: Interim report. *Institute for Strategic Dialogue*. Retrieved from https://www.isdglobal.org/wp-content/uploads/2020/06/An-Online-Environmental-Scan-of-Right-wing-Extremism-in-Canada-ISD.pdf

Detroit Free Press. (2019a, September 9). *Michigan church, Islamophobic pastor blasted for plans to host anti-Muslim 9/11 event*. Retrieved from https://www.freep.com/story/news/nation/2019/09/09/anti-muslim-911-event-bloomfield-hills-baptist-church-michigan/2265688001/

Detroit Free Press. (2019b, September 10). *Bloomfield church cancels anti-Muslim 9/11 event after backlash*. Retrieved from https://www.freep.com/story/news/local/michigan/oakland/2019/09/10/bloomfield-hills-baptist-church-muslim/2272674001/

Detroit Metro Times (2019, September 10). *Bloomfield Hills church cancels Islamophobic 9/11 event after backlash*. Retrieved from https://www.metrotimes.com/news-hits/archives/2019/09/10/bloomfield-hills-church-cancels-islamophobic-9-11-event-after-backlash

el-Aswad, el-S. (2013). Images of Muslims in Western scholarship and media after 9/11. *Digest of Middle East Studies, 22*(1), 39–56.

el-Aswad, el-S. (2019). *The quality of life and policy issues among the Middle East and north African countries*. Cham, Switzerland: Springer.

el-Aswad, el-S., Sirgy, M., Estes, R., & Rahtz, D. (2020, December 17). Global jihad and international media use. In *Oxford research encyclopedia of communication*. Oxford University Press. https://doi.org/10.1093/acrefore/9780190228613.013.1151

Elfrink, T. (2020, August 19). 'Great going': Trump praises right-wing activist Laura Loomer after her Florida GOP primary win. *Washington Post*. Retrieved from https://www.washingtonpost.com/nation/2020/08/19/trump-laura-loomer-primary-gop/

European Commission. (2020). *The EU Code of conduct on countering illegal hate speech*. online. Retrieved from https://ec.europa.eu/info/policies/justice-and-fundamental-rights/combatting-discrimination/racism-and-xenophobia/eu-code-conduct-countering-illegal-hate-speech-online_en and https://ec.europa.eu/info/sites/info/files/aid_development_cooperation_fundamental_rights/assessment_of_the_code_of_conduct_on_hate_speech_on_line_-_state_of_play__0.pdf

Faithconnector Event Flyer. (2019). *9/11 Forgotten? Is Michigan Surrendering to Islam*. Retrieved from https://faithconnector.s3.amazonaws.com/tilproject/files/jarvis_flyer_2019_-sept_11th_-_2019_eventp.pdf

Fox 2 News. (2019, September 5). '*Proud Islamophobe' pastor hosts anti-Muslim event on 9/11 at Bloomfield Hills church*. Retrieved from https://www.fox2detroit.com/news/proud-islamophobe-pastor-hosts-anti-muslim-event-on-9-11-at-bloomfield-hills-church

Fung, B. (2021, March 25). Facebook, Twitter and Google CEOs grilled by Congress on misinformation. *CNN Business*. Retrieved from https://www.cnn.com/2021/03/25/tech/tech-ceos-hearing/index.html

Gallup. (2020). *Bias in others' news a greater concern than bias in own news*. Retrieved from https://news.gallup.com/poll/319724/bias-others-news-greater-concern-bias-own-news.aspx

Garz, M. (2014). Good news and bad news: Evidence of media bias in unemployment reports. *Public Choice, 161*, 499–515.

Gerbner, G., Gross, L., Morgan, M., & Signorielli, N. (1980). The "mainstreaming" of America: Violence profile no. 11. *Journal of Communication, 30*(3), 10–29.

Givetash, L. (2018, November 22). Laura Loomer banned from Twitter after criticizing Ilhan Omar. *NBC News*. Retrieved from https://www.nbcnews.com/tech/security/laura-loomer-banned-twitter-after-criticizing-ilhan-omar-n939256

Government of Canada. (2019a, July 17). *Building a foundation for change: Canada's anti-racism strategy 2019–2022*. Retrieved from https://www.canada.ca/en/canadian-heritage/campaigns/anti-racism-engagement/anti-racism-strategy.html

Government of Canada. (2019b, July 28). *Constitution Act, 1982*. Retrieved from https://perma.cc/2SZZ-TRYJ

Hammoud, A., & Manoogian, M. (2019, September 4). Hammoud and Manoogian stand against Islamophobia. *Michigan House Democrats*. Retrieved from https://housedems.com/hammoud-and-manoogian-stand-against-islamophobia/

Henry, F., & Tator, C. (2015). Racist discourse in Canada's English print media. *Canadian Race Relations Foundation* Retrieved from https://www.crrf-fcrr.ca/en/resources/research-projects/item/23532-racist-discourse-in-canadas-english-print-media-en-gb-1

Hersch, G. (2016). *Measuring well-being for public policy: Doing without theory* (Ph.D. thesis). University of California, San Diego. Retrieved from https://escholarship.org/uc/item/42c4b7f5.

Isaacs, A. (2018a). The Real Founders of Fake News? American Islamophobes. *The Nation*. Retrieved, 31 July, from *Tom Dispatch*: *A Regular Antidote to the mainstream Media* https://www.thenation.com/article/real-founders-fake-news-american-islamophobes/

Isaacs, A. (2018b). Giving a Pass to Anti-Muslim Bigotry Islamophobia Enters the Government, Is Incorporated into the Law, and Becomes Increasingly Acceptable in America. Retrieved, 10 May, from *Tom Dispatch: A Regular Antidote to the mainstream Media http://www.tomdispatch.com/post/176434/tomgram%3A_arnold_isaacs%2C_promoting_islamophobia_in_america/#more*

Klonick, K. (2018). The new governors: The people, rules, and processes governing online speech. *Harvard Law Review, 131*, 1598–1670. Retrieved from https://harvardlawreview.org/wp-content/uploads/2018/04/1598-1670_Online.pdf

Levin, A., & Dingell, D. (2019, September 5). *Levin and Dingell condemn planned Anti-Muslim events in Bloomfield Hills.* Retrieved from https://debbiedingell.house.gov/news/documentsingle.aspx?DocumentID=1875

Lynch, J. (2008). *Debates in peace journalism.* Sydney University Press.

Lynch, J. (2014). *A global standard for reporting conflict.* Routledge.

Media Matters. (2011, March 29). *Right-wing media attacked Muslim advocates for giving Muslims common legal advice.* Retrieved from https://www.mediamatters.org/daily-caller/right-wing-media-attacked-muslim-advocates-giving-muslims-common-legal-advice

Media Matters. (2017, February 8). *When discussing Trump's Muslim ban, cable news excluded Muslims.* Retrieved from https://www.mediamatters.org/donald-trump/when-discussing-trumps-muslim-ban-cable-news-excluded-muslims

Media Matters. (2019, August 7). *Right-wing extremism in America is a real threat. Conservative media downplaying the problem only makes it worse.* Retrieved from https://www.mediamatters.org/fox-news/right-wing-extremism-america-real-threat-conservative-media-downplaying-problem-only-makes

Muslim Advocates. (2020, August 19). *Muslim Advocates responds to anti-Muslim bigotry from Marjorie Taylor Greene and Laura Loomer.* Retrieved from https://muslimadvocates.org/2020/08/muslim-advocates-responds-to-anti-muslim-bigotry-from-marjorie-taylor-greene-and-laura-loomer/

National Council of Canadian Muslims. (2019, May 9). *Brief on online hate: Legislative and policy approaches.* Retrieved from https://www.nccm.ca/nccm-presents-before-house-of-commons-standing-committee-on-justice-and-human-rights-on-online-hate/

Open Letter. (2016). *We reject hate and anti-Muslim bigotry: An open letter to our constituents and the American people from elected officials across the United States.* Retrieved from https://drive.google.com/file/d/0BzQcoSYZoBLfNFRlSzZPczl0VWc/view

Osterbur, M. (2020). Hate crime policy in the United States. In *Oxford research encyclopedia of politics.* Oxford University Press. https://doi.org/10.1093/acrefore/9780190228637.013.1220

Payne, J. (2017, August 20). *Mass celebration of diversity overwhelms anti-Islam rally at city hall.* Retrieved October 22, 2018, from https://vancouversun.com/news/local-news/anti-immigration-rally-at-vancouver-city-hall

People for the American Way. (2016, September 29). *500+ Local elected officials pledge to combat xenophobia, anti-Muslim attacks.* Retrieved from https://www.pfaw.org/press-releases/500-local-elected-officials-pledge-to-combat-xenophobia-anti-muslim-attacks/

Phillips, W. (2018, May 3). The oxygen of amplification: Better practices for reporting on extremists, antagonists, and manipulators online. *Data & Society Research Institute.* Retrieved from https://datasociety.net/wp-content/uploads/2018/05/3-PART-3_Oxygen_of_Amplification_DS-1.pdf

Power, G., Murphy, S., & Coover, M. (1996). Priming prejudice: How stereotypes and counter-stereotypes influence attribution of responsibility and credibility among ingroups and outgroups. *Human Communication Research, 23*(1), 36–58.

Right Wing Watch. (2011). *The right wing playbook on anti-Muslim extremism.* Retrieved from https://www.rightwingwatch.org/report/the-right-wing-playbook-on-anti-muslim-extremism/

Rosen, G. (2021, March 22). How we're tackling misinformation across our apps. *Facebook.* Retrieved from https://about.fb.com/news/2021/03/how-were-tackling-misinformation-across-our-apps/

Ryan, M. (2021). Running on racism: Far-right congressional candidates in the 2020 elections, and those who lean that way. *Right Wing Watch.* Retrieved from https://www.rightwingwatch.org/report/running-on-racism-far-right-congressional-candidates-in-the-2020-elections-and-those-who-lean-that-way/

Shearer, E. (2021, January 12). More than eight-in-ten Americans get news from digital devices. *Pew Research Center: Fact tank*. Retrieved from https://www.pewresearch.org/fact-tank/2021/01/12/more-than-eight-in-ten-americans-get-news-from-digital-devices/

Shearer, E., & Mitchell, A. (2021, January 12). News use across social media platforms in 2020. *Pew Research Center*. Retrieved from https://www.journalism.org/2021/01/12/news-use-across-social-media-platforms-in-2020/

Southern Poverty Law Center (2011, June 17). *The anti-Muslim inner circle*. Retrieved from https://www.splcenter.org/fighting-hate/intelligence-report/2011/anti-muslim-inner-circle

Southern Poverty Law Center (2017, August 24). *Ten ways to fight hate: A community response guide*. Retrieved from https://www.splcenter.org/20170814/ten-ways-fight-hate-community-response-guide

Southern Poverty Law Center. (2018, April 15). *Hate crimes, explained*. Retrieved from https://www.splcenter.org/20180415/hate-crimes-explained

Southern Poverty Law Center. (2020). *Hate map*. Retrieved from https://www.splcenter.org/hate-map

Stucke, M. E. (2008). Better competition advocacy. *St. John's Law Review, 82*(3), 951–1036. Retrieved from https://scholarship.law.stjohns.edu/cgi/viewcontent.cgi?article=1081&context=lawreview

Stucke, M. E., & Grunes, A. P. (2009). Toward a better competition policy for the media: The challenge of developing antitrust policies that support the media sector's unique role in our democracy. *Connecticut Law Review, 42*(1), 101. Retrieved from https://heinonline.org/HOL/LandingPage?handle=hein.journals/conlr42&div=6&id=&page

The White House. (2021a, January 20). *Proclamation on ending discriminatory bans on entry to the United States*. Retrieved from https://www.whitehouse.gov/briefing-room/presidential-actions/2021/01/20/proclamation-ending-discriminatory-bans-on-entry-to-the-united-states/

The White House. (2021b, January 20). *Executive order on advancing racial equity and support for underserved communities through the federal government*. Retrieved from https://www.whitehouse.gov/briefing-room/presidential-actions/2021/01/20/executive-order-advancing-racial-equity-and-support-for-underserved-communities-through-the-federal-government/

U.S. Code. (2021, March). *47 USC 230: Protection for private blocking and screening of offensive material*. Retrieved from https://uscode.house.gov/view.xhtml?req=(title:47%20section:230%20edition:prelim)

U.S. Department of Justice. (2020). *Section 230 — Nurturing innovation or fostering unaccountability? Key takeaways and recommendations*. Washington, DC. Retrieved from https://www.justice.gov/file/1286331/download

United Nations. (1966). International covenant on civil and political rights. *Office of the High Commissioner for Human Rights*. Retrieved from https://www.ohchr.org/en/professionalinterest/pages/ccpr.aspx

United Nations. (2014). Developing national action plans against racial discrimination: A practical guide. *Office of the High Commissioner for Human Rights*. Retrieved from https://www.ohchr.org/Documents/Publications/HR-PUB-13-03.pdf

United Nations News (2019, September 18). *International convention on the elimination of all forms of racial discrimination*. Retrieved from https://tbinternet.ohchr.org/_layouts/15/treatybodyexternal/Download.aspx?symbolno=CERD/C/ISL/CO/21-23&Lang=En

Vosoughi, S., Roy, D., & Aral, S. (2012). The spread of true and false news online. *Science, 359* (6380), 1146–1151. https://doi.org/10.1126/science.aap9559. Retrieved from http://science.sciencemag.org/content/359/6380/1146

Walker, J. (2018, June 29). Hate speech and freedom of expression: Legal boundaries in Canada. *Library of Parliament, Ottawa, Canada*. Retrieved from https://perma.cc/8JPB-BMJ9

Waltman, M. S., & Mattheis, A. A. (2017, September 26). Understanding hate speech. In *Oxford research encyclopedia of communication*. Oxford University Press. https://doi.org/10.1093/acrefore/9780190228613.013.422

Chapter 9
Education Policy

9.1 Introduction

Anti-Islamophobia and anti-discrimination have to be made a central focus of education policies of North American educational systems given the multiple ways in which many educational institutions and schools produce and reproduce structural anti-Muslim racism. This chapter focuses on the education policies implemented in the U.S. and Canada to combat Islamophobia and related discriminatory actions in schools. Although indicators show that Muslims in North America have an average of 13.6 years of schooling, which is higher than the average of 5.6 years Muslim adults have globally (Pew Research Center, 2016), several studies have documented unfair and inequitable treatment of Muslim minority students in North American schools (Asvat & Malcarne, 2008; Bakali, 2015; Douglass, 2009; Ghonaim, 2019; Hodge et al., 2016; Kazi, 2016; Kulkarni, 2020; Kunst, 2012; Niyozov & Plum, 2009; Zaidi, 2019; Zine, 2001).

Muslim minority students as well as children of other minorities are protected by the United Nations. In 1989, the United Nations Convention on the Rights of the Child (CRC) ensured that all children receive an adequate education. In article 28 of the CRC, governments were directed to recognize the rights of all children to education as well as to make primary education compulsory and free. In addition, article 30 of the CRC stated that in nations that have ethnic, religious or linguistic minorities, children belonging to such minorities have the right to enjoy their own culture, to profess and practice their own religion, or to use their own language (United Nations Human Rights, 1989).

This chapter is concerned with two core objectives. On the one hand, it aims to reveal the negative impact of Islamophobia and discrimination on students' overall well-being and academic achievement. On the other hand, it addresses policies, particularly those that deal with Muslim minorities, that seek to reform the education system and eliminate biases. Improving educational outcomes, moreover, requires understanding the impact of educational policies on pupils' learning. This study

el-S. el-Aswad, *Countering Islamophobia in North America*, Human Well-Being Research and Policy Making, https://doi.org/10.1007/978-3-030-84673-2_9

proposes that anti-Islamophobia and anti-discrimination policies, among other education policies are underscored as key factors in the guidelines and efforts aimed at improving educational environments.

Undoubtedly, uneven distribution of educational and economic benefits has a negative impact on the quality of life and educational progress of minorities in North America. Studies that examine minority groups and technology indicate that education and economics are major factors causing the widening information gap between majority and minority populations of North America (Dawson & Chatman, 2001). In addition, there is a critical issue pertaining to broader conflicts over the role of religion in public schools in that the religious interests of students, parents, administrators and teachers often clash and lead to discrimination (Pew Research Center, 2019).

Researchers maintain that experiencing discrimination can cause stress responses akin to post-traumatic stress disorder. Students who experience anti-Muslim racism and discrimination in school are more likely to have negative attitudes about school, low self-esteem, lower academic motivation and performance, tendencies to avoid interactions with majority members, and are at increased risk of dropping out of school (Broman, 1997; Brown, 2015; Dei et al., 1997; el-Aswad, el-S., 2006; Saleem & Ramasubramanian, 2017).

Quality of life and well-being is the main objective of social-public policy overall in the sense that social, health, educational, economic, domestic, and national policy issues represent great concern to scholars, government officials, policy makers for their citizens (American Educational Research Association, 2013; Birkland, 2016; Brown, 2015). Effective education policies are viewed here as a means of enhancing the overall well-being of all people, Muslims and non-Muslims. When considering educational policies, it is worthy to mention that the fourth objective of the United Nations' Sustainable Development Goals is to "ensure inclusive and equitable quality education and promote life-long learning opportunities for all" (United Nations, 2018).

It is necessary to improve the quality of education at all levels by eliminating discrimination in schools, updating curricula about Muslim culture, increasing funding for minority groups, recruiting and training highly qualified instructors, building reliable educational resources and facilities, and improving administrative systems that appreciate equal treatment of all educators, employees and students. Serious and well-executed policies regarding strategies for eliminating or reducing Islamophobia and discrimination in North American educational and school systems must be implemented without causing negative outcomes that might affect the civil society or prevent decision makers from presenting effective policy options.

9.2   Education and Islamophobia

The following sections discuss the impact of Islamophobia, anti-Muslim racism and related discriminatory attitudes and actions on the well-being and educational achievements of Muslim students in American and Canadian schools.

9.2.1   The U.S.

The U.S. "government has never declared—and our system has never enshrined in the Constitution—a right to education, or healthcare, or a living wage… While we might pass policies to address the problems that arise when dealing with these policy matters, we generally do not deal with them as matters of right. In the United Sates, one cannot claim that the failure of federal government to provide education, healthcare, or many other things violates a right stated or implied by the Constitution" (Birkland, 2016 p.10). However, the U.S. national policy toward education is maintained through legislation and federal court rulings, which explain rights pertaining to the school setting (Jonson-Reid, 2015; Lieberman & McLaughlin, 1982). The U.S. public education system includes programs beginning from early childhood through adulthood. Although federal policies related to each sector of this public educational system continue to function, most operational management is controlled by state and local authorities (Jonson-Reid, 2015).

Public high schools in the U.S. existed prior to 1900, but only about 6% of the population attended them. By 1929 all states had enacted compulsory attendance laws that included high school education. By the mid-1930s, most states embraced kindergarten. However, compulsory attendance policy varies by state with required entry at ages 5 to 7 and allowed exit at ages 16 to 18. Although public education has served low-income students, the proportion of preschool to 12th-grade students who are poor has multiplied (Jonson-Reid, 2015).

Some policymakers argue that education can only be promoted and improved by using market forces to compel low-performing schools to improve. This idea motivates leaders of federal policy to encourage charter schools, offering vouchers to allow some families in low-functioning systems to move their children to better schools. Therefore, states have begun to oversee some forms of private and charter schools. These schools receive public financing but are created and run independently by outside organizations or individuals. As of 2011–2012, there were nearly 6000 charter schools in the United States (Jonson-Reid, 2015). Despite the increase in private schools and private business interests in education, "these programs have not worked well for marginalized groups" (Ryan, 2018 p.5). It is interesting to observe that marginalized populations such as ethnic minorities, including religious groups view their access to schooling as a fundamental component of their guarantees as citizens and human beings (Bajaj & Kidwai, 2016).

The problem is that white privilege, discrimination and racism are embedded in the fabric of American history and society (Kulkarni, 2020; Leonardo, 2009; Shealey et al., 2005). Scholars have discussed several reasons for the existence of disproportionate representation of minority students, including systemic racism present in school systems and the intersections of race with poverty and health (Kulkarni, 2020). Within this racial orientation, Islamophobia and religious discrimination are serious threats for the education and public health of Muslim communities. Islamophobia and acts of discrimination against Muslim minorities have occurred not only in the U.S mainstream society, but also in public schools (U.S. Commission on Civil Rights, 2014).

The U.S. Department of Justice (2016 p.12) stated, "Federal laws, including Title IV of the Civil Rights Act of 1964 (Title IV), prohibit religious discrimination in educational institutions. Yet despite these protections, students of all ages and grade levels too often find themselves bullied or harassed because of their religious beliefs." However, in a roundtable, organized by the U.S. Department of Justice, participants "noted that there still remains confusion about when the prohibition on discrimination based on race, color, or national origin in Title VI of the Civil Rights Act of 1964 (Title VI), which pertains to discrimination in Federally-funded programs or activities, may be implicated in situations where there is religious discrimination that is closely tied to race, color, or national origin" (U.S. Department of Justice, 2016 p.15). This confusion was expressed earlier in a report provided by the U.S. Commission on Civil Rights that referred to "the significant gap in American civil rights protections wherein laws do not prohibit religious discrimination in the federally-assisted educational programs and activities as they protect students from discrimination on the basis of race, color, national origin, sex, disability, and even membership in patriotic youth organizations. This prevents the Department of Education from protecting students from various forms of religious bigotry, affecting many Muslim and Sikh students, particularly in recent years" (U.S. Commission on Civil Rights, 2014 pp. 16–17). Additionally, the Council on American-Islamic Relations (2017 p.26) evoked the U.S. Congress to "Amend Title VI of the Civil Rights Act of 1964" as it "does not prohibit discrimination on the basis of religion".

Paul Findley, expressing his early experience as a child attending Presbyterian Sunday School in Jacksonville, Illinois, said, "Our teacher... told us that uneducated, primitive, violent people lived in desert areas of the Holy Land and worshiped a 'strange God'... I remember that she called them Mohammadans and kept repeating, 'they aren't like us'" (Findley, 2001 p. 19). Furthermore, a study concerning teaching about Islam showed that materials and contents of social studies textbooks, from the 1970s and 1980s dealing with topics of Islam and Muslims could not be characterized as fair or accurate as they contained misinformation about the Qur'an, the Prophet Muhammad, and the teaching of Islam (Douglass, 2009).

Because of biased attitudes and practices that promoted Islamophobia, schools have become fertile grounds for bullying Muslim children, youth, and those perceived to be Muslim (Bajaj et al., 2016). Bullying has been one of the serious problems within American schools based on race, religion and sexual orientation (Wang et al., 2009). In March 2010, "Muslim Mothers Against Violence conducted a survey of 78 Muslim male and female youth between 12 and 17 years of age in Northern Virginia. . . 80 percent responded that they had been subjected to bigoted taunts and epithets and harassment" (U.S. Commission on Civil Rights, 2014 p.114). According to the Institute for Social Policy and Understanding (2017), 42% of American Muslims who had children in K–12 public school, reported harassment and bullying of their children because of their religion, compared with 23% of Jews, 20% of Protestants, 6% of Catholics, and 10% of the general public. In addition, one in four Muslim bullying incidents involved a teacher or other school official. Research has shown that discrimination from teachers has a negative impact on students' academic motivation (Brown, 2015).

In an interview with Amir Aswad, a successful attorney, graduated from the University of Chicago, he recalled his difficult experience he had during high school in Dearborn, Michigan. He said, "I remember feeling isolated—feeling as if I never really belonged to either Arab-Muslim or American community. Among my white classmates, I was a 'terrorist,' 'haji' or 'camel.' My Arab and Muslim acquaintances cut me no slack. To them, I was 'whitey' or 'sour cream.' Lacking a sense of belonging with both groups, I felt like an Arab or Muslim among Americans and an American among Arabs or Muslims."

A study, focusing on indicators of school crime and safety in the U.S. public schools in 2009, found that about 28% of students (ages 12–18) "reported having been bullied at school during the school year" (Robers et al., 2012 p. v). In 2015, 46% of public education students in the U.S. were part of a racial or ethnic minority group, compared to about 33% in the late 1990s (Jonson-Reid, 2015). The Council on American-Islamic Relations-California (2019) conducted a survey in 2018–2019, reviewing approximately 1500 Muslim students between the ages of 11 and 18, enrolled in public and private schools statewide. The survey revealed that 40% of respondents reported that students at school were bullied for being Muslim, which is double the national statistic for students being bullied at school. Concerning gender-based differences, the survey found that 44% of female respondents reporting being bullied compared to 37% of male respondents. Regarding age-based differences, the survey indicated that high school-age student respondents were bullied at a higher rate than those in lower grades, with 48% of 12th-grade respondents reporting being bullied, the highest rate based on age/grade (Council on American-Islamic Relations-California, 2019).

Additionally, Americans with relatively low levels of educational attainment tend to be more negative in their views about Muslims and Islam than those with higher levels of educational attainment (Pew Research Center, 2017). The predicament here is that despite the dominate stereotype Americans have about Muslims being a threat to America or being anti-America (Braunstein, 2017; Russel, 2013), this particular stereotype received less negative views from Americans compared with other stereotypes. Table 9.1 shows that the indicator, "the majority of Muslim Americans are anti-America," received less negative views from Americans with different levels of education: high school (31%), university level (27%), and college/university graduate (14%) than the indicator, "Islam is not part of mainstream American society," which received the most negative views from Americans among the three

Table 9.1 Views of Islam and Muslims based on Americans' levels of education

Level of Education	Islam encourages violence more than any other religion %	Muslim Americans are extremists %	The majority of Muslim Americans are anti-America %	Islam is not part of mainstream American society %	Islam and democracy are not compatible %
High school or less	42	43	31	52	49
College/ university	44	37	27	50	45
College/ university graduate	32	23	14	47	38

Source: Pew Research Center (2017): U.S. Muslims concerned about their place in society

levels of education: high school (52%), university level (50%), and college/university graduate (27%).

Due to ignorance and an Islamophobic ideology, a 14-year-old Sudanese Muslim student, Ahmed Mohamed, was punished by a school in Irving, Texas, in 2015 because of his homemade clock that was perceived by teachers, administrators, and police as a bomb (Huseman, 2015; Washington Post, 2015). Ahmed, who once built a Bluetooth speaker for a friend, was a gifted and brilliant student. Yet, instead of praising Ahmed's potential creativity, the school, assumed that he was a danger to other students and handed him to police who transported him in handcuffs to a juvenile detention center (Huseman, 2015). In 2007, a second-grade Iraqi-American boy, at a school in Phoenix, Arizona, was called "Osama Bin Laden" by his classmates. However, his teacher thought he was claiming to be Bin Laden and called the FBI. In turn, FBI agents called his father. On another occasion, when the same boy "wore traditional Saudi clothing for a class assignment, he was made fun of. Students told him to 'go hijack a plane and run into a building.' They said, 'You are a terrorist. Your mom is a terrorist. Your dad is a terrorist. You have to go back to your country'" (American-Arab Anti-Discrimination Committee Research Institute, 2008 p. 57). In 2015, at Broward School in Florida, a 14-year-old Muslim student of Lebanese and Moroccan descent, was bullied by his teacher calling him a "raghead Taliban" and "terrorista," which means terrorist in Spanish, in front of whole class (Afshar, 2015). In Texas, a Middle School teacher called a 12-year-old student a terrorist in front of his peers. The teacher, however, was placed on leave (Rahman & George, 2016). Another incident relates to a boy, at a school in California, who walked up to a 17-year-old girl at lunch-time and shouted, "Her father is bin Laden! She's going to blow up the school...She has a bomb under her sweater! Everybody run, this jihad girl is going to kill us!" (American-Arab Anti-Discrimination Committee Research Institute, 2008 p.56). It is to be noted that harassment based on one's social identity, particularly religion, race and gender, has significant harmful mental health and social effects for targeted youth (American Educational Research Association, 2013).

Islamophobia and related actions of bullying have reached higher levels of education in North America as well. According to the American Educational Research Association (2013 p.48), the rates of bullying, including harassment or discrimination, among faculty and staff of North American universities "range from 32% to 52% in the United States and Canada."

An example of Islamophobia in American universities is presented in David Horowitz's infamous book (2006), *The Professors: The 101 Most Dangerous Academics in America* in which he attacked Muslim scholars, accusing them of spreading false information and extremist ideologies as well as misleading students. The book, however, has been refuted and criticized by a study entitled "Facts Count," organized by the Free Exchange on Campus, which is a coalition of ten groups including the American Association of University Professors (Jaschik, 2006). According to "Facts Count," Horowitz's book is sloppy and full of false information. In addition, Horowitz was not concerned with the students he claimed he was aiming to protect, but was actually trying to punish professors whose views he doesn't like. Further, the tone and format of his book brought to mind a McCarthy-era blacklist style and an obstruction of free speech rights and academic freedom (Jaschik, 2006).

The U.S. Commission on Civil Rights (2014 p.106) stated that Muslim parents of college students do not want them to engage in constitutionally protected activities due to fear of surveillance. But, this "climate of fear has also impacted political activities on college campuses, especially in California where outside influences have had a detrimental impact on student free expression."

This hostile environment has resulted in calls to murder Muslims in universities, in particular by Jerry Falwell Jr., the president of Liberty University and an advisor to former President Trump. During a speech at the Liberty University, hosting thousands of students, Falwell encouraged students to kill Muslims. He was not simply advocating for self-defense, but explicitly encouraging thousands of people to open fire on Muslims should they visit his college campus. Falwell said, "I just wanted to take this opportunity to encourage all of you to get your gun permit. We offer a free course... Let's teach them a lesson if they Muslims ever show up here" (Bailey, 2015, quoted in Walker, 2019 p.22).

Although the issue of Islamic schools in North America is beyond the scope of this study, the earliest Islamic schools in North America were part of the Nation of Islam revival project. The establishment of these schools was an act of protest against the absence of fair and equal educational opportunities in American society as well as in the American educational system. However, in Canada, there are no Nation of Islam schools, as the Nation of Islam did not establish any schools outside the United States (Tiflati, 2021).

Despite discriminatory and Islamophobic events and occurrences within the U.S educational environment, Muslims have similar levels of education as Americans overall. About 31% of American Muslims have college or postgraduate degrees, equivalent to that of U.S. adults as a whole (31%). Muslim immigrants are, on average, more highly educated than both U.S.-born Muslims and the U.S. public as a

Table 9.2 Level of education of Muslims compare to other faith groups

Level of Education	Less than high school	High school graduate	Less than 4 year-college	4 year-college (Bachelor)	Graduate school
Muslim	7%	27%	27%	26%	11%
Catholic	NA%	26%	23%	35%	11%
Protestant	4%	31%	23%	27%	12%
Jewish	3%	12%	20%	32%	31%
Non-affiliated	3%	20%	34%	23%	15%
General Public	3%	25%	26%	28%	14

Source: Adapted with modification from Institute for Social Policy and Understanding (2017)
Note: Numbers do not add up to 100% because remaining respondents did not provide a response to this question

whole. To be specific, 38% of foreign-born Muslims have at least a college degree compared with 21% of Muslims born in the U.S. and with 31% of the U.S. general public. However, this might reflect the U.S. immigration policies that give preference to highly educated immigrants (Pew Research Center, 2017).

The Institute for Social Policy and Understanding, ISPU (2017) has reached similar results in its comparative study of levels of education among diverse faith groups. For example, one of the significant findings of the ISPU's study, shown in Table 9.2, is that American Muslims are comparable with Protestants and the general public in educational attainment.

9.2.2   Canada

In Canada, education is a provincial responsibility as there is no federal government presence in schooling as is the case in the U.S. While there are a great many similarities in the provincial and territorial education systems across Canada, there are significant differences in curriculum, assessment, and accountability policies among the jurisdictions that express the geography, history, language, culture, and corresponding specialized needs of the populations served (Council of Ministers of Education, Canada, n.d.; Government of Canada, 2020). However, the Council of Ministers of Education, Canada (CMEC) has provided direction on how all children should be able to access inclusive education in Canada (Sider, 2020).

In 2020, both Canada and the U.S. rated closely together internationally on the domains indicated by the Human Development Index (HDI) and the Educational Index. Table 9.3 shows that the Human Development Index (HDI) of Canada was 0.929, while that of the U.S. was 0.926, achieving, respectively global ranks of 16 and 17 (out of 189 countries). For the Educational Index, Canada's score was 0.894, while the U.S. was 0.900 (United Nations Development Programme, 2020).

Table 9.3 Human Development Index and Educational Index of Canada and the U.S

Country	HDI value	HDI rank (out of 189 countries)	Educational Index
Canada	0.929	16	0.894
U.S.	0.926	17	0.900

Source: Adapted with modification form United Nation Development Programme (2020)

As in the U.S., Muslim students in Canada face racism, as well as Islamophobia, and they are singled out and discriminated against based on their gender, race, and religious identity (Hindy, 2016; Zine, 2001). In 2009, the Ontario Ministry of Education (2009 p.8) noted "a documented increase in reported incidents of anti-Black racism, antisemitism, and Islamophobia in Canada." In addition, advanced technology has been used for cyberbullying and hate propaganda on the Internet in Canadian schools (Ontario Ministry of Education, 2009; Wade & Beran, 2011). Other studies focusing on schools in Toronto revealed that after the tragic events of 9/11, incidents of religious-based bullying and harassment in schools had unprecedently increased. Incidents reported ranged from verbal abuse and joking about identity or faith to physical threat, violence, and the destruction of property (Wang et al., 2009; Zine, 2004).

Harassment can include racial harassment, religious harassment, gender harassment, sexual harassment, and other forms of cultural bias (Meyer, 2020). Examples of incidents of harassment and bullying against students in Canada included a teacher asking a student to change his name (Muhammed) because it was not a good name. A student whose name was "Usama" was called "Bin Laden" by other students, with refence to the terrorist Usama Bin Laden. Schoolgirls wearing hijabs were depicted as terrorists and suffered from having stones thrown at them as they walked to and from school. Even parents were stressed because of the harassment they faced when coming to the schoolyard to pick up their children (Zine, 2004). The politics of veiling in Canadian schools and society represents the contested notion of gender identity in Islam. For girls who adhere to Islamic dress codes that visibly designate them as Muslims, such as wearing the hijab or headscarf, problems of ethno-religious subjugation in the form of Islamophobia are particularly alarming. Studies that underscore the impact of gendered Islamophobia have shown that Muslim women who wear the hijab suffer discrimination in both the school and workplace (Hindy, 2016; Zine, 2006). For example, girls were removed from a Montreal high school for wearing the hijab (Hills, 2019; Todd, 1999). Additionally, several studies have revealed instances of Islamophobia and racism existing in Canadian universities (Alizai, 2017).

9.3   Policies Countering Islamophobia and Discrimination in Educational Institutions

Providing a fair and equitable education has been a major issue facing the North American public education system (U.S. Department of Education, 2003). However, in response to the startling spread of Islamophobic incidents targeting Muslim students, several government and NGOs organizations have provided policies and initiatives that seek to counter Islamophobia and discrimination in schools, on the one hand, and promote inclusive education, on the other. Education policies that counter Islamophobia in schools are supposed to bring about not only good quality of life and success to Muslim students, but also healthy and equitable environment to schools. The following sections address education policies in the U.S and Canada.

9.3.1   The U.S.

Education policies in the U.S. have progressed and advanced over the last hundred years to deal with a considerable array of policy issues, including the establishment of a general system of primary and secondary education, the warranting of equity and admission for students, the improvement of academic outcomes, the preparation of youth for postsecondary education, and the training of youth for the workforce (Jonson-Reid, 2015).

In 2010, the U.S. Department of Education issued the *"Dear Colleague Letter: Harassment and bullying"* stating, "While Title VI does not cover discrimination based solely on religion, groups that face discrimination on the basis of actual or perceived shared ancestry or ethnic characteristics may not be denied protection under Title VI on the ground that they also share a common faith" (U.S. Department of Education, 2010 p.5). The letter also stated, "even when bullying or harassment is not a civil rights violation, schools should still seek to prevent it in order to protect students from the physical and emotional harms that it may cause" (U. S. Department of Education, 2010 p.1).

In 2015, the U.S. Department of Education released a *letter to educational leaders regarding discrimination and harassment based on race, religion, or national origin*, urging them to uphold nondiscrimination policies and ensure that public schools and institutions of higher education would be free from discrimination and harassment based on race, religion, or national origin. The letter addressed the potential challenges that may be faced by students who were especially at risk of harassment, including those who were, or were perceived to be Muslim, Middle Eastern, or Arab, among other minorities in the U.S. The letter referred to several policies and resources used to assist school officials, educators, students, families, and communities in promoting more positive school climates. One of these resources is a website entitled *Stopbullying.gov* (n.d.), an official website of the United States government, which serves as a clearinghouse for all Federal anti-bullying resources and information about State laws and model policies to stop bullying and protect children (U.S. Department of Education, 2015).

In addition, The U.S. Department of Education (2016) issued a series of actions and guidelines that would confront discrimination and promote inclusive school environments. These actions and guidelines included the establishment of a new website on religious discrimination, an updated civil rights complaint form, an expanded survey of America's public schools on religious-based bullying, technical assistance for schools, and an outreach on confronting religious harassment in education.

According to the U.S. Department of Education (2016), the Department's Office for Civil Rights (OCR) launched a page on its website with information about federal laws that protect students from discrimination involving their religion. This online page is entitled *Religious Discrimination* (U.S. Department of Education, n.d.). The page links to OCR policy guidance, noteworthy case resolutions, and resources in multiple languages and from other federal agencies. It is interesting to observe that the OCR, within its online complaint form, has stated that that it can investigate complaints regarding racial, ethnic or national origin discrimination involving religion, reaffirming that students, parents, and persons of all faiths can file such complaints with the OCR even though the laws OCR enforces do not expressly address religious discrimination in education (U.S. Department of Education, 2016).

Additionally, several policies such as the Family Educational Rights and Privacy Act (FERPA) and the No Child Left Behind Act emphasize the family's right to information and appeal regarding special education eligibility and placement, discipline, and school choice (Jonson-Reid, 2015).

In 2020, the U.S. Department of Education published its *Guidance on constitutionally protected prayer and religious expression in public elementary and secondary schools*, providing comprehensive policies and guidelines that include the following:

- Schools should have well-publicized policies prohibiting harassment and procedures for reporting and resolving complaints that will alert the school to incidents of harassment.
- Students have the right to engage in religious activity or study religious materials with fellow students during recess, the lunch hour, or other non-instructional time to the same extent that they may engage in secular or nonreligious activities.
- It would be lawful for schools to excuse Muslim students from class to enable them, for example, to fulfill their religious obligations to pray during Ramadan.
- Students should not engage in religious harassment of others.
- A school is responsible for addressing harassment incidents about which it knows or reasonably should have known.
- State and local school districts should provide teachers and students with guidance to address bullying and harassment as well as to combat religious discrimination in schools.
- A school should provide training or other interventions not only for the harassers or perpetrators, but also for the larger school community, to ensure that all

students, their families, and school staff can recognize harassment if it recurs and know how to respond.

- While disciplining the perpetrators is likely a necessary step, it often is insufficient. A school's responsibility is to eliminate the hostile environment created by the harassment, address its effects, and take steps to ensure that harassment does not recur.
- While school authorities may impose rules of order and pedagogical restrictions on student activities, they should not discriminate against student prayer or religious perspectives in applying such rules and restrictions
- While schools enjoy substantial discretion in adopting policies relating to student dress and school uniforms, they should not single out religious attire in general, or attire of a particular religion, for prohibition or regulation.
- If a school makes exceptions to the dress code for nonreligious reasons, it must also make exceptions for religious reasons.
- Schools should not favor or disfavor students on the basis of their religious affiliations.

In addition to education policy provided by the U.S. Department of Education and local school districts, NGOs and researchers have contributed to this important domain of education policy (Shafer, 2016). For example, one researcher suggested that North American government and education authorities should apply Germany's experience in designing curriculum in which Islamic instruction is effectively placed on equal footing with similarly state-approved ethics training in the Protestant and Catholic faiths (Zaidi, 2019).

Another example pertains to Seyfi Kenan (2005) who has focused on the pedagogical policy of a curriculum entitled *(Re)embracing Diversity in New York City Public Schools: Educational Outreach for Muslim Sensitivity* developed by New York City schools in the following months of 9/11. The curriculum's core policy or objective was to improve the well-being of New York City school children belonging to Arab and Muslim minorities, who "were subjected to several instances of verbal and physical harassment and attacks due to the anti-Muslim backlash that followed the tragic events of 9/11" (Kenan, 2005 p. 173–174). The curriculum supported educators' efforts to foster tolerance and multiplicity in order to nurture the healing process of recuperating the well-being of all school children. The curriculum contained three modules with twelve lessons focusing on such topics as eliminating all forms of discrimination against Muslim students, understanding Islam and its contribution to civilization, embracing diversity in American society, debating civil rights and homeland security, and raising students' critical understanding through the promotion of interpersonal and intercultural dialogue based on tolerance and respect for ethnic and religious diversity (Kenan, 2005).

9.3.2 Canada

The Canadian Charter of Rights and Freedoms, 1982 confirmed education on an equal basis for all students. Section 15 (Equality Rights) assured equal rights and protection for every individual without discrimination based on race, national or ethnic origin, color, religion, sex, age or mental or physical disability (Canadian Encyclopedia, 2020; Canadian Legal Information Institute, 2021).

However, Canada does not have a federal department or national system of education. The Ministry of Education of each province is the governmental office in charge of education and is responsible for the development of education policies, legislation and regulations (Zine, 2008). Accordingly, the process of policies starts with a province establishing its education policies, then, boards develop or advance the policies in line with the requirements of provincial policies, and finally school principals implement the board policies (Government of Canada, 2020). The issue here is that the Ministry of Education of a province and local school boards work together to create policies that give direction for how certain procedures and practices in schools need to take place. These policies take the form of policy statements, guidelines, or memorandums (Ghonaim, 2019; Ontario Ministry of Education, 2013).

As far as education in Canada is a provincial responsibility, the focus here is on Ontario, which is the largest province in Canada, with a population of approximately 13 million and home of 582,000 Muslims (4.6% of the province's population), forming the largest Muslim community in Canada. Among Canadian cities, Toronto has the largest population of Muslims, at just over 424,900 (Statistics Canada, 2011). In the Ontario publicly-funded education system, schools are governed by district school boards, which are administered by the Ontario Ministry of Education. As of 2019–2020, there were 31 English public-school boards, 29 English Catholic school boards, 4 French public-school boards, and 8 French Catholic school boards. Additionally, there were 2,056,058 students and "3,967 elementary and 877 secondary schools in Ontario" (Ontario Ministry of Education, 2021).

The Ontario Ministry of Education has issued several policies or program memoranda to support equity, student achievement, and positive school climates. In 1993, the Ministry issued the Policy Program Memorandum (PPM) No. 119, *development and implementation of school board policies on antiracism and ethnocultural equity*, which went beyond a broad focus on multiculturalism and race relations to "focus on identifying and changing institutional policies and procedures, as well as individual behaviors and practices that may be racist in their impact" (Ontario Ministry of Education, 2013 p.2). In 2009, the Policy/Program Memorandum No. 119, *developing and implementing equity and inclusive education policies in Ontario schools,* broadened the scope of No. 119 (1993), to promote a system-wide approach to identifying and removing discriminatory biases and systemic barriers that helped to ensure that all students would feel welcomed and accepted in school life (Ontario Ministry of Education, 2013).

In 2013, the Ministry's new guidelines of *developing and implementing equity and inclusive education policies in Ontario schools: Guidelines for Policy Development and Implementation* provided the following board policies:

- School Boards and school leaders must be responsive to the diverse nature of Ontario's communities.
- School Boards are expected to take appropriate steps to provide religious accommodation for students and staff.
- School boards and schools are expected to provide leadership that is committed to identifying and removing discriminatory biases and systemic barriers to learning.
- Boards and their schools should use inclusive curriculum and assessment practices and effective instructional strategies that reflect the diverse needs of all students and the learning pathways that they are taking.
- School board policies must be comprehensive and must cover the prohibited grounds of discrimination set out in the Ontario Human Rights Code (Ontario Human Rights Commission (OHRC), 2013). The code prohibits discrimination on any of the following grounds: race, color, ancestry, place of origin, citizenship, ethnic origin, disability, creed (e.g., religion), sex, sexual orientation, gender identity, gender expression, age, family status, and marital status.

Although the aforementioned guideline of 2013 prohibits all forms of discrimination, it does not particularly mention problems of Islamophobia or anti-Muslim sentiments targeting Muslim students. This particular issue has been addressed in subsequent policies.

In 2014, the Ontario Ministry of Education provided policies against Islamophobia and discrimination stating that an "improved awareness of the negative impact on students' lives of discriminatory behavior and attitudes, including racism, Islamophobia and other forms of discrimination, can help education leaders, trustees, and staff change individual behavior and institutional practices to eliminate systemic barriers" (Ontario Ministry of Education, 2014 p.30). It also stated that the policies "must be ongoing to ensure that our schools continue to provide caring, inclusive, safe, and accepting environments that support the achievement and well-being of every student" (Ontario Ministry of Education, 2014 p.5). Eliminating discrimination and establishing an equitable and inclusive education system require commitment from all education partners including the ministry, school boards, and schools. And all students, parents, and other members of the school community are welcomed and respected. The Ontario Ministry of Education (2014, p. 6) confirmed that education "is a key means of fostering social cohesion, within an inclusive society where diversity is affirmed in a framework of common values that promote the well-being of all citizens."

Despite these progressive policies issued by the Ontario Ministry of Education and local school boards, there is a concern related to the implementation of these policies to all schools, not just some of them Hindy, 2016). Researchers suggest that developing an anti-Islamophobic pedagogy may effectively reduce or completely eliminate Islamophobia into the next generation (Zaidi, 2019). Ontario school boards need to advocate acceptance of Islamic dress and have clear consequences for any harassment by intolerant persons. Teachers should be advised to be "observant of male–female relations in student seating and group work" (Ghonaim, 2019 p.17). Additionally, Ontario school boards should offer anti-Islamophobia workshops for teachers and provide lesson plans and other curricula resources to support teachers in teaching against Islamophobia in the classroom (Hindy, 2016; Zine, 2004).

Canadian NGOs and civil society have played an important role in providing policies and recommendations to improve education, in general, and help minorities and Muslim students, in particular. For instance, the National Council of Canadian Muslims (2019), in collaboration with the Islamic Social Services Association (ISSA) has prepared a guide to help educators address concerns arising from the spread of Islamophobia and its impact on children and youth. To be more specific, it provides the following selected practical recommendations:

- Canadian government should partner with Canadian Muslim communities to create an effective strategy to combat extremist narratives.
- Community stakeholders must work together to find new approaches to teach about tolerance and acceptance as well as to promote diversity and multiculturalism.
- Provincial ministries of education should ensure that teachers are using the resources to ensure curricula are taught through a lens that allows young people to identify stereotypes and to challenge popular mis-conceptions.
- Mental health professionals need to be involved in the efforts to address the emotional and mental impact that religious-based discrimination and bullying has on Muslim students.
- Special attention should be paid to Muslim girls who wear the religious garb or veil (hijab), as they are frequent targets for hate and physical harm.

9.4   Conclusion

Education enables people to exercise influence within and beyond the nation's borders through participation in policies and decisions taken on local and global measures (el-Aswad, el-S., 2019). The dilemma here is that despite the common challenge of discrimination and extremism in religion can be overcome only through education (Crane, 2010), there are religious discrimination inside educational systems of the most advanced and free countries. This chapter has focused on two core objectives. First, to address the negative impact of Islamophobia and discrimination on students' overall well-being and academic achievement in North America. Second, to highlight education policies designed and implemented by Canada and the U.S. to reform their education systems, specifically in dealing with minorities, including Muslim students. Education policies and guidelines for schools and educators aiming at countering Islamophobia and discrimination against Muslims have been underscored in this study.

This study has shown that it is imperative to advance the quality of education of Muslim students at all levels in North America and other nations by eliminating discrimination and Islamophobia in schools, updating curricula about Muslim culture, recruiting and training highly qualified instructors, increasing funding for minority groups, building reliable educational resources and facilities, and improving administrative systems that appreciate equal treatment of all educators, administrators, staff, and students. This study has demonstrated that for both Canada and the U.S., all children should be able to attend school regardless of socio-economic condition, religion, cultural background, political position, gender, skin color, language, sexual orientation, geographical context, or physical, emotional, or cognitive ability. However, there are shortcomings in fighting Islamophobia and anti-Muslim racism in North American schools. North American educational systems must recognize that minority populations are mostly bicultural, creating an exceptional backdrop of socio-cultural and emotional issues to which these systems must be prepared to respond (Cross et al., 1989).

The U.S. federal government needs to develop adequate cross-cultural communication skills as well as to explore new education policies to communicate information about discrimination including that found in the use of social media, online platforms and video. It also needs to find novel ways of distributing school guidance to reach students, parents or families, and teachers. Media education is being identified as an essential part of the school curriculum worldwide (Watt, 2008).

Although Canada has developed policies and programs that fight discrimination and support inclusive education through the Council of Ministers of Education and both the Ministry of Education and school borders of each province, there is still a real need for more effective approaches and attitudes for countering Islamophobia in schools in ways similar to what was aforementioned.

Islamophobia or religious discrimination against Muslim students in schools is not only a violation of academic freedom and ethical principles, but also has negative impact on the overall well-being of Muslim students. Discrimination, poverty and economic ill-being at the family and school levels lead to meager educational opportunities and outcomes. Educators and policymakers still need to balance local, state, and federal guideline, management, and accountability. They should also balance attention to students belonging to minority groups and education of entire schools (Jonson-Reid, 2015).

Internationally, the Organization for Security and Cooperation in Europe [OSCE]/Democratic Institutions and Human Rights [DIHR], the Council of Europe and the UNESCO (2011) have provided policies and guidelines for educators on countering intolerance and discrimination against Muslims with a special focus on addressing Islamophobia through education. These guidelines are intended for a wide audience, including education policymakers and officials, teacher trainers, teachers, principals and head teachers, staff in teacher unions and professional associations, and members of NGOs. The following are selected policies and recommendations offered by these organizations (OSCE/ODIHR, Council of Europe, & UNESCO, 2011 pp., 23–28):

- Teachers are responsible not only for teaching about the subject matter, but also for promoting mutual respect and understanding among the students. They should react to any expressions of anti-Muslim views or use of stereotypes.
- Portrayals of Islam and Muslims—and of all religions and their adherents—are to be accurate, fair and respectful.
- A human rights-based approach to education should be implemented in order to give students and teachers a reliable framework within which to assess behaviors and attitudes in a school setting as well as to guarantee the right to respect in the learning environment.
- The curriculum should be developed with the active participation of bodies representative of the minorities in question.
- Schools should seek to provide opportunities for discussion about stereotypes and portrayals of Muslims.
- Schools should monitor, in co-operation with all educational stakeholders, manifestations of intolerance against any group on an ongoing basis, in order to take preventive and protective action as needed and to avoid any escalation.
- Teaching about religions—including Islam—can contribute to understanding and to reducing intolerance and discrimination.

In addition, the author suggests the following broad policies and recommendations that are applicable to both the U.S and Canada:

- Schools should consult minority communities, including Muslims, about needed curricula and other educational needs.
- Students, teachers, and school administrators should learn about broader lessons of religious freedom, respect for differences, and inclusivity.
- Educators and administrators should recognize that the issue of targeting Muslim students goes beyond local schools, to be linked to broader socio-cultural issues associated with negative stereotypes of Muslims.
- Teachers should know how to prevent students from holding negative and stereotypical views of Muslims.
- Stakeholders, including governments, should take steps to better understand the underlying biases that shape students' negative stereotypes about different religions.
- The focus should be on mentoring students and scholars to include anti-Islamophobia and anti-racist research and action they might be involved in.
- Design anti-Islamophobia programs and encourage Muslims to be involved in workshops through which they express their views about Islam.
- Design curriculum and *academic coursework* focusing on educating students about Islamic history, values, traditions (*halal* food, costumes and olfactory, for example).

One of the most important recommendations that might effectively reduce or eliminate an Islamophobic environment in schools is to increase cultural competency not only in educational systems and schools, but also in the entire society. Cultural competence "is a set of congruent behaviors, attitudes, and policies that come together in a system, agency, or among professionals and enable that system, agency, or those professionals to work effectively in cross-cultural situations" (Cross et al., 1989 p.13). In this particular context, the concept of culture "implies the integrated pattern of human behavior that includes thoughts, communications, actions, customs, beliefs, values, and institutions of a racial, ethnic, religious, or social group" (Cross et al., 1989 p.13). Culture is viewed as providing explanations of core features of educational policy and administration (Bromley, 2016). Finally, it is important to build an educational environment where all students, regardless of their faith and ethnic background, are treated as persons of dignity and equal worth.

References

Afshar, P. (2015, March 7). Broward teacher accused of calling her student 'raghead Taliban' gets 5-day suspension. *Miami Herald*. Retrieved from http://www.miamiherald.com/news/local/community/broward/article15046943.html

Alizai, H. (2017). Impact of Islamophobia on post-secondary Muslim students attending Ontario universities. *Electronic Thesis and Dissertation Repository*. Retrieved from https://ir.lib.uwo.ca/etd/4716

American Educational Research Association. (2013). *Prevention of bullying in schools, colleges and universities: Research report and recommendations*. AERA. Retrieved from https://www.aera.net/Portals/38/docs/News%20Release/Prevention%20of%20Bullying%20in%20Schools,%20Colleges%20and%20Universities.pdf

American-Arab Anti-Discrimination Committee Research Institute. (2008). *Report on hate crimes and discrimination against Arab Americans: 2003-2007*. ADC Publications. Retrieved from https://archive.mbda.gov/sites/mbda.gov/files/migrated/files-attachments/20032007ReportonHateCrimesandDiscriminationAgainstArabAmericans.pdf

Asvat, Y., & Malcarne, V. L. (2008). Acculturation and depressive symptoms in Muslim university students: Personal-family acculturation match. *International Journal of Psychology, 43*(2), 114–124. https://doi.org/10.1080/00207590601126668

Bailey, S. P. (2015, December 5). Jerry Falwell Jr.: "If more good people had concealed-carry permits, then we could end those" Islamist terrorists. *Washington Post*. Retrieved from https://www.washingtonpost.com/news/acts-of-faith/wp/2015/12/05/liberty-university-president-if-more-good-people-had-concealed-guns-we-could-end-those-muslims/

Bajaj, M., Ghaffar-Kucher, A., & Desai, K. (2016). Brown bodies and xenophobic bullying in US schools: Critical analysis and strategies for action. *Harvard Educational Review, 86*, 481–505. Retrieved from https://meridian.allenpress.com/her/article-abstract/86/4/481/32201/Brown-Bodies-and-Xenophobic-Bullying-in-US-Schools?redirectedFrom=fulltext

Bajaj, M., & Kidwai, H. (2016). Human rights and education in South Asia. In K. Mundy, A. Green, R. Lingard, & A. Verger (Eds.), *Handbook of global education policy* (pp. 206–223). Wiley-Blackwell.

Bakali, N, (2015). Challenging anti-Muslim racism through a critical race curriculum in Quebec secondary schools. Critical Intersections in Education, 3: 19-24. Retrieved from file:///Users/elaswad/Downloads/Challenging_Anti-Muslim_Racism_Through_a.pdf

Birkland, T. A. (2016). *An introduction to the policy process: Theories, concepts, and models of public policy making*. Routledge.

Braunstein, R. (2017). Muslims as outsiders, enemies, and others: The 2016 presidential election and the politics of religious exclusion. *American Journal of Cultural Sociology, 5*(3), 355–372. https://doi.org/10.1057/S41290-017-0042-X

Broman, C. L. (1997). Race-related factors and life satisfaction among African Americans. *Journal of Black Psychology, 23*(1), 36–49.

Bromley, P. (2016). Policy and administration as culture: Organizational sociology and cross-national education trends. In K. Mundy, A. Green, R. Lingard, & A. Verger (Eds.), *Handbook of global education policy* (pp. 470–489). Wiley-Blackwell.

Brown, C. S. (2015). *The educational, psychological, and social Impact of discrimination on the immigrant child*. Migration Policy Institute. Retrieved from https://www.migrationpolicy.org/sites/default/files/publications/FCD-Brown-FINALWEB.pdf

Canadian Encyclopedia. (2020, March 2). *Canadian charter of rights and freedoms*. Retrieved from https://www.thecanadianencyclopedia.ca/en/article/canadian-charter-of-rights-and-freedoms

Canadian Legal Information Institute. (2021). *The Constitution Act, 1982: Part I Canadian charter of rights and freedoms*. Retrieved from https://www.canlii.org/en/ca/laws/stat/schedule-b-to-the-canada-act-1982-uk-1982-c-11/latest/schedule-b-to-the-canada-act-1982-uk-1982-c-11.html

Council of Ministers of Education, Canada (n.d.). *Over 50 years of Pan-Canadian leadership in education*. Retrieved from https://cmec.ca/299/Education-in-Canada-An-Overview/index.html

Council on American-Islamic Relations-California (2017). *Civil rights report 2017: Islamophobia in educational institutions*. Retrieved from http://www.islamophobia.org/images/2017CivilRightsReport/2017-Empowerment-of-Fear-Final.pdf

Council on American-Islamic Relations-California (2019). *Singled out: Islamophobia in the classroom and the impact of discrimination on Muslim students*. Retrieved from https://ca.cair.com/wp-content/uploads/2019/11/2019-Bullying-Report.pdf

Crane, R. D. (2010). Islamophobia, mimetic warfare and the bugaboo of Shari'a compliance: Counter-strategies for common ground. *Arches Quarterly, 4*(7), 54–61.

Cross, T. L., Bazron, B. J., Dennis, K. W., & Isaacs, M. R. (1989). *Towards a culturally competent system of care*. CAASP Technical Assistance Center.

Dawson, E. M., & Chatman, E. A. (2001). Reference group theory with implications for information studies: A theoretical essay. *Information Research, 6*(3) Retrieved from http://informationr.net/ir/6-3/paper105.html#ref4

Dei, G. J., Mazzuca, J., McIsaac, E., & Zine, J. (1997). *Reconstructing dropout: A critical ethnography of the dynamics of black students' disengagement from school*. University of Toronto Press.

Douglass, S. L. (2009). Teaching about religion, Islam, and the world in public and private schooling curricula. In Y. Y. Haddad, F. Senzai, & J. I. Smith (Eds.), *Educating the Muslims of America* (pp. 85–108). Oxford University Press.

el-Aswad, el-S. (2006). The dynamics of identity reconstruction among Arab communities in the United States. *Anthropos: International Review of Anthropology and Linguistics, 101*, 111–121.

el-Aswad, el-S. (2019). *The quality of life and policy issues among the Middle East and North African countries*. Springer.

Findley, P. (2001). *Silent no more: Confronting America's false images of Islam*. Amana Publications.

Ghonaim, F. (2019). Inclusion of Muslim students in Ontario public education: A qualitative inquiry of elementary school principals. *Electronic Thesis and Dissertation Repository*. Retrieved from https://ir.lib.uwo.ca/cgi/viewcontent.cgi?article=8396&context=etd

Government of Canada. (2020). *Education in Canada*. Retrieved from https://www.canada.ca/en/immigration-refugees-citizenship/services/new-immigrants/new-life-canada/enrol-school.html

Hills, T. T. (2019). The dark side of information proliferation. *Perspectives on Psychological Science, 14*(3), 323–330.

Hindy, N. (2016). Examining Islamophobia in Ontario public schools. *The Tessellate Institute*. Retrieved from http://tessellateinstitute.com/wp-content/uploads/2016/11/Examining-Islamophobia-in-Ontario-Public-Schools-1.pdf

Hodge, D. R., Zidan, T., & Husain, A. (2016). Depression among Muslims in the United States: Examining the role of discrimination and spirituality as risk and protective factors. *Social Work, 61*(1), 45–52.

Huseman J. (2015, September 16). Schools in Irving, Texas feared Islam well before they thought Ahmed Mohamed's Clock was a bomb. *Slate*. Retrieved from http://www.slate.com/blogs/schooled/2015/09/16/ahmed_mohamed_s_school_it_was_afraid_of_islam_well_before_it_thought_a_clock.html

Institute for Social Policy and Understanding. (2017). *American Muslim poll 2017: Muslims at the crossroads: A monograph on effective services for minority children who are severely emotionally disturbed*. Retrieved from https://www.ispu.org/american-muslim-poll-2017/

Jaschik, S. (2006, May 9). Fact-checking David Horowitz. *Inside Higher Ed*. Retrieved from https://www.insidehighered.com/news/2006/05/09/fact-checking-david-horowitz

Jonson-Reid, M. (2015, July 2). Education policy. In *Oxford research encyclopedia of social work*. Oxford University Press. https://doi.org/10.1093/acrefore/9780199975839.013.121

Kazi, N. (2016, September 18). Teaching against Islamophobia in the age of terror. *Chronicle of Higher Education*. Retrieved from https://www.chronicle.com/article/teaching-against-islamophobia-in-the-age-of-terror/

Kenan, S. (2005). Reconsidering peace and multicultural education after 9/11: The case of educational outreach for Muslim sensitivity curriculum in New York City. *Educational Sciences: Theory and Practice, 5*(1), 172–180.

Kulkarni, S. S. (2020, June 30). Racial and ethnic disproportionality in special education programs. In *Oxford research encyclopedia of education*. Oxford University Press. https://doi.org/10.1093/acrefore/9780190264093.013.1242

Kunst, J. R. (2012). Coping with islamophobia: The effects of religious stigma on Muslim minorities' identity formation. *International Journal of Intercultural Relations, 36*(4), 518–532.

Leonardo, Z. (2009). The colour of supremacy: Beyond the discourse of 'white privilege'. In E. Taylor, D. Gillborn, & G. Ladson-Billings (Eds.), *Foundations of critical race theory in education* (pp. 261–276). Routledge.

Lieberman, A., & McLaughlin, M. (1982). *Policy making in education*. University of Chicago Press.

Meyer, E. J. (2020, October 27). Gender and bullying. In *Oxford research encyclopedia of education*. Oxford University Press. https://doi.org/10.1093/acrefore/9780190264093.013.1320

National Council of Canadian Muslims (2019). *Helping students deal with trauma related to geopolitical violence & Islamophobia*. Retrieved from https://www.toronto.ca/wp-content/uploads/2019/04/97e4-Geopolitical-Violence-and-Islamophopia.pdf

Niyozov, S., & Plum, G. (2009). Teachers' perspectives on the education of Muslim students: A missing voice in Muslim education research. *Curriculum Inquiry, 39*, 637–677. https://doi.org/10.1111/j.1467-873X.2009.00463.x

Ontario Human Rights Commission. (2013). *Guide to your rights and responsibilities under the Human Rights Code*. Retrieved from http://www.ohrc.on.ca/en/guide-your-rights-and-responsibilities-under-human-rights-code-0

Ontario Ministry of Education. (2009). Realizing the promise of diversity: Ontario's equity and inclusive education strategy. Retrieved from http://www.edu.gov.on.ca/eng/policyfunding/equity.pdf

Ontario Ministry of Education. (2013). *Developing and implementing equity and inclusive education policies in Ontario schools*. Retrieved from http://www.edu.gov.on.ca/extra/eng/ppm/119.pdf

Ontario Ministry of Education. (2014). *Equity and inclusive education in Ontario schools: Guidelines for policy development and implementation: Realizing the promise of diversity*. Retrieved from http://www.edu.gov.on.ca/eng/policyfunding/inclusiveguide.pdf

Ontario Ministry of Education. (2021). *Ontario education facts*. Queen's Printer for Ontario. Retrieved from http://www.edu.gov.on.ca/eng/educationfacts.html

OSCE/ODIHR, Council of Europe & UNESCO. (2011). *Guidelines for educators on countering intolerance and discrimination against Muslims: Addressing Islamophobia through education.* Retrieved from https://www.osce.org/files/f/documents/4/2/84495.pdf

Pew Research Center. (2016, December 13). *Religion and education around the world.* https://www.pewforum.org/2016/12/13/religion-and-education-around-the-world/

Pew Research Center. (2017, July 26), *U.S. Muslims concerned about their place in society, but continue to believe in the American Dream.* Retrieved from https://www.pewforum.org/2017/07/26/findings-from-pew-research-centers-2017-survey-of-us-muslims/

Pew Research Center. (2019, October 3). *Religion in the public schools.* Retrieved from https://www.pewforum.org/2019/10/03/religion-in-the-public-schools-2019-update/

Rahman, F., & George, C. (2016, April 1). Teacher placed on leave after allegedly calling 12-year-old 'terrorist'. *Houston Chronicle.* Retrieved from http://www.houstonchronicle.com/neighborhood/fortbend/news/article/Teacher-placed-on-leave-after-allegedlycalling-7223910.php .

Robers, S., Zhang, J., Truman, J., & Snyder, T. (2012). *Indicators of school crime and safety: 2011 (NCES 2012-002/NCJ 236021).* National Center for Education Statistics, U.S. Department of Education, and Bureau of Justice Statistics, Office of Justice Programs, U.S. Department of Justice. Retrieved from https://nces.ed.gov/pubs2012/2012002rev.pdf

Russel, W. F. (2013). *Islam: A threat to civilization.* First Edition Design Pub..

Ryan, J. (2018). Introduction: Cases for inclusion. In D. Griffiths & J. Ryan (Eds.), *Case studies for inclusive educators and leaders* (pp. 1–10). Word & Deed.

Saleem, M., & Ramasubramanian, S. (2017). Muslim Americans' responses to social identity threats: Effects of media representations and experiences of discrimination. *Media Psychology, 22*(3), 373–393. https://doi.org/10.1080/15213269.2017.1302345

Shafer, L. (2016, November 23). Dismantling Islamophobia. *Usable Knowledge.* Retrieved from https://www.gse.harvard.edu/news/uk/16/11/dismantling-islamophobia

Shealey, M. W., Lue, M. S., Brooks, M., & Mccray, E. (2005). Examining the legacy of Brown: The impact on special education and teacher practice. *Remedial and Special Education, 26*(2), 113–121. https://doi.org/10.1177/07419325050260020601

Sider, S. (2020, August 27). Policies that foster education for all: Implications for economically wealthy nations. In *Oxford research encyclopedia of education.* Oxford University Press. https://doi.org/10.1093/acrefore/9780190264093.013.1027

Statistics Canada (2011). *Immigration and ethnocultural diversity in Canada.* Retrieved from https://www12.statcan.gc.ca/nhs-enm/2011/as-sa/99-010-x/99-010-x2011001-eng.pdf

Stopbullying, gov. (n.d.). *Prevention: Learn how to identify bullying and stand up to it safely.* Retrieved from https://www.stopbullying.gov

Tiflati, H. (2021). *Islamic schooling and the identities of Muslim youth in Quebec: Navigating national identity, religion, and belonging.* Taylor & Francis.

Todd, S. (1999). Veiling the "other," unveiling ourselves: Reading media images of the hijab psychoanalytically to move beyond tolerance. *Canadian Journal of Education, 23*(4), 438–451.

U.S. Commission on Civil Rights. (2014). *Federal civil rights engagement with Arab and Muslim American communities.* Washington, DC. Retrieved from https://www.usccr.gov/pubs/docs/ARAB_MUSLIM_9-30-14.pdf

U.S. Department of Education. (2003, July 28). *Dear colleague letter: First amendment.* Retrieved from https://www2.ed.gov/about/offices/list/ocr/firstamend.html

U.S. Department of Education. (2015, December 31). *Letter to educational leaders regarding discrimination and harassment based on race, religion, or national origin.* Retrieved from https://www2.ed.gov/policy/gen/guid/secletter/151231.html

U.S. Department of Education. (2016, July 22). *U.S. Department of Education takes actions to address religious discrimination.* Retrieved from https://www.ed.gov/news/press-releases/us-department-education-takes-actions-address-religious-discrimination

U.S. Department of Education. (2020, January 16). *Guidance on constitutionally protected prayer and religious expression in public elementary and secondary schools.* Retrieved from https://www2.ed.gov/policy/gen/guid/religionandschools/prayer_guidance.html

U.S. Department of Education. (n.d.). *Religious discrimination*. Retrieved from https://www2.ed.gov/about/offices/list/ocr/religion.html

U.S. Department of Education: Office for Civil Rights. (2010, October 26). *Dear colleague Letter: Harassment and bullying*. Retrieved from https://www2.ed.gov/about/offices/list/ocr/letters/colleague-201010.pdf

U.S. Department of Justice. (2016). *Combating religious discrimination today: Final report*. Washington, DC. Retrieved from https://www.justice.gov/crt/file/877936/download

United Nations. (2018). *The sustainable development goals 2015–2030*. United Nations Association of Philadelphia. Retrieved from http://una-gp.org/the-sustainable-development-goals-2015-2030/

United Nations Development Programme. (2020). *Human development index*. Retrieved from http://hdr.undp.org/en/indicators/103706

United Nations Human Rights. (1989). *Convention on the rights of the child*. Retrieved from https://www.ohchr.org/en/professionalinterest/pages/crc.aspx

Wade, A., & Beran, T. (2011). Cyberbullying: The new era of bullying. *Canadian Journal of School Psychology, 26*, 44–61.

Walker, N. (2019, August 28). Political contempt and religion. In *Oxford research encyclopedia of politics*. Oxford University Press. https://doi.org/10.1093/acrefore/9780190228637.013.1156

Wang, J., Iannotti, R., & Nansel, T. (2009). School bullying among US adolescents: Physical, verbal, relational and cyber. *Journal of Adolescent Health, 45*(4), 368–375.

Washington Post. (2015, September 16) *'They thought it was a bomb': 9th-grader arrested after bringing a home-built clock to school*. Retrieved from https://www.washingtonpost.com/news/morning-mix/wp/2015/09/16/they-thought-it-was-a-bomb-ahmed-mohamed-texas-9th-grader-arrested-after-bringing-a-home-built-clock-to-school/

Watt, D. (2008). Challenging islamophobia through visual media studies: Inquiring into a photograph of Muslim women on the cover of Canada's National News magazine. *Studies in Media & Information Literacy Education, 8*(2), 1–14.

Zaidi, R. (2019, January 25) Islamophobia and education. *Oxford research encyclopedia of education*. : Oxford University Press. https://doi.org/10.1093/acrefore/9780190264093.013.231. https://oxfordre.com/view/10.1093/acrefore/9780190264093.001.0001/acrefore-9780190264093-e-231

Zine, J. (2001). Muslim youth in Canadian schools: Education and the politics of religious identity. *Anthropology & Education Quarterly, 32*(4), 399–423.

Zine, J. (2004). Anti-islamophobia education as transformative pedagogy: Reflections from the educational front lines. *American Journal of Islam and Society, 21*(3), 110–119. https://doi.org/10.35632/ajiss.v21i3.510

Zine, J. (2006). Unveiled sentiments: Gendered islamophobia and experiences of veiling among Muslim girls in a Canadian Islamic School. *Equity & Excellence in Education, 39*, 239–252.

Zine, J. (2008). *Canadian Islamic schools: Unravelling the politics of faith, gender, knowledge, and identity*. University of Toronto Press.

Chapter 10
Human Rights Policy

10.1 Introduction

It is interesting to observe that "cross-cultural misunderstanding occurs when persons, holding specific worldviews, interpret and judge the behaviors of people belonging to another culture as if they were holding the same worldviews" (el-Aswad, el-S., 2012, p. 148). Because of this cross-cultural misunderstanding, Muslims in North America have faced many civil rights challenges both before and since 9/11, including hate crimes, discrimination, harassment, bullying, interrogation, improper questioning at borders, and law enforcement policies among other biased and unjust practices. Ironically, it is some liberal democratic states such as the U.S. and Canada, acclaiming the importance of the rule of law and the protection of human rights, that have been seen to undermine those protections (Steinback, 2011).

This chapter proposes that Islamophobia, an irrational fear of Muslims, has become a real and *rational* fear that Muslims experience due to frightening and vicious attacks on their human rights as well as on their lives. Islamophobia is viewed here as a fundamental human rights abuse and violation of human dignity (Abadi, 2018; el-Aswad, el-S., 2013a). Within this broader scope, "Islamophobia is a civil society problem and not only a Muslim issue" (Bazian, 2018, p. 70).

In a nutshell, this chapter critically examines policies of North American governments and NGOs showing both the positive and negative sides of their policies in fighting Islamophobia. Countering Islamophobia in North America depends on multiple agencies including governments, political parties, think tanks, and NGOs or advocacy organizations, taking a steadfast stand against forms of racism and discrimination, including Islamophobia. In addition, the chapter provides recommendations that might help both policymakers and ordinary North American Muslims effectively combat Islamophobia and enjoy a peaceful and healthy life. Ordinary Muslims also become responsible for defending their human rights since people who are not aware of their civil rights are unlikely be able to shield them.

© The Author(s), under exclusive license to Springer Nature Switzerland AG 2021   173
el-S. el-Aswad, *Countering Islamophobia in North America*, Human Well-Being
Research and Policy Making, https://doi.org/10.1007/978-3-030-84673-2_10

Islamophobia has resulted in Muslims' ill-being, as represented in their being victims of human rights violation, social instability, economic inequality, unemployment, lack of social services, deterioration of health care, and negative representation in the media. Islamophobia has created a climate of fear that has impacted Muslims' well-being as well as their human and political rights. Protecting people's rights is guided by the understanding of human rights in terms of international human rights law and appreciating the distinction between binding legal obligations on governments and the broader issues of ethics, politics, and social change (el-Aswad, el-S., 2005, 2019; Hannum, 2019).

The following sections address efforts of selected government and NGOs or advocacy organizations that have launched plans, initiatives or programs directed toward securing Muslims' human rights as well as fighting Islamophobia and racism. Examples of the outcomes of these efforts are provided. However, before proceeding, it might be helpful to refer to what is meant by human rights.

10.2   Human Rights

The concept of rights is included in the United Nation's nonbinding Universal Declaration of Human Rights (UDHR), adopted by the United Nations General Assembly in 1948. The UDHR identifies the rights of individuals in 30 distinct articles. According to the first article, "All human beings are born free and equal in dignity and rights. They are endowed with reason and conscience and should act towards one another in a spirit of brotherhood" (United Nations, 2015, p. 4). Human rights include, for example, the right to life and liberty; freedom from slavery and torture; freedom of thought, conscience and religion; freedom of opinion and expression; the right to take part in the government; the right to work and education; and the right to rest and leisure. Everyone is entitled to these rights, without discrimination or being subjected to arbitrary arrest, detention or exile (United Nations, 2015). Additionally, there is what is known as the international human rights law that determines the obligations of Governments to promote and protect human rights and fundamental freedoms of individuals or groups (United Nation, 2021).

From these statements, it is clear that the concept of human rights encompasses multiple and interconnected magnitudes of political rights, civil rights, social, economic, and cultural rights, in addition to rights of development and freedom from poverty (Anderson & Murdie, 2017). Hence, human rights constitute a holistic subject matter addressed by interdisciplinary fields including, for instance, political science, sociology, anthropology, law, economics, history, and psychology (Morgan, 2009). Additionally, NGOs and civic society, protecting and supporting human rights, include academic institutes, social movement organizations, think tanks advocacy groups, religious organizations, interest groups, voluntary organizations, political action committees, and philanthropic foundations, to name but a few.

Human rights are addressed here within the outline of issues discussed in previous chapters, particularly those pertaining to social, religious, and political disadvantages of North American Muslims caused by Islamophobia and other forms of discrimination and racism. Human rights of Muslim minorities in North America are inseparable from human rights of other minorities, nationally, regionally and globally. Violations and desecrations of minority rights are generally structural in nature, as discriminatory practices are constructed in political, social and economic systems to deny fundamental rights (Price, 2012).

The rest of this chapter seeks to answer this question: What policies and guidelines have the government's agencies, and NGOs, including advocacy organizations, used to secure human rights and religious freedom of Muslim minorities in North America?

10.3 Government Agencies

Full understanding of human rights situations requires comprehension of the domestic factors and features of governments and bureaucracies. One of the main objectives here concerns the abuses of the human rights of citizens of a specific state by governmental actors from this state. Human rights abuses are means that political leaders use to try to hold on to political power (Anderson & Murdie, 2017; el-Aswad, el-S., 2016; Ritter, 2014). However, the violation of human rights causes internal and domestic conflict (Thoms & Ron, 2007; Center for American Progress 2011a, 2011b, 2015). The following sections address the human rights policies institutionalized by governments of the U.S. and Canada.

10.3.1 The United States

Despite the Religious Freedom Restoration Act, enacted by the U.S Congress in 1993 as a measure to protect the rights of religious individuals and communities that may be troubled by government activity (Congress Gov., 1993), violation of Muslims' human rights and religious freedoms has increased particularly since the tragic events of 9/11. Muslim minorities have faced physical abuses and social discrimination while the right of freedom of expression has been used as a justification for assaulting and attacking Muslims (el-Aswad, el-S., 2013b). The "Civil Rights Division of the U.S. Department of Justice reports that allegations of abuse include: telephone, internet, and face-to-face threats; minor assaults; vandalism; shootings; and bombings of homes, businesses, and places of worship" (Moore, 2012, p. 92).

According to the Human Rights Watch (HRW), in 2019 the U.S. continued to move backwards on human rights as the Trump administration (2017–2021) rolled out inhumane immigration policies and promoted false narratives that disseminated Islamophobia, racism, and discrimination (Human Rights Watch, 2017, 2021a). The

Trump administration "has openly transformed anti-Muslim bigotry into govern-ment policy, appointing known anti-Muslim extremists to government positions" (Mitchell, 2017, p. 50). In general, the U.S. continues to have the highest reported criminal incarceration rate in the world, with 2.2 million people in jails and prisons, in addition to 4.5 million on probation and parole as of 2017 (Human Rights Watch, 2020a). In many cases, however, the government, especially its executive branch, has been one of the main causes behind the violation of human rights in the name of combatting terrorism, particularly when the government's Islamophobes call them-selves *terrorism experts*. The "U.S. government has spent $40 million on spreading misinformation about American Muslims" (U.S. Commission on Civil Rights, 2014, p. 18). Notably, democracy is often theorized not only in terms of free elections, but also in terms of constraints on an executive's power (Anderson & Murdie, 2017).

The U.S. government's Islamophobic actions, including a Muslim ban, unjustified counter radicalization, racial profiling of Muslims, and propaganda against Muslim places of worship, such as mosques, are viewed by the judicial system, policy advocates, scholars, and law makers as unconstitutional and a violation of religious freedom (Moore, 2012). In addition, the U.S. "federal government's 'counter-radicalization' efforts create a danger of creating a government-approved 'Official Islam,' which adversely impacts religious freedom and potentially violates the Establishment Clause" (U.S. Commission on Civil Rights, 2014, p. 44) of the First Amendment that prohibits the government from establishing a religion (United States Courts, n.d.). According to the Muslims in America policy poll, conducted by Emgage (2020), over 80% of American Muslims responded that civil rights policies were of the most urgent concern for them, while 65% stated that healthcare was another top policy priority. Over 45% of Muslim respondents reported they would like to see policy changes in the areas of religious discrimination (Emgage, 2020).

The following is an example of one of the academic institutions that uncovered incidents of desecration of Muslims' human rights executed by governments. To be more specific, a report, issued by the Center for Human Rights and Global Justice (School of Law, New York University), stated that since the events of 9/11, the U.S. government, in the name of counter-terrorism, has targeted Muslims in the U.S. by sending paid, untrained informants into mosques and Muslim communities. Such a policy has led to the unwarrantable prosecution of more than 200 individuals in terrorism-related cases. Specifically, the report examined three high-profile ter-rorism prosecutions in which.

> government informants played a critical role in instigating and constructing the plots that were then prosecuted. In all three cases, the FBI or New York City Police Department (NYPD) sent paid informants into Muslim communities or families without any particular-ized suspicion of criminal activity. Informants... work for a government-conferred bene-fit—say, a reduction in a preexisting criminal sentence or a change in immigration status—in addition to fees for providing useful information to law enforcement, creating a dangerous incentive structure... [T]he government's informants held themselves out as Muslims and looked in particular to incite other Muslims to commit acts of violence. The government's informants introduced and aggressively pushed ideas about violent jihad and, moreover, actually encouraged the defendants to believe it was their duty to take action against the

United States. In two of the three cases, the government relied on the defendants' vulner-
abilities—poverty and youth, for example—in its inducement methods. In all three cases, the
government selected or encouraged the proposed locations that the defendants would later be
accused of targeting. In all three cases, the government also provided the defendants with, or
encouraged the defendants to acquire, material evidence, such as weaponry or violent
videos, which would later be used to convict them...The defendants in these cases were
all convicted and are facing prison sentences of 25 years to life (Center for Human Rights
and Global Justice, 2011, p. 2).

Similar patterns of the violation of American Muslims' human rights are
documented in a report by the U.S. Commission on Civil Rights (2014) in which
different government agencies have been criticized by both government and NGOs
professionals and experts. Even the U.S. countering violent extremism (CVE) programs have been counterproductive, dehumanizing Muslim communities and imper-
iling their human rights (Waheed, 2018).

In general, and within this anti-human rights climate, Americans have provided
low and negative ratings in their evaluation of several core human rights and
democratic principles. For example, there has been a decline in the number of both
Republicans and Democrats who say the phrase "the rights and freedoms of all
people are respected" describes the country well. In 2020, only 52% of Republicans
said the rights of all people are respected, down from 60% since 2018, compared to
30% of Democrats who said the same; there has been an 8-point decline since 2018.
More than 85% of Americans said it is very important that the rights and freedoms of
all people are respected (Pew Research Center, 2020a). Likewise, the share of
Americans who said the phrase, "people are free to peacefully protest" describes
the country very or somewhat well has fallen from 73% to 60%, with the decline
occurring almost entirely among Democrats. Consequently, in 2020, 79% of Democrats said significant changes in the structure of government are needed, compared
with 41% of Republicans (Pew Research Center, 2020a). According to a recent poll
survey, conducted by Gallup as part of its annual poll surveys performed in January
of each year, 27% of Americans were satisfied with how government was working in
2021, compared to 43% in 2020, a decrease of 16 points. A mere 18% of Americans
reported being satisfied with the nation's moral and ethical climate, down by more
than half from 47% in 2002 and lagging behind the prior low of 32% in 2020
(Gallup, 2021).

It is worthy to note that the aforementioned report of the U.S. Commission on
Civil Rights, issued in September 2014, provided one of the most positive policy
plans toward the recognition of American Muslims' civil rights. The report focused
on "actions taken by the federal government to address, prevent and eradicate
violations of civil rights laws against the Arab and Muslim-American communities"
(U.S. Commission on Civil Rights, 2014, p. 5). The following are selected policy
recommendations provided by the U.S. Commission on Civil Rights (2014):

- Federal government agencies, including the U.S. Department of Justice (DOJ),
  the Federal Bureau of Investigations (FBI) and the U.S. Department of Homeland
  Security (DHS), among other agencies, should expand their outreach efforts to
  the American Muslim community.

- Federal agencies should collaborate with local government agencies and advocacy groups that regularly engage and serve the diverse American Muslim community.
- Federal agencies should continue local outreach efforts with Muslim communities, but forbid all offices engaging in such outreach from sharing information gained through such efforts for investigative or surveillance purposes.
- The U.S. Department of Justice (DOJ) should conduct a thorough investigation of how Muslims are being interrogated and searched at the border and prohibit Customs and Border Patrol officers from asking questions related to First Amendment-protected activity (i.e., freedom of religion, speech, press, assembly, and petition).
- Government engagement efforts should be *de-securitized* to holistically focus on the host of social, economic, and political factors that affect the vitality of Arab and Muslim communities.
- Government engagement programs should be subject to citizen and Congressional oversight to ensure stated objectives are in fact met and government resources are not wasted.

It is interesting to observe and appreciate several positive actions made by the U.S. government. A report entitled *combating religious discrimination today*, issued by the U.S. Department of Justice (2016), referred to a community engagement initiative planned to promote religious freedom, challenge religious discrimination, and enhance the U.S. Department of Justice's efforts to combat religion-based hate violence. The report acknowledged that "individuals from less familiar religious communities, particularly those that are—or are perceived to be—Muslim, experience higher levels of religious discrimination and harassment once hired" (U.S. Department of Justice, 2016, p. 17). In addition, the initiative focused on protecting people and places of worship from religion-based hate crimes, countering anti-Muslim rhetoric, and addressing unlawful barriers that interfere with the construction of places of worship. With reference to an issue related to constructing mosques in the U.S., the report stated, "discrimination against houses of worship and religious congregations remains a serious and growing problem" (U.S. Department of Justice, 2016, p. 23).

Unfortunately, while the government demands the initiative's guidelines to be respected and followed, many American Muslims believe that local and federal agencies have not implemented these guidelines since Islamophobia, discrimination, and violation human rights have intensified. Therefore, on March 7, 2019, the U.S. House of Representatives of the 116th Congress (2019–2020), passed the resolution (H. Res. 183), condemning anti-Semitism and anti-Muslim discriminations and all forms of racism, hateful expressions, and bigotry against all minorities as contrary to the values of the United States. This resolution acknowledged the harm suffered by Muslims and others from the harassment, discrimination, and violence that result from anti-Muslim racism. In addition, the resolution encouraged all public officials to confront the reality of anti-Semitism, Islamophobia, racism, and other forms of bigotry to ensure that the U.S. lives up to the principles of tolerance, religious freedom, and equal protection of human rights (Congress Gov., 2019). It seems that such an outstanding resolution supports the statement of the U.S. Commission on Civil Rights (2014, p. 18) that there "is a need to highlight American Muslims' contributions since the attack [of 9/11] in protecting the nation, and in partnering with government and law enforcement to ensure a safer society, and in preserving civil liberties within their communities."

On February 4, 2021, the U.S. House of Representatives sanctioned Marjorie Taylor Greene, a House Representative Republican from Georgia, depriving her of her right to participate on the Education and Budget Committees for endorsing conspiracy theories, Islamophobia, racist dogma and violence against Democratic politicians (BBC News, 2021; The Hill, 2021). With reference to Muslim Congresswomen, Greene said the 2018 U.S. congressional midterm elections ushered in an Islamic invasion of the U.S. government, (BBC News, 2021). It is acknowledged that in democratic states, citizens have more institutionalized channels through which to get their grievances heard by the regime (Anderson & Murdie, 2017). The U.S. Supreme Court had earlier ruled 8–1 in favor of a young Muslim woman who has sued retailer Abercrombie & Fitch when the Islamophobic owner of the store failed to hire her because she wore a headscarf in observance of her religion (de Vogue, 2015; Naylor, 2015).

10.3.2 Canada

Concerning government agencies in Canada, the government of Prime Minister Justin Trudeau has made notable efforts to advance human rights, advocating for a pluralistic society that respects the rights of immigrants, people with disabilities and other minorities. Canada is a diverse, multi-cultural democracy that enjoys a global reputation as a defender of human rights and a strong record on key civil and political rights protections guaranteed by the Canadian Charter of Rights and Freedoms (Human Right Watch, 2020b).

Cross-culturally, a survey, conducted in 2020 by the Pew Research Center (2020b), measuring the indicators of "promoting human rights" and "promoting patience" across globally advanced economies, concluded that for the indicator of "promoting human rights," Canada, with the score of 78%, performed better than the U.S. (70%). Likewise, for the indicator of "promoting peace," Canada, with the score of 82%, performed better than the U.S. (72%).

Despite this progress, the Canadian government grapples with serious human rights issues related to the continued confinement of immigration detainees in jails, including Muslims, and a prison law that does not stop prolonged solitary incarceration (Human Rights Watch, 2020b). Furthermore, the Canada Border Services Agency remained the only major law enforcement agency in the country without some form of independent civilian oversight (Human Rights Watch, 2021b).

Canada is still facing other longstanding human rights challenges. For example, in 2017, the most commonly cited religious identity related to complaints of discrimination in Canada on the basis of religion was Muslim (40%). Of these complaints, "7% raised systemic issues such as racial profiling by police, limited access to religious programs for Indigenous inmates, unfair treatment of Muslim travelers at borders, and denial of banking services based on national or ethnic origin" (Canadian Human Rights Commission, 2017, p. 7). According to Canadian Human Rights Act, discrimination includes all discriminatory practices based on race, national or ethnic origin, color, religion, age, sex, sexual orientation, gender identity or expression (Government of Canada, n.d.). Islamophobia is used in Canada to justify ever-increasing state interference in the private and public spheres of Muslims (Cader & Kassamali, 2012). In June 2019, the Canadian province of Quebec passed Bill 21 preventing certain categories of public employee from wearing religious symbols at work. Teachers, judges, police officers, among other civil servants, are prohibited from wearing symbols of their faith, including hijabs and turbans, in the workplace. The controversial law also prohibits anyone with religious face coverings from receiving government services, including healthcare and public transit (Human Rights Watch, 2020b).

Issues such as human rights, privacy rights, civil liberties, religious freedom, immigration, combatting terrorism, and national security are often debated and decided by the government without participation of Canadian Muslims. For instance, in June 2020, Human Rights Watch research found that Canada failed to develop adequate policies to assist and repatriate more than 40 Canadians, including Muslims, unlawfully detained in life-threatening conditions, prisons and camps for the Islamic State (ISIS) suspects and their families in northeast Syria. However, none of the Canadian Muslims has been charged with any crime or brought before a judge to review the legality and necessity of their detention. In addition, during 2019–2020, children were placed in detention to accompany their detained parents (Human Rights Watch 2021a, 2021b). This pattern of human rights violation occurred two decades ago in what is known as Arar's civil case, drawing a broad and global consideration, in which both Canada and the U.S. were involved (Institute for Research on Public Policy, 2008).

Maher Arar, a Canadian Muslim and father of two children, was travelling home to Canada after visiting his wife's family in Tunisia in 2002. While changing planes at New York City's JFK airport, he was detained and held for 12 days by U.S. authorities. He was then transferred secretly, via Jordan, to Syria, where he was held in degrading and inhumane conditions, interrogated, and tortured for a year. The CIA was involved in Arar's detention in Syria. Maher was given an Immigration and Naturalization Service (INS) issued document stating that he was inadmissible into the United States because he belonged to an organization designated as a foreign terrorist organization, namely, al-Qa'ida (Amnesty International Canada, 2017).

According to Amnesty International Canada (2017), Arar was neither involved in terrorist activities nor associated with the al-Qa'ida terrorist group. There was no evidence indicating the Mr. Arar committed any offense or implicated in terrorist activity. The dilemma is that the U.S. decision to detain Arar relied on inaccurate information about him that had been provided by Canadian officials. Canadian officials had not acted quickly enough to get Mr. Arar out of Syria and leaked false information which tarnished Mr. Arar's reputation upon his return (Amnesty International Canada, 2017; Canadian Encyclopedia, 2016; Craddock, 2008). The Arar commission concluded that the potential for the infringement of the human rights of innocent Canadian Muslims is higher in national security enforcement due to the stricter scrutiny to which members of these groups are subjected (National Council of Canadian Muslims, 2016b).

NGOs and advocacy organizations, such as the Amnesty International Canada that intervened, defended Arar's civil case, pushing the Canadian government to settle the case in January 2007. The Canadian government apologized to Maher Arar and his family for the terrible ordeal they suffered, paying him nearly $10 million in compensation. Mr. Arar also called on the U.S. to "come clean" and acknowledge "the deficiencies and inappropriate conduct that occurred in this case" (Center for Constitutional Rights, n.d., p. 9).

10.4   NGOs and Advocacy Organizations

The literature on the impact of non-government organizations (NGOs) and non-state groups on protecting Muslim human rights and countering Islamophobia is largely scant. It has been confirmed that international and domestic NGOs play a central role in most advocacy networks of civil society (McEntire et al., 2015; Murdie, 2009). A healthy civil society is a "set of institutions and social norms that make pluralism a civil process of persuasion and reconciling of differences" (Snyder & Ballentine, 1996, p. 9).

While mainstream messages can be issued from the government, they can also be from non-government organizations that are part of civil society. When civic institutions establish bridges between different ethnic groups, there will be peace or at least a less violent engagement between individuals of these groups (Varshney, 2001). And if good civic organizations serving the economic, social and cultural needs of different communities exist, the support for collective peace tends to be strong and well expressed (Varshney, 2001).

In addressing NGOs or advocacy organizations, some studies focus only on Muslim civic interest groups (Cury, 2016), but this chapter broadens the scope to include both Muslim and non-Muslim organizations as active agents for protecting civil rights and fighting Islamophobia. In other words, in their efforts to combat Islamophobia and to provide significant insights to Muslims' human rights, both Muslims and non-Muslims have established institutions and organizations equipped with cyber communication and online facilities. While some of these organizations aim at developing education and religious or spiritual awareness, others are more concerned with human rights and democratic issues (Moore, 2012).

Currently, a considerable number of American and Canadian Muslim organizations are calling on all levels of their governments to address systemic racism and combat Islamophobia as well as to protect Muslims' human rights and religious practices (Adams, 2017). Anti-Islamophobia organizations work through public lectures, online writings or texts, public-political pressure, op-eds, interviews, and lawsuits (Council on American-Islamic Relations, 1997). Organizations work toward addressing the drivers and causes of Islamophobia and anti-Muslim racism, providing solutions and recommendations. However, it is be noted that unlike Muslim advocacy organizations that focus on the Muslim minority, non-religiously affiliated advocacy organizations address diverse minorities, but the attention here is given to their handling of human rights of Muslims in North America.

The NGOs in the U.S. include, for example, the Council on American–Islamic Relations (CAIR), Muslims for American Progress (MAP), the Arab–American Anti-Discrimination Committee (ADC), the Muslim Public Affairs Council (MPAC), the Institute for Social Policy and Understanding (ISPU), the Carter Center, the Center for American Progress (CAP), the Islamic Society of North America (ISNA), the Muslim American Society (MAS), the Association of Muslim Social Scientists in North America (AMSS), the Islamic Center of Detroit (ICD), the Islamic Supreme Council of America (ISCA), the Islamic Cultural Institute (ICI), and the Southern Poverty Law Center (SPLC).

The NGOs in Canada include, for instance, the National Council of Canadian Muslims (NCCM), the Canadian Muslim Union (CMU), the Muslim Association of Canada (MAC), the Canadian Anti-Hate Network (CAN), Amnesty International Canada (AIC), the Canadian Civil Liberties Association (CCLA), the Canada Centre for Community Engagement and Prevention of Violence, and the Canadian Muslim Forum (CMF), to mention but a few.

Out of these advocacy organizations, two organizations from the U.S. namely the Council on American–Islamic Relations (CAIR) and Carter Center; and another two from Canada, the National Council of Canadian Muslims and the Canadian Anti-Hate Network are examined. The reasons for focusing on these particular organizations are as follows:

- First, they represent different Muslim and non-Muslim views and approaches in handling issues of civic rights;
- Second, they represent certain different local and national concerns in their dealing with Islamophobia and Muslim human rights;
- Third, they provide distinct policies and recommendations to policymakers, political leaders and those interested in countering Islamophobia and anti-Muslim racism;
- Fourth, problems of Islamophobia and Muslims' human rights are not viewed in this study as confined to Muslims, but rather embrace, and are entrenched in, entire civil societies in both the U.S and Canada;
- Fifth, defending Muslim communities is a solemn task that shows sincere cooperation of multiple elements and forces of civil society.

The following subsections focus on differing Muslim and non-Muslim advocacy organizations from the U.S as well as from Canada.

10.4.1   The United States

One of the most influential non-governmental organizations in the U.S is the Council on American–Islamic Relations (CAIR), founded in 1994. As an anti-Islamophobia network, the CAIR is considered the largest non-profit Muslim civil rights and advocacy organization in the United States that has established a *counter-Islamophobia project* (2018a), proposing three practical and effective policies.

First, it specifies and designates prejudicial organizations that manufacture and disseminate Islamophobia, showing how much they violate Muslims' human and civil rights. For example, it identified more than 70 organizations comprising the U.S. Islamophobia network of which more than 30 groups form an inner core network whose purpose is to promote hatred of Islam and Muslims. (Council on American–Islamic Relations, 2018b).

Second, it uncovers ideologies and funding resources of Islamophobia organizations, documenting most if not all anti-Muslim hate crimes and incidents of prejudice, including harassment, bullying and bias in schools. Hate crimes are criminal attacks against persons or property, and/or incidents that can be charged as such under proper state or federal law. For instance, the Council on American-Islamic Relations (Council on American–Islamic Relations, 2017) indicated that the number of hate crimes in the first half of 2017 spiked to 91% (or 134 hate crimes) as compared to the same time period in 2016 (or 70 hate crimes).

Third, it works to raise Muslims' awareness of the danger of such atrocious organizations by establishing the project of "Know Your Rights," which is a guide that informs Muslims about their rights in dealing with law enforcement, discrimination, employment, education, travel, and peaceful protest among other civil rights. People can download the guide in multiple languages including Arabic, Bengali, Bosnian, Farsi, Somali, Urdu, and English (Council on American-Islamic Relations, n.d.).

In addition, CAIR invites and encourages people to work cooperatively to counter all forms of racism and Islamophobia. Countering Islamophobia, a system of a religious and racial animosity, requires committed action and resources. For example, for the purpose of combating Islamophobia, the Council on American-Islamic Relations (2019) founded another project entitled *anti-prejudice tools* that includes policies and recommendations directed to both American Muslim individuals and American Muslim institutions.

Policies and recommendations to American Muslim individuals include several actions that can be summed as follows:

- **Be active in community life and get involved in neighbors as well as with** community leaders, representing different cultural, religious, and ethnic groups, and community sectors (such as schools, associations, unions, businesses, and so like) to assess current initiatives and determine future needs and policies.
- Be active in political life and get involved in state and national elections.
- **Document and report all acts of Islamophobia and anti-Muslim discrimination.**

- Speak out in a clear and sophisticated way condemning any form of racism and bigotry.
- Exercise self-control when confronted by hate of offence and behave assertively and politely.
- **Support** and collaborate with **local, national, and regional Muslim organizations** whose work is to protect human rights and counter Islamophobia.
- Turn negative incidents into positive solutions. For instance, if a place of worship is vandalized, work to bring communities together to collectively repair it, showing cohesion and solidarity (Council on American–Islamic Relations, 2019).

Regarding policies and recommendations to American Muslim Institutions, they include the following:

- Expose the Islamophobes through unified efforts. Although Islamophobes are small in number and they do not represent the majority of the public, they can mislead the general public by providing misinformation. Muslim institutions should unify their efforts in exposing and refuting all manufactured misinformation about Islam.
- **Empower communities through civic engagement. Institutions should provide civic participation training for those who are interested in improving the impact of the ideas and efforts concerned with civil and human rights.**
- Support law enforcement and the protection of individual rights and national security to ensure that civil and constitutional rights of all Americans are protected.
- Provide positive alternatives to anti-Islamophobic events by forming community groups that promote mutual understanding.
- **Invest in community development by establishing systematic and comprehensive programs to educate interested Americans about Islam in the form of classes in mosques based on a nationally established curriculum. This also includes participation in the development of Muslim colleges that can produce graduates who think based on Islamic values and act in the American pluralistic and constitutional context**
- **Re-introduce Islam by promoting books, movies and art produced by objective people or by Muslims. Institutions should urge scholars and communications experts to counter and correct the narratives that misrepresent Islam, such as Quranic verses quoted out of context, mistreatment of women, or certain terms such as 'jihad' and 'shari'a.'**

Another influential non-profit, nongovernmental organization is the Carter Center, founded in 1982 by former U.S. President Jimmy Carter and his wife, Rosalynn, in partnership with Emory University, to advance peace and health worldwide. The Carter Center has established a *human rights program* whose goal is to enhance and protect human rights by supporting individuals, communities and nations striving to attain the civil, political, economic, social, and cultural rights and responsibilities acknowledged by the United Nations' Universal Declaration of Human Rights (Carter Center, 2021).

The former U.S. President, Jimmy Carter whose center published a guidebook on countering Islamophobia in 2018, stated,

I have watched with concern the unprecedented rise of anti-Muslim hate crimes and hate speech. From surveillance and imprisonment, with fewer procedural safeguards against anti-Muslim legislation, Muslims have been subjected to discriminatory and unconstitutional practices. Such actions not only infringe on the freedom of Muslims to practice their faith, but also marginalize them as engaged citizens... We must use the laws that enshrine human and civil rights to combat Islamophobia as they have been used to combat other forms of discrimination (Carter, 2018, p. 4).

The Carter Center's guide of *countering the Islamophobia industry* offers robust, public-facing operational policies that help policymakers and anti-Islamophobia activists to sustain and secure Muslims' civil and human rights. Selected policies and recommendations from this guide are presented in the following:

- The responsibility to counter Islamophobia falls on everyone who aspires to defend human and constitutional rights.
- Apply scientific research studies to identify patterns of Islamophobia and hate crimes and appropriate legal responses to them.
- Conduct a wide-ranging assessment of Islamophobia industry, in terms of its ideology, agenda, working system and level of activity, to determine its weak points to be contested and fought.
- Islamophobic industry and Islamophobes must be exposed, banished and downgraded in all domains of civil society.
- Establish or collaborate with a well-coordinated human rights group or alliance that counters Islamophobia aided by teamwork of advocacy organizations and communities. The alliance must develop a mechanism for swift response to Islamophobia propaganda.
- Moral support must be given to individuals and organizations fighting Islamophobia, particularly those defending marginalized Muslim women.
- Work diligently to refute the false association made by Islamophobes between terrorism and Muslims to justify their attacks on Muslims. This means that it is important to disassociate countering Islamophobia from combating all forms of terrorism and violent extremism not related to anti-Muslim racism.
- Highlight the work of unrecognized ant-Islamophobia activists who work persistently while being attacked by Islamophobes.
- Assist mosques to become a community resource for non-Muslims through open houses and interfaith engagement.
- Develop financial structures and endowments for funding the human rights alliance and other groups combating Islamophobia industry, recognizing that the latter is well-funded
- Equality of all individuals or citizens, regardless to race, religion, ethnicity and/or color, must be protected by law. Those who violate the law, Muslims and non-Muslims, are held accountable for their actions (Almontaser, 2018, pp. 99–102; Bazian, 2018, pp. 65–72).

10.4.2   Canada

In Canada, the National Council of Canadian Muslims (NCCM), formerly (before July 6, 2013) called the Canadian Council on American-Islamic Relations (CAIR. CAN), was founded in 2000 (National Council of Canadian Muslims, 2013). The NCCM, an independent, non-partisan and non-profit advocacy organization, is a leading voice for Muslim civic engagement and the promotion of human rights. The NCCM works to counter Islamophobia, build mutual understanding between Canadians, promote the public interests of Canadian Muslim communities, protect the constitutional rights of Canadian Muslims, and support the rights of all Canadians. The NCCM has been fighting all forms of bigotry, racism and Islamophobia (National Council of Canadian Muslims, 2013). In addition, the NCCM monitors legal developments and intervenes at Canadian national courts, particularly before the Supreme Court of Canada, in cases that impact fundamental rights and freedoms (National Council of Canadian Muslims, n.d.-a).

The NCCM challenged Canadian security agencies in their efforts to carry on the profiling of Canadians Muslims on the basis of fighting terrorism and radicalization. The NCCM's Human Rights Department monitors and responds to violations of human rights and civil liberties, and provides dedicated services in challenging the discrimination and harassment that Canadian Muslims face (National Council of Canadian Muslims, n.d.-b). In March 2015, the NCCM called for Bill C-51, the Anti-terrorism Act-2015, to be repealed on the basis that it increased the risk of violating the rights of innocent Canadians while failing to enhance national security. Canadian Muslims are more likely than others to find themselves targeted by national security investigations. The NCCM states that it has always supported the government's responsibility to ensure national security, but Canadian Muslims believe that national security policy fails to abide by the standards established in the Canadian Charter of Rights and Freedom that forms part of Canadian Constitution. Canadian Muslims expect the Charter to protect them as much as it protects any other Canadians (National Council of Canadian Muslims, 2016b, 2017). The following are recommendations provided by the NCCM in response to the Bill C-51or anti-terrorism Act-2015:

- Community-based engagement and solutions are the best defense against human rights abuse as well as against radicalization as Canadian Muslim communities and community leaders have been at the forefront of confronting radicalization to criminal violence.
- There is a need for coordinated national support of grassroots' activities in areas like counselling, deradicalization, repurposing initiatives, education, and social media messaging.
- Partake in public consultations and work with the federal government at the grassroots partnership level to develop and implement a national coordinated strategy for community-based policies.

- Parliamentary National Security Committee should maintain an ongoing discourse with civil society to ensure the work of the national security institutions is cognizant of the social impact it produces.
- End no-fly list as Canadian Muslims and their families are the most adversely affected by that list, damaging their personal and professional interests.
- Provide consistent information sharing between government departments and agencies.
- Repeal the previous government's torture directives, which permit the use and sharing of information with foreign regimes that practice torture (Council of Canadian Muslims, 2016b; Stevenson, 2016).

It is worthy to point out that in 2017, the House of Commons approved and passed Motion 103 (M-103), condemning Islamophobia and all forms of systemic racism and religious discrimination as well as calling the government to quell the increasing public climate of hate and fear (House of Commons, 2017). Notwithstanding this strong M-103, Canadian Muslims, including Iqra Khalid who introduced the Motion, have been continues targets of Islamophobia and racism (Gunter, 2017; Parry, 2017).

The NCCM has addressed critical issues related to racism and Islamophobia, particularly at the Canada Border Services Agency Act (CBSA). The NCCM states that there are over 500 allegations of misconduct by CBSA officers filed between 2018 and 2019. Currently, the CBSA has no independent, external civilian oversight. The following recommendations seek to ensure that racial discrimination is not active on the border. The suggested policy recommendations are:

- Ensure that CBSA officers who engage in misconduct in an off-duty capacity can be investigated by the oversight body.
- As complainants may be afraid to file complaints to the oversight body, ensure that civil society organizations have standing to make complaints.
- Ensure that the oversight body can hear complaints regarding CBSA policies and procedures.
- Develop a clear workplan and require regular reviews to be submitted to Parliament on steps taken to change the culture of discrimination and harassment at the by the Canada Border Services Agency Act (National Council of Canadian Muslims, 2020).

Additionally, the NCCM collaborates with other Canadian advocacy organizations and welcomes their efforts to provide policies that protect Muslim human rights. For example, the NCCM, in collaboration with other organizations, has provided the Canadian government with recommendations for countering Islamophobia (National Council of Canadian Muslims, 2016a, 2017, 2018). According to these recommendations, the government should:

- Recognize the need to suppress and control the increasing public climate of hate and fear. Canada Border Services Agency Act.
- Condemn Islamophobia and all forms of systemic racism and religious discrimination.

- Request that the Standing Committee on Canadian Heritage undertake a study on how the government could develop an official approach to reducing or eliminating systemic racism and religious discrimination including Islamophobia in Canada, while ensuring a community-centered focus with a holistic response through evidence-based policy-making.
- Eliminate racial discrimination and inequality, particularly in dealing with minorities.
- Establish an *Anti-Racism Directorate* within the Department of Canadian Heritage to develop and lead a *national action plan against racism.*
- Collect data to contextualize hate crime reports and to conduct primary assessments to improve civil, social and political positions of Muslims and other minorities

Another active NGO in Canada, is the Canadian Anti-Hate Network (CAN), a new independent, nonprofit organization concerned with issues pertaining to human rights and countering all forms of racism and Islamophobia driven by hate groups (Canadian Anti-Hate Network, n.d.). The Canadian Anti-Hate Network's advisory committee is composed of court-recognized experts, researchers, and academics dealing with hate crimes. For example, Barbara Perry stated that replicated threat assessment narratives and reports published by federal agencies make little or no reference to the threat driven by right-wing extremists (Perry, 2017).

The Canadian Anti-Hate Network has relationships with institutes and organizations fighting for human rights nationally and internationally, such as the Southern Poverty Law Center (2020). The mandate of the CAN is to monitor, research, and counter hate groups, including Islamophobia by providing education and information on hate groups to the public, media, researchers, courts, law enforcement, and community groups (Canadian Anti-Hate Network, n.d.).

Specifically, the policy of the Canadian Anti-Hate Network is to track hate groups and anti-Muslim organizations and, in collaboration with other advocacy groups, advise and urge the Canadian government to dismantle all these dangerous hate groups both online and offline. The Canadian Anti-Hate Network provides policymakers, who want to understand organized grassroots hate in Canada, with information about the size and activities of these sinister networks whose number exceeds 300, based on Barbara Perry's estimate (Balgord & Smith, 2021; Boutilier, 2019; Canadian Anti-Hate Network, 2019). In 2019, the government of Canada banned two white supremacist, neo-Nazi organizations; Blood & Honor and Combat 18 (Casey, 2020; Global News, 2019).

Additionally, the Canadian Anti-Hate Network and other advocacy organizations called on the federal government to establish a national action plan on designating and dismantling other white supremacists and extreme right-wing groups such as the Atomwaffen Division and The Base as terrorist entities, threatening Canadian Muslim community amongst other racialized communities (Canadian Anti-Hate Network, 2020, 2021). Such a call was effective particularly after members of white supremacy organizations were involved in the storming of the U.S. Capitol on January 6, 2021. Designated terrorist groups may face serious troubles including travel or flight restrictions and economic sanctions that weaken their financial support, among other restrictions (Canadian Anti-Hate Network, 2021).

It is worthy to refer to an ethnographic fieldnote that relates to a North American Muslim who has been involved in human rights activities. This person is Amir Aswad, and Arab-Muslim American successful attorney, graduated from the University of Chicago, who, in an interview, recounted, "I used to perceive myself as a nobody: neither Arab-Muslim nor American. But after different experiences and worldviews in the field of human rights, I've come to realize that I can, and have the right to, be both equally. Among 'pure' Arabs-Muslims, I can lean on my Egyptian roots, make jokes, and socialize. Among White Americans, I can lean on my Scottish and Canadian heritage and blend right in. People may have perceived me as an outsider, but the real blow was that I regarded myself as one. That's a blow that hard to recover from. It took me my entire life."

10.5   Conclusion

This chapter has examined some of the human rights policies issued and implemented by North American governments and NGOs to secure the human rights and religious freedom of Muslim minorities, disclosing both the positive and negative features of these policies. Furthermore, the chapter has reviewed, assessed and provided plans and recommendations that might help policy makers, political leaders, and ordinary North American Muslims to effectively counter Islamophobia, conserve their civil rights, and enjoy healthy and prosperous life.

This study has focused on policies and actions taken by North American governments, mainly of the U.S and Canada, to address, prevent and eradicate violations of civil rights laws against Muslim minorities. Although there are genuine efforts made by North American governments to counter anti-Muslim racism, unfortunately, Islamophobia persists. Particularly, this study has observed that there is a sort of discrepancy between federal or international laws of human rights and the actual practices of governments' official agencies that in many cases violate human rights and spread fear and anxiety among Muslims. Essentially, this is a critique of the federal governments' abuse and mistreatment of Muslims' human rights; however, the main objective of this critique is to urge governments' institutions and agencies to become better in honoring the laws and respecting the civil rights of all citizens. Compelling laws and impartial implementation of such laws addressing and dealing with Islamophobia, hate crimes, and discrimination are powerful tools of governments in their effort to dismantle hate groups and protect civil rights and civil society.

Although the focus here is to address Islamophobia and systemic racism at the federal level, it is important to stress the fact that any effective method of countering Islamophobia and religious discrimination requires cooperation across all levels of North American governments.

Advocacy organizations and their leaders in the U.S and Canada are active agents of human rights. Despite the fact that there are numerous, active NGOs, this study has focused on four differing Muslim and non-Muslim organizations in the U.S. and Canada respectively, namely the Council on America-Islamic Relations, the Carter Center Institute, the National Council of Canadian Muslims and Canadian Anti-Hate Network. Additionally, this chapter has shown how Islamic organizations, reflecting the diversity and pluralism of Muslim communities in North America, have embarked on momentous tasks to counter the human rights challenges faced by these communities. Although some of these organizations are more concerned with human rights and democratic issues, while others focus on religious freedom, education and spiritual awakening, the shared objective of most of them is fighting Islamophobia. Another shared purpose of these organizations is that they serve as bridges or intermediaries between North American governments and diverse Muslim communities.

Despite the energetic activities and positive outcomes of anti-Islamophobia organizations in defending Muslims' human rights, their efforts need to be supported and amplified to more effectively address, confront or uproot, Islamophobia and anti-Muslim organizations. In a word, civil liberties protection and promotion of cultural and religious diversity in North America need to be improved and promoted. Public officials should also speak out against Islamophobia stereotypes in mainstream popular culture.

This chapter proposes that both the governments and NGOs of North America should intensify their fight against white supremacist, far-right groups and other terrorist or extremist groups that hurt not only Muslims, but all citizens. North American progress in the domains of fostering human rights and religious tolerance must not be obstructed by poorly informed agents or those with extremist ideologies.

References

Abadi, H. (2018). The Carter Center works to understand and counter the rise of islamophobia. In *Countering the islamophobia industry: Toward more effective strategies* (pp. 5–7). The Carter Center. Retrieved from https://www.cartercenter.org/resources/pdfs/peace/conflict_resolution/countering-isis/cr-countering-the-islamophobia-industry.pdf

Adams, C. (2017, February 8). Canadian Muslim community calls on government to combat Islamophobia. *Vice News*. https://www.vice.com/en/article/595v3a/canadian-muslim-community-calls-on-government-to-combat-islamophobia

Almontaser, D. (2018). Islamophobia: From challenge to opportunity. In *Countering the Islamophobia industry: Toward more effective strategies* (pp. 99–102). The Carter Center. Retrieved from https://www.cartercenter.org/resources/pdfs/peace/conflict_resolution/countering-isis/cr-countering-the-islamophobia-industry.pdf

Amnesty International Canada. (2017). *The case of Maher Arar*. Retrieved from https://www.amnesty.ca/legal-brief/case-maher-arar

Anderson, J., & Murdie, A. (2017, May 24). *What helps protect human rights: Human rights theory and evidence*. Oxford Research Encyclopedia of Politics. https://doi.org/10.1093/acrefore/9780190228637.013.513.

Balgord, E., & Smith, P. (2021, February 24). How many hate groups are there in Canada. *Canadian Anti-Hate Network*. Retrieved from https://www.antihate.ca/how_many_hate_groups_are_there_in_canada

Bazian, H. (2018). Countering Islamophobia is a civil society responsibility. In *Countering the islamophobia industry: Toward more effective strategies* (pp. 65–72). The Carter Center. Retrieved from https://www.cartercenter.org/resources/pdfs/peace/conflict_resolution/countering-isis/cr-countering-the-islamophobia-industry.pdf

BBC News. (2021, February 5). *Marjorie Taylor Greene: US House votes to strip Republican of key posts*. Retrieved from https://www.bbc.com/news/world-us-canada-55940542

Boutilier, A. (2019, March 6). Researchers to probe Canada's evolving far-right movements. *Toronto Star*. Retrieved from https://www.thestar.com/politics/federal/2019/03/06/researchers-to-probe-canadas-evolving-far-right-movements.html

Cader, F., & Kassamali, S. (2012, February 1). Islamophobia in Canada: A primer. *New Socialist: Ideas for Radical Change*. Retrieved from http://newsocialist.org/islamophobia-in-canada-a-primer/

Canadian Anti-Hate Network. (2019 July 29). *Hate groups find foothold on east coast*. Retrieved from https://www.antihate.ca/hate_groups_find_foothold_on_east_coast

Canadian Anti-Hate Network. (2020, February 26). *State of hate: Canada 2020*. Retrieved from https://www.antihate.ca/state_of_hate_canada_2020

Canadian Anti-Hate Network. (2021, February 3). *Atomwaffen division, the Base, Proud Boys, and Russian imperial movement added to the Canadian terrorism list*. Retrieved from https://www.antihate.ca/atomwaffen_division_the_base_white_power_groups_added_canada_terror_list?utm_campaign=newsletter_feb_9&utm_medium=email&utm_source=antihate

Canadian Anti-Hate Network. (n.d.). *About us: Exposing and stopping hate*. Retrieved from https://www.antihate.ca/about

Canadian Encyclopedia. (2016). *Maher Arar case*. Retrieved from https://www.thecanadianencyclopedia.ca/en/article/maher-arar-case

Canadian Human Rights Commission. (2017, November 20). *Private members' motion M-103, systemic racism and religious discrimination*. Retrieved from https://www.chrc-ccdp.gc.ca/eng/content/private-members-motion-m-103-systemic-racism-and-religious-discrimination

Carter, J. (2018). Forward. *Countering the islamophobia industry: Toward more effective strategies* (p. 4). The Carter Center. Retrieved from https://www.cartercenter.org/resources/pdfs/peace/conflict_resolution/countering-isis/cr-countering-the-islamophobia-industry.pdf

Carter Center. (2021). *Human rights program*. Retrieved from https://www.cartercenter.org/peace/human_rights/index.html

Casey, L. (2020, October 5). Human rights groups ask Ottawa for plan to deal with white supremacy in Canada. *CBC News*. Retrieved from https://www.cbc.ca/news/canada/toronto/ont-white-supremacy-call-out-1.5751057

Center for American Progress. (2011a). *Fear, Inc. The roots of the Islamophobia network in America*. Retrieved 26 August, from https://www.americanprogress.org/issues/religion/reports/2011/08/26/10165/fear-inc/

Center for American Progress. (2011b). *Understanding Sharia law*. Retrieved March 31, from https://www.americanprogress.org/issues/religion/reports/2011/03/31/9175/understanding-sharia-law/

Center for American Progress. (2015). *Fear, Inc. 2.0: The Islamophobia network's efforts to manufacture hate in America*. Retrieved February 11, from https://www.americanprogress.org/issues/religion/reports/2015/02/11/106394/fear-inc-2-0/

Center for Constitutional Rights. (n.d.). *The story of Maher Arar: Rendition to torture*. Retrieved from https://ccrjustice.org/files/rendition%20to%20torture%20report.pdf

Center for Human Rights and Global Justice. (2011). *Targeted and entrapped: Manufacturing the "homegrown threat" in the United States*. NYU School of Law. Retrieved from https://chrgj.org/wp-content/uploads/2016/09/targetedandentrapped.pdf

Congress Gov. (1993). H.R.1308 – Religious Freedom Restoration Act of 1993. Retrieved from https://www.congress.gov/bill/103rd-congress/house-bill/1308

Congress Gov. (2019). H.Res.183 – Condemning anti-Semitism as hateful expressions of intolerance that are contradictory to the values and aspirations that define the people of the United States and condemning anti-Muslim discrimination and bigotry against minorities as hateful expressions of intolerance that are contrary to the values and aspirations of the United States. Retrieved from https://www.congress.gov/bill/116th-congress/house-resolution/183/text

Council on American-Islamic Relations. (1997). *The state of Muslim civil rights in the United Sates: Unveiling prejudice.* Retrieved from https://www.cair.com/wp-content/uploads/2020/08/1997-The_Status_of_Muslim_Civil_Rights_in_the_United_States_1997.pdf

Council on American-Islamic Relations. (n.d.). *Know your rights.* Retrieved from https://www.cair.com/know_your_rights/

Council on American–Islamic Relations. (2017, October 11). *2017 on track to becoming one of the worst years ever for anti-Muslim hate crimes.* Retrieved from http://www.islamophobia.org/articles/209-2017-on-track-to-becoming-one-of-the-worst-years-ever-for-anti-muslim-hate-crimes.html

Council on American–Islamic Relations. (2018a). *Counter-Islamophobia project.* Retrieved from http://www.islamophobia.org

Council on American–Islamic Relations. (2018b). *U.S. Islamophobia Network: Islamophobic organizations.* Retrieved from http://www.islamophobia.org/islamophobic-organizations.html

Council on American–Islamic Relations. (2019, May 13). *Anti-prejudice tools.* Retrieved from http://www.islamophobia.org/blog/anti-prejudice-tools.html#edn2

Craddock, E. (2008). *Torturous consequences and the case of Maher Arar: Can Canadian solutions cure the due process deficiencies in U.S. removal proceedings.* Retrieved from https://core.ac.uk/download/pdf/216737259.pdf

Cury, E. (2016). Muslim American integration and interest group formation: A historical narrative. *Diaspora Studies, 10*(1), 81–96.

de Vogue, A. (2015, June 1). *SCOTUS rules in favor of Muslim woman in suit against Abercrombie and Fitch.* Retrieved from CNN (video). Retrieved from https://www.cnn.com/2015/06/01/politics/supreme-court-abercrombie-fitch-headscarf/index.html

el-Aswad, el-S. (2005). Review of Islam in urban America: Sunni Muslims in Chicago. *Digest of Middle East Studies, 14*(1), 78–81.

el-Aswad, el-S. (2012). *Muslim worldviews and everyday lives.* AltaMira. Press.

el-Aswad, el-S. (2013a). Images of Muslims in Western scholarship and media after 9/11. *Digest of Middle East Studies, 22*(1), 39–56.

el-Aswad, el-S. (2013b). Muslim Americans. In C. E. Cortés (Ed.), *Multicultural America: A multimedia encyclopaedia* (pp. 1525–1530). Sage.

el-Aswad, el-S. (2016). Political challenges confronting the Islamic world. In H. Tiliouine & R. J. Estes (Eds.), *The state of social progress of Islamic societies: Social, economic, political, and ideological challenges* (pp. 361–377). Springer.

el-Aswad, el-S. (2019). *The quality of life and policy issues among the Middle East and North African countries.* Springer.

Emgage. (2020, August). *Muslims in America policy poll.* Retrieved from https://emgageusa.org/wp-content/uploads/2020/08/Muslims-in-America-Policy-Poll-Final.pdf

Gallup. (2021, February 4). *U.S. satisfaction sinks with many aspects of public life.* Retrieved from https://news.gallup.com/poll/329279/satisfaction-sinks-aspects-public-life.aspx?utm_source=alert&utm_medium=email&utm_content=morelink&utm_campaign=syndication

Global News. (2019, June 26). *Canada adds neo-Nazi groups Blood & Honour, Combat 18 to list of terror organizations.* Retrieved from https://globalnews.ca/news/5432851/canada-adds-neo-nazi-groups-blood-honour-and-combat-18-to-list-of-terror-organizations/

Government of Canada. (n.d.). *Canadian Human Rights Act (R.S.C., 1985, c. H-6).* Retrieved from https://laws-lois.justice.gc.ca/eng/acts/h-6/page-1.html

Gunter, L. (2017, February 19). The harassment of Khalid is wrong, but doesn't justify M-103. *Toronto Sun*. Retrieved from https://www.torontosun.com/2017/02/19/the-harassment-of-khalid-is-wrong-but-doesnt-justify-m-103

Hannum, H. (2019). *Rescuing human rights: A radically moderate approach*. Cambridge University Press.

House of Commons. (2017, March 23). *Private members' business M-103 (systemic racism and religious discrimination)*. Retrieved from https://www.ourcommons.ca/Members/en/votes/42/1/237

Human Rights Watch. (2017). *Hate crimes against Muslims in US continue to rise in 2016*. Retrieved from https://www.hrw.org/news/2017/05/11/hate-crimes-against-muslims-us-continue-rise-2016#

Human Rights Watch. (2020a). *United States: Events of 2019*. Retrieved from https://www.hrw.org/world-report/2020/country-chapters/united-states#

Human Rights Watch. (2020b). *Canada: Event of 2019*. Retrieved from https://www.hrw.org/world-report/2020/country-chapters/canada#

Human Rights Watch. (2021a). *US: Trump's actions fuel Capitol riot*. Retrieved from https://www.hrw.org/news/2021/01/06/us-trumps-actions-fuel-capitol-riot

Human Rights Watch. (2021b). *Canada: Events of 2020*. Retrieved from https://www.hrw.org/world-report/2021/country-chapters/canada

Institute for Research on Public Policy. (2008). *Arar: The affair, the inquiry, the aftermath*. Retrieved from https://irpp.org/research-studies/arar-the-affair-the-inquiry-the-aftermath/

McEntire, K. J., Leiby, M., & Krain, M. (2015). Human rights organizations as agents of change: An experimental examination of framing and micromobilization. *American Political Science Review, 109*(3), 407–426.

Mitchell, E. A. (2017). Reducing a threat to a nuisance: A holistic strategy to counter Islamophobia. In *Countering the islamophobia industry: Toward more effective strategies* (pp. 46–54). The Carter Center. Retrieved from https://www.cartercenter.org/resources/pdfs/peace/conflict_resolution/countering-isis/cr-countering-the-islamophobia-industry.pdf).

Moore, A. (2012). American Muslim minorities: The new human rights struggle. *Human Rights & Human Welfare: An Online Journal of Academic Literature Review*, 91–99. Retrieved from https://www.du.edu/korbel/hrhw/news/digest.html and http://www.du.edu/korbel/hrhw/researchdigest/minority/Muslim.pdf.

Morgan, R. (2009). Human rights research and the social sciences. In R. Morgan & B. Turner (Eds.), *Interpreting human rights: Social science perspectives* (pp. 1–30). Routledge.

Murdie, A. (2009). The impact of human rights NGO activity on human right practices. *International NGO Journal, 4*(10), 421–440.

National Council of Canadian Muslims. (2013, July 6). CAIR.CAN evolves – Introducing the National Council of Canadian Muslims (NCCM). Retrieved from https://www.nccm.ca/introducing-the-national-council-of-canadian-muslims-nccm/

National Council of Canadian Muslims. (2016a, December 5). *Canadian Muslim organizations call for government action to counter growing islamophobia*. Retrieved from https://www.nccm.ca/canadian-muslims-call-for-government-action-to-counter-growing-islamophobia/

National Council of Canadian Muslims. (2016b, December 14). *Brief to the Standing Committee on Public Safety and National Security with respect to: Our security, our rights national security green paper, 2016*. Retrieved from https://mk0nccmorganizadbkcm.kinstacdn.com/wp-content/uploads/2016/12/NCCM_BRIEF_RE_Green_Paper_14Dec2016_FINAL.pdf

National Council of Canadian Muslims. (2017, November 6). *Government must take "concrete steps" to address human rights concerns inside CSIS*. Retrieved from https://www.nccm.ca/nccm-government-must-take-concrete-steps-to-address-human-rights-concerns-inside-csis/

National Council of Canadian Muslims. (2018, February 1). *NCCM welcomes heritage committee's recommendations on islamophobia and systemic discrimination*. Retrieve from https://www.nccm.ca/nccm-welcomes-heritage-committees-recommendations-on-islamophobia-and-systemic-discrimination/

National Council of Canadian Muslims. (2020, October). *NCCM policy paper: CBSA oversight.* Retrieved from https://mk0nccmorganizadbkcm.kinstacdn.com/wp-content/uploads/2020/10/CBSA-Policy-Paper-9.pdf

National Council of Canadian Muslims. (n.d.-a). *Public advocacy.* Retrieved from https://www.nccm.ca/programs/public-advocacy/

National Council of Canadian Muslims. (n.d.-b). *Defending rights: Charter of rights and freedoms.* Retrieved from https://www.nccm.ca/programs/defending-rights/

Naylor, B. (2015, June 1). Supreme Court rules for woman denied Abercrombie & Fitch job over headscarf. *NPR.* Retrieved from https://www.npr.org/sections/thetwo-way/2015/06/01/411213623/supreme-court-rules-for-woman-denied-abercrombie-fitch-job-over-headscarf#:~:text=The%20Supreme%20Court%20has%20ruled,for%20hire%20by%20an%20interviewer

Parry, T. (2017). Police offer extra protection to MP Iqra Khalid following threatening messages. *CBC News.* Retrieved from https://www.cbc.ca/news/politics/khalid-police-protection-messages-islamophobia-1.3989476

Perry, B. (2017, September 13). Canada has seen an increase in right-wing extremism over the past year: Policy-makers and practitioners seem ill-prepared to deal with it. *Policy Options.* Retrieved from https://policyoptions.irpp.org/magazines/september-2017/the-threat-of-right-wing-extremism/

Pew Research Center. (2020a, September 2). *In views of U.S. democracy, widening partisan divides over freedom to peacefully protest.* Retrieved from https://www.pewresearch.org/politics/2020/09/02/in-views-of-u-s-democracy-widening-partisan-divides-over-freedom-to-peacefully-protest/?utm_source=Pew+Research+Center&utm_campaign=0f3ef94846-Weekly_2020_09_05&utm_medium=email&utm_term=0_3e953b9b70-0f3ef94846-400057377

Pew Research Center. (2020b, September 21). *International cooperation welcomed across 14 advanced economies.* Retrieved from https://www.pewresearch.org/global/2020/09/21/international-cooperation-welcomed-across-14-advanced-economies/

Price, J. R. (2012). Introduction: Minority rights. *Human Rights & Human Welfare: An Online Journal of Academic Literature Review, 3–5.* Retrieved from https://www.du.edu/korbel/hrhw/news/digest.html and https://www.du.edu/korbel/hrhw/researchdigest/minority/Introduction.pdf

Ritter, E. H. (2014). Policy disputes, political survival, and the onset and severity of state repression. *Journal of Conflict Resolution, 58*(1), 143–168.

Snyder, J., & Ballentine, K. (1996). Nationalism and the marketplace of ideas. *International Security, 21*(2), 5–40. https://doi.org/10.2307/2539069

Southern Poverty Law Center. (2020). *White nationalist group posed as VICE reporters while identifying D.C. protesters.* Retrieved from https://www.splcenter.org/hatewatch/2020/06/04/white-nationalist-group-posed-vice-reporters-while-identifying-dc-protesters

Steinback, R. (2011). *Jihad against Islam.* Southern Poverty Law Center: Intelligence report, 142. Retrieved from http://www.splcenter.org/get-informed/intelligence-report/browse-all-issues/2011/summer/jihad-against-islam

Stevenson, V. (2016, January). *Organization puts callout for Canadians affected by no-fly lists.* National Council of Canadian Muslims. Retrieved from https://www.nccm.ca/nccm-callout-for-canadians-no-fly-list/

The Hill. (2021, February 4). *House votes to kick Greene off committees over embrace of conspiracy theories.* Retrieved from https://thehill.com/homenews/house/537445-house-votes-to-kick-greene-off-committees-over-embrace-of-conspiracy-theories?rnd=1612480554

Thoms, O. N. T., & Ron, J. (2007). Do human rights violations cause internal conflict? *Human Rights Quarterly, 29*(3), 674–705.

U.S. Commission on Civil Rights. (2014). *Federal civil rights engagement with Arab and Muslim American communities.* Washington, DC. Retrieved from https://www.usccr.gov/pubs/docs/ARAB_MUSLIM_9-30-14.pdf

U.S. Department of Justice. (2016). *Combating religious discrimination today: Final report.* Washington, DC. Retrieved from https://www.justice.gov/crt/file/877936/download

United Nations. (2015). *Universal declaration of human rights.* Retrieved from https://www.un.org/en/udhrbook/pdf/udhr_booklet_en_web.pdf

United Nations. (2021). *Human rights.* Retrieved from https://www.un.org/en/sections/issues-depth/human-rights/

United States Courts. (n.d.). *First amendment and religion.* Retrieved from https://www.uscourts.gov/educational-resources/educational-activities/first-amendment-and-religion

Varshney, A. (2001). Ethnic conflict and civil society: India and beyond. *World Politics, 53*(3), 362–398. Retrieved from https://cridaq.uqam.ca/IMG/pdf/varshney_civil_society_copy_1_Jacques_Bertrand.pdf

Waheed, M. (2018). Countering violent extremism: Harming civil rights and hurting communities based on a false promise of success. In *Countering the islamophobia industry: Toward more effective strategies* (pp. 40–45). The Carter Center. Retrieved from https://www.cartercenter.org/resources/pdfs/peace/conflict_resolution/countering-isis/cr-countering-the-islamophobia-industry.pdf

Chapter 11
Concluding Thoughts: Counter-Islamophobia Policies

11.1 Introduction

The existence of the phenomenology of Islamophobia in North America has become increasingly central in the determination of domestic and international policies. The objective of this final chapter is to show to what extent understanding the drivers of ideologies and activities of Islamophobia help governments and policy makers generate sociocultural plans aimed at implementing a set of policies and interventions designed to effectively counter Islamophobia and enhance the well-being of both Muslim and non-Muslim communities. Policy makers should not ignore the menace and danger staged by Islamophobes' ideologies and actions.

By providing the necessary information of the drivers and motivations of Islamophobes, North American governments, civil societies and policymakers can design effective plans and policies to counter the discriminatory ideology of Islamophobic agents. In other words, to counter Islamophobes' ideologies and actions, they must first be identified, subsequently examined, and ultimately addressed. Moreover, policy strategies and plans to combat Islamophobia must be multidimensional, informed, far-reaching, and well organized to be effective. Additionally, the chapter provides ideas and recommendations for long-term policies aimed at reducing or eliminating the rising tide of Islamophobic racism. The goal, of course, is not only to help protect and enhance the well-being of Muslims in North America but also to ensure social justice and the propagation of human rights.

This monograph has provided evidence showing that North American Muslims have experienced negative sentiment caused by a number of interrelated quality-of-life factors triggered by Islamophobia. These factors have included economic drivers, as evidenced by disparities in economic resources between Muslims and Western or non-Muslim communities; political factors, as reflected in the exclusion of Muslims from mainstream civil and political affairs; religious drivers, as manifested by increased Western vilification of Islamic beliefs and values; cultural causes, as mirrored in the perceived indifference of North American culture and

Western prejudice against Muslims; and media factors, as represented by the prov-ocation of North American media against Muslims. This is alarming in that the rapidly growing Muslim communities in North America, composed mostly of young people, becomes negatively impacted across several dimensions.

Islamophobia has been viewed in this research as both a driver and consequence of anti-Muslim sentiment. The industry of Islamophobia embraces socio-political and media propaganda as well as activities driven by group dynamics, motivations and actions carried out by individuals and organizations, directed by economic, political, cultural, religious, ideological, and media drivers.

Notions of market supply and demand, as used in the examination of terrorist organizations (Krueger, 2003, 2007; Iannaccone, 2006; el-Aswad, el-S. 2019; Sirgy et. al., 2019), have been similarly applied here. Like terrorist organizations, many organizations espousing Islamophobia are run in ways similar to that of a firm. The supply side includes economic charges and expenses. For example, individuals or groups of people offer their services to Islamophobia organizations thus promoting their ideology. The demand side of the Islamophobia market includes multiple components such as economic, political, religious, cultural, ideological, and media drivers, among other factors that have been elaborated on in previous chapters. The policy here is to identify ideological and political agendas so as to respond effec-tively and demand full responsibility from those who act motivated by these agendas.

The main motivations for running and sustaining the Islamophobia industry are profound commitments to religious, cultural, social or political causes. This study proposes that the long-term remedy to the problem of religious fanaticism and far-right extremism in North America depends on altering market conditions, with particular emphasis on altering the *demand* side which Islamophobes and their organizations seek to perpetuate. Although the dismantling of economic resources, finance, funding, and other material capacities of the Islamophobia groups might be relevant, the most important and effective strategy to counter Islamophobia is by focusing on the demand and designing effective interventions to treat the drivers and causes that generate and breed anti-Muslim racism. This is to say, policies "should target causes rather than consequences" (Sirgy et. al., 2019, p. 152).

11.2   Drivers of Islamophobia and Projected Policies for Counter-Islamophobia

Public policy, aiming to affect a vast portion of the public, determines the process through which a government acts to improve people's quality of life and deal with the needs of its citizens via plans and actions as defined by its laws and constitution (Birkland, 2016; O'Donnell et al., 2014). Concurrently, social policy refers to the plans or programs designed by the political system and the private sector to solve public problems confronting the society as well as to achieve the objectives pursued by the greater population (el-Aswad, el-S., 2016b, 2019). The development of interventions to enhance quality of life and well-being presupposes that policy makers understand the causes or drivers of Islamophobia.

Anti-Islamophobia is an essential thesis for scholars, policymakers, political leaders, advocacy organizations, and interfaith movements (el-Aswad, el-S., 2007). By providing policy makers with the necessary information of the drivers and motivations of Islamophobes, governments and civil societies can design long-term objectives for effective plans and policies to counter Islamophobia. As afore-mentioned, Islamophobia is a socio-political activity driven and carried out by individuals and small groups, motivated by specific factors and drivers. These factors, mentioned earlier, include economic, political, religious, cultural, ideolog-ical, and media drivers. These drivers will be discussed in the following sections within the framework of projected policies designed to combat Islamophobia.

11.2.1   Economic Driver, Disparity and Counter-Islamophobia Policies

Despite the economic prosperity of North America, Islamophobia has negatively impacted Muslims' economic activities (Lean, 2017; Love, 2017; Statistics Canada, 2019). This book has highlighted the fact that for North American Muslims, the consequences of Islamophobia have been serious and have led to such occurrences as income disparities, poverty, and unemployment. Communities experiencing patent income disparities tend to score lower on quality-of-life measures than communities with less income disparities (el-Aswad, el-S., 2019). The economic drivers of Islamophobia indicate economic factors or, put differently, institutional-ized Islamophobia is both a driver and an outcome of the economics reflected in wide-ranging inequalities between Muslims and non-Muslim communities living in North America.

Islamophobia has created not only economic disparity, but also socio-economic anxiety. This economic disparity in the U.S. has grown since 2020, a year discerned by unprecedented challenges associated with the Corona virus (COVID-19) pan-demic and the economic crisis that it has created (Boushey & Park, 2021). A new poll conducted by Gallup between January 4 and 15, 2021 revealed that the overall quality of life of Americans declined 17 percentage points from 84% in January 2020 to 67% in January 2021 (Table 11.2). Additionally, the indicator of "opportu-nity for a person in this nation [U.S.] to get ahead by working hard," declined 14 percentage points from 72% in January 2020 to 58% in January 2021 (Gallup, 2021). Even the indicator of "size and influence of major corporations" declined 16 percentage points from 41% in 2020 to 26% in 2021 (Gallup, 2021). It is to be noted that 29% of Muslims were underemployed compared with 12% of other American adults (Pew Research Center, 2017). This lower income is also reflected in Canada where Muslims earned $53,800 on average in 2016, compared with an average employment income of no less than $63,000 for people in all other religious affiliation categories (Statistics Canada, 2019).

If Islamophobia is viewed within a market framework enticing potential employees to pursue careers in attacking Muslims (leading to negative consequences), it would be perspicacious of the governments or public and private sectors of both Canada and the U.S. to provide well designed policy to address this issue. Policy could include supporting unemployed Muslim minorities, particularly among young adults who represent about 28% of American Muslims (el-Aswad, el-S., 2013b). Globally, Muslims, with a median age of 23, are younger than the overall global population, with a median age of 28 (Pew Research Center, 2012). Also, policy makers should recommend creating other more appealing and productive options of employment for those who are willing to stop serving Islamophobes.

Islamophobia and hate activities necessitate plans, policies and actions from policymakers and advocates to counter all forms of prejudice, injustice and discrimination directed at Muslims. Governments should promote economic well-being and quality of life by facilitating small businesses for young people, supporting investment, offering compensation for those who lost their jobs, reducing corruption among government employees, and developing new strategies for improving economic activities (Table 11.3). Such economic policies may reduce the economic injustice toward underprivileged Muslims and weaken business-leader Islamophobes who might lose their employees or assistants when they are offered decent and non-violent oriented occupations.

11.2.2 Political Driver, Exclusion and Counter-Islamophobia Strategies

The relationship between Islamophobia and political factors is mirrored in the exclusion of Muslims from mainstream civil and political affairs in North America. Islamophobia is imbricated in wider racial politics and becomes "an emblematic expression of contemporary biopolitical racism" (Tyrer, 2013, p. 21). Islamophobia and racism harm North American minorities as it excludes Muslims and other marginalized groups from mainstream political affairs. Islamophobia is designed and intended to prevent Muslims from making positive contributions to their communities or the countries in which they live (Hayoun, 2013).

Although the Islamophobia industry is driven by a small network of individuals and institutions, the extent of their reach and consequences of their programs engenders the anti-Muslim hate within easily led groups of people who, once adopting their Islamophobic propaganda, join their ranks. However, the dominant group, including far-right politicians and business tycoons, benefit more by subjugating minorities (Levin, 1975). Islamophobes have managed to attach Islamophobia to the designation of right-wing populism that has become synonymous with other systematic organizations of hatred (Lean, 2017). Islamophobia in North America involves white supremacists, who, like far-right groups, depict Islam as a backward, inferior and false religion. White supremacy has been woven not only into the policies of the U.S. government, but also into its economy and education (Jonson-Reid, 2015; West, 2020).

Islamophobes, boosting racist aggression against Muslims, seek to influence political outcomes by embracing strong political views and imposing an extremist ideology through violent means. The Islamophobes' policies are based on maintaining their monopoly of power. Political leaders, most notably the former U.S. president Donald Trump, have been involved in the anti-Muslim and anti-Arab Islamophobia industry by, for example, declaring and supporting a discriminatory travel ban, preventing individuals from Muslim majority countries from entering the U.S. Notably, this travel ban was revoked by President Biden (The White House, 2021), and is considered a significant step in countering Islamophobia.

The profiling by government officials often increases public suspicion of American Muslims, giving permission to private actors to think that they can handle security issues in their own way. After 9/11, fear of government surveillance created an anxiety over freedom of expression and freedom of association on college campuses and congregations for American Muslims (U.S. Commission on Civil Rights, 2014). According to Gallup (2021), the political indicator measuring Americans' satisfaction "with how the government system is working," declined 16 percentage points from 43% in January, 2020 to 27% in January, 2021 (Table 11.2). Also, in Canada, discriminatory policies and practices by government agencies have fortified anti-Muslim sentiment and official use of profiling has sent a message to the larger community that a person who fits a certain physical or religious description might be suspect (Perry & Poynting, 2006).

Islamophobia is a political and ideological form of racism leading to violence against Muslims (Sheehi, 2011) and counter-Islamophobia is its political response. Internationally, the international human rights law determines the obligations of Governments to promote and protect human and political rights as well as fundamental freedoms and civil rights of individuals or groups (United Nation, 2021). Governments should be held accountable for human rights violations against Muslims globally. Islamophobia challenges Muslims not only in North America, but also worldwide (el-Aswad, el-S., 2016a).

This monograph has shown that North American Muslims are becoming politically active in various domains, notwithstanding their being socially marginalized and viewed as radicalized. Scholars and policymakers should work together to fight and change Islamophobic and stereotypical images of Muslim Americans being depicted, perhaps intentionally so, as politically passive people. The politically oriented Islamophobia industry must be exposed and recognized in all domains of civil society. Therefore, more efforts are needed to support public and political policies that provide initiatives to combat Islamophobic propaganda targeting Muslims (Table 11.3). Policy makers must offer comprehensive options to neutralize the Islamophobes' appeal for the most politically susceptible targets. In addition, federal agencies should collaborate with local government agencies and advocacy groups that engage and serve diverse Muslim communities throughout North America.

11.2.3   Religious Drivers and Counter-Islamophobia Policies

North America represents a flourishing religious marketplace for the Islamophobia industry in which religious drivers are represented in extreme religiosity and ignorance of Islam (el-Aswad, el-S., 2013a, c). Islamophobia is viewed here as an ideology used by politicians and right-wing extremist groups for achieving political gains by promoting hatred against Islam and Muslims. It might be helpful to draw a distinction between the concept of religious worldview and that of ideology to better understand the religious driver underlying the Islamophobia industry. Worldview "is based on assumptions concerning the structure of the universe. It includes the society as well as the human and nonhuman beings and forces, both perceptible and imperceptible, that constitute the integrated parts of the universe or cosmos" (el-Aswad, el-S., 2012, p. 1). Worldview, then, indicates a belief system comparable to a meaning system, patterns of thought, and perceptual framework and related symbolic actions. On the contrary, ideology, a subcategory of worldview accentuating asymmetrical relations of power, implies certain political orientations related particularly to power, authority and domination (el-Aswad, el-S., 2002, 2012).

This distinction is important as it highlights the ideological assumptions of Islamophobia adopted by a politically oriented small group of militant Christians in North America. The distinction is also useful in making a comparison between Islamophobia organizations and jihadist terrorist organizations in which convergence of extreme religious and ideological perspectives between them can be traced. Both of them are minorities that do not represent Christianity and Islam. They divide the world into opposing components of good and evil, eliminating the possibility of neutrality. As Islamist jihadis view jihad as the sole way for establishing an Islamic State (el-Aswad, el-S. et al., 2020), militant Christians, driven by power and domination, believe what some authors call the "Christian jihad" as the right way for establishing a "Christian nation" in which church is married to state, contrary to modern secular values (Diab, 2007). However, in its worldview, Christianity "warns against dominating or exploiting others" (Valk, 2012, p. 164). The human, notwithstanding conditions of race, religion, ethnicity and/or color, is not to be surrendered or sacrificed for purposes of personal or national gain (Valk, 2012). In political and public spheres in the U.S., evidence indicates that white evangelical and Republican identities are fused together (Lewis, 2019). Table 11.1 elucidates this comparison.

Both militant Christians sustaining Islamophobia organizations and jihadist terrorist organizations are driven by a "religiosity" that includes doctrinal, experiential, ritualistic, ideological, intellectual, creedal, communal, moral, as well as the cultural components of personal involvement in religion (el-Aswad, el-S., 2019). In short, religious extremism is an example of some of the fundamental features of religiosity.

Several researchers of religious studies have concluded that white Christians, particularly white evangelical Protestants, embrace and spread negative attitudes about racial, ethnic and religious minorities, including Muslims, in addition to instigating class-based anxieties, and Islamophobia (Gorski, 2017; Jones, 2020). These researchers maintained that white supremacist ideology is deeply entrenched

Table 11.1 Comparison between Islamophobic extremist and Jihadist terrorist organization

	Islamophobia organizations	Jihadist terrorist organizations
1	Driven by radical ideology, not overarching Christian worldviews	Driven by radical ideology, not overarching Islamic worldviews
2	Christian fanaticism (Christian far-right)	Muslim fanaticism (*Salafi*)
3	Using communications technologies and videos to spread their ideologies, locally and globally	Using communications technologies and videos to spread their ideologies, locally and globally
4	Run by small militant groups that do not represent Christianity	Run by small militant groups that do not represent Islam
5	Followers of radical Evangelism	Followers of radical Wahhabism
6	Christian *jihadists* believe that they are exclusively chosen by, and fight for, God	Islamist *jihadists* believe that they are exclusively chosen by, and fight for, Allah
7	Fight against atheists	Fight against atheists *kuffār* (Sing., *kāfir*)
8	Attack Muslims or perceive Muslims as being a threat	Attack Westerners and/or perceive them as a destructive (imperial/colonial) power
9	Attack their citizens (e.g., North American Muslims) for not following their ideology	Attack their citizens (Muslims) for not following their ideology
10	Attack Muslims; perceive them in terms of corruption/oppression	Attack Westerners; perceive them in terms of decadence
11	Believe in the apocalyptic fight against the Antichrist (Christian convention)	Believe in the apocalyptic fight against the Antichrist (Islamic convention)
12	Disseminate and carry out violence	Disseminate and carry out violence
13	Violation of human rights	Violation of human rights

Source: Compiled by the author

within white Christian theology (Jones, 2020). The Rev. David McAllister-Wilson, President of Wesley Seminary, "challenged Evangelicals to take the lead in Christian engagement with Islam. He suggested that they are the most able to understand the experience of being Muslim in America simply because a number of other Christians speak as disparagingly about them as they do about Muslims" (Johnston, 2016, p. 170). In brief, evangelical Christians, or at least some of them, are the most antagonistic towards Muslims depicting Islam and the Islamist movement as enemies who incite war against Judeo-Christianity (Braunstein, 2017; Todd, 2011).

Such negative attitudes have impacted North American Muslims. For instance, in the U.S., 61% of Muslims, more than any other faith group, reported experiencing religious discrimination (Institute for Social Policy and Understanding, 2017). In Canada, when Muslims were compared with other immigrants in the country, they fell behind in many different areas, including, for example, economy and health issues (Kazemipur, 2014). The dilemma here is that Muslims feel they are situated between extreme religiosity of militant white supremacists and the extreme secularism of a capitalist society. This problem might be explained by the declining impact of moderate organized religion on American society. For example, Table 11.2 shows that the indicator of "the influence of organized religion" in the U.S. declined 11 percentage points from 59% in January 2020 to 48% in January 2021 (Gallup, 2021).

Table 11.2 Recent indicators of Americans' quality of life and satisfaction

Indicators of quality of life and satisfaction	2020%	2021%	Change pct. pts.
The overall quality of life	84	67	−17
The opportunity for a person in this nation to get ahead by working hard	72	58	−14
The influence of organized religion	59	48	−11
The size and power of the federal government	38	31	−7
Our system of government and how well it works	43	27	−16
The size and influence of major corporations	41	26	−15
The moral and ethical climate	32	18	−14

Source: Adopted with modification from Gallup (2021). *U.S. satisfaction sinks with many aspects of public life*

Regarding the driver of the zealous religiosity among both radical or conservative Christians and Muslims, policy makers and religious leaders should advocate religious moderation and reflection, and expose the dangers of radicalism and extremism. The foremost problems of discrimination and extremism in religion can be surmounted through education (Crane, 2010; Jonson-Reid, 2015). Therefore, it is necessary to improve the quality of education at all levels by eliminating discrimination in schools, updating curricula about Muslim culture, increasing funding for minority students, recruiting and training highly qualified instructors, establishing robust educational resources and facilities, and improving administrative systems that value equal treatment of diverse educators, administrators and students. In addition, policy makers should develop policies and strategies aimed at modifying the framework of Christian extremists' religiosity (Table 11.3).

Countering Islamophobia requires plans and actions from all North Americans, Muslims and non-Muslims, who can engage in religious dialogue. It is worthy to point out that Paul Findley, a Christian politician said, "All my life I had heard about the Judeo-Christian ethic, but no one spoke about the Judeo-Christian-Islamic ethic" (Findley, 2001, p. 4). Muslim and non-Muslim leaders should work together to increase dialogue, understanding, and peace. However, policy makers and religious leaders should not stigmatize or marginalize religious extremists (Muslim or Christian), rather they should dialogue with them and assure them that their fears are exaggerated and inappropriate (Diab, 2007) and encourage them to see similarities rather than imagined extreme and irresolvable differences.

Government and NGOs should organize campaigns and conferences on the topic of religious tolerance aiming to promote contact between different faith groups. There is an urgent demand to replace the destructive discourse of the "clash of civilizations" (Huntington, 1993) in favor of a new constructive discourse of "dialogue between civilizations." This objective can be achieved through effective interaction, collaboration, and exchange of ideas. These policies might lead to better understanding, cooperation, and respect between Muslims and non-Muslims.

Table 11.3 Drivers of islamophobia, outcomes and counter-islamophobia policies

Drivers	Outcomes	Counter Islamophobia (Policies and Recommendations)
Economic factors	Income inequality-disadvantage of Muslim minority	Reduce inequalities in economic well-being within and across North American countries
	Unemployment-immigration/travel ban targeting Muslims	Create entrepreneurship programs and support legal immigration
		Provide employment opportunities
Political drivers	Violation of Muslims' human rights	Reform government institutions recognition of Muslims' civil rights
	Exclusionary and prejudiced political systems	Nation-building policies supporting democratic systems and civil liberties
Religious drivers	Increased religious extremism among conservative Christians Protestants (evangelical)	Advocate religious moderation and expose the danger of extremism religiosity
	Lack of tolerance toward Muslim minorities	Promote religious tolerance among conservative and radical Christians and other faith groups
Cultural drivers	Stigma and stereotypes of Muslims due to lack of knowledge of Muslims' diverse cultures	Cultural dialogue and mutual respect Muslims work to spread correct knowledge about Islam Increase cultural competency
	Discrimination against Muslims by Western/North American (far-right groups)	Protection of the dignity of Muslims Civil and advocacy organizations fighting discrimination
	Discrimination against Muslim students in school systems	Reform of educational systems
Media drivers	North America's media bias against Muslims	Establish online anti-media bias campaigns Launch online media-educational programs refuting Islamophobia

Source: Compiled by the author

11.2.4   Cultural Drivers and Counter-Islamophobia Strategies

This subsection tackles the underlying ideology shared by Islamophobes, as revealed in their cultural activities and propaganda so as to provide effective counter-policies for North American governments and civil society.

There is a complex and intricate relationship between culture and religion in such a way that religious commitment shapes cultural membership in North American life (Stewart et al., 2017). Cultures driven by extreme religious outlook, prejudice, and biased ideology spawn an unhealthy social environment (Allport, 1979). Culturally, white supremacy is one of the cultural drivers (Fiedler, 2016) behind the spread of Islamophobia. White supremacy and white privilege exist at the micro level of the person and the macro level of society and culture. At the national level, the "Unites

States is where racism, white supremacy and white privilege run rampant" (Sullivan, 2019, p. 4). While not all white supremacists identify as Christian, the extreme behavior of some religiously unaffiliated white supremacists may be seen as a reactionary and secularized version of white Christian nationalism (Gorski, 2017; Jones, 2020). Although Canada is consistent in maintaining multiculturalism and a liberal-democratic society, anti-Muslim sentiment is growing and spreading due to the view of Islam by a non-Muslim population as incompatible with democracy.

Additionally, this monograph has shown that there are cultural factors that are critical to the generation of Islamophobia and cultural divergence in North America, namely ignorance of Islam and discrimination against Muslims. Incidents of culture-based discrimination include, for instance, police brutality based on racial group, social or class divisions, and anti-Islamic bullying (Baldwin, 2017). Among cultural factors that trigger discriminatory attitudes against Muslims in North America are authoritarianism, patriotism, fear, and misinformation about Islam. From an author-itarian point of view, the cultural attitudes and behaviors of Muslims do not show a full conformity with the ideological orientations of North American authoritarian elites, who, in turn, develop discriminatory views and actions against Muslims. By the same token, white-nationalist patriotic people in North America are likely to embrace and implement actions of discrimination against Muslims, viewing them as non-nationalistic citizens (Kalkan et al., 2009).

Because of the fear of Islam, Muslims are depicted in North America as cultural enemies (el-Aswad, el-S., 2006). In the U.S., for example, 58% of Americans say there is more discrimination against Muslims than against any other religious group (Pew Research Center, 2009). This cultural predicament displayed by ignorance of Islam and discrimination against Muslims, results in fear and negative consequences for both the Muslim minority and mainstream society. It is alarming to observe, according to Gallup (2021), that the indicator of the "moral and ethical climate" in the U.S. declined 14 percentage points from 32% in January 2020 to 18% in January 2021 (Table 11.2).

There is a need for policymakers and regular citizens to adopt a quality of life and cultural competence approach that includes not only awareness, knowledge, and skills at the interpersonal level about diverse cultures, but also policies and structures at the institutional and systemic level, which enable people and organizations to work effectively in cross-cultural situations. Culturally competent agencies recognize the relationship between policy and practice, and implement policies that improve inclusion services to diverse minority groups (Cross et al., 1989).

Policymakers should spare no time resisting Islamophobia and improving Muslim and non-Muslim relations in North America based on reliable and practical policies. Muslims of North America should offer clarification about their heritage and to teach non-Muslims about their religion, Islam, in an attempt to discourage intolerance and injustices towards them. In response to these efforts, North American mainstream citizens should objectively educate themselves about Islam and Islamic culture. They also should make trustworthy efforts to become more familiar with Muslim minority and community outreach groups in their communities to be able to develop more favorable, tolerant, and inclusive views about Islam and Muslims (Table 11.3).

In both Canada and the U.S. anti-Islamophobia advocacy organizations have urged authorities to shut down white supremacist organizations for violating human rights and spreading Islamophobia (Cader and Kassamali, 2012). Policymakers and political leaders should include in their policies some reliable measurements indicating to what extent governments of both Canada and the U.S. have responded to the requests of anti-Islamophobia advocacy organizations.

11.2.5   Media Drivers and Counter-Islamophobia Policies

Several North American media outlets have falsely framed Muslims as felons, fanatics, terrorists, criminals, and killers. The core objective of biased media is to work to keep the fear of terrorism and Islamophobia alive. Many aspects of global media, driven by far-right groups and neoconservatives, have focused on what is known as fear of the other and the war on terror, rendering all Muslims a suspect community. Conservative and far-right media outlets, including, for example, Fox News and Breitbart News, have adopted an anti-Islam ideology and conspiracy theory (Benkler et al., 2017) that have had a negative impact on North American society.

In terms of the marketplace, media coverage of Islamophobia is exceptionally profitable. Because stereotypes appeal to and are easily processed by wide-ranging consumers, media misrepresentations of racial and ethnic groups enable good revenue and profits (Dixon et al., 2019). Stereotypes influence consumer emotions, and these emotions then mediate the relationship between stereotype activation and subsequent consumer cognitions (Babin et al., 1995). Islamophobia, then, can be viewed as a marketable product that American consumers are willing to "buy" or buy into.

Media (mis)representations of Muslims impact North American's images of and attitudes towards Muslims (el-Aswad, el-S., 2011). In other words, media play a critical role in the creation and maintenance of Islamophobic stigma and negative images impacting the way majority group members in North America perceive and treat Muslims.

Media portrayals of Muslims in North America affect their well-being as well as their perception about being accepted or rejected in the mainstream cultures. These media images generate stereotypes which distance Muslims from the rest of North America, inciting emotion and fear among Americans and Canadians and causing cultural and political polarization in which Muslims are depicted as aliens and threatening 'others' (Tutt, 2013). This pattern of media bias has been documented by researchers: about 17% of American Muslims cited negative portrayals of Muslims in the media, including movies and television shows and 15% mentioned stereotyping of Muslims driven by Donald Trump's megaphonic rhetoric and disdainful policies toward Muslims (Pew Research Center, 2017).

This monograph has highlighted two approaches for combating biased media and Islamophobia. One approach proposed that policies providing guidelines and restrictions on biased media offer solutions, while the other recommended an open marketplace of ideas, allowing full freedom of expression (Walker, 2018). Concerning the important role played by media in society, any reliable reform must involve advancing a competitive market place of ideas with cost-effective measures to combat Islamophobia and media bias (Stucke, 2008). Scholars have reported that increased competition in the news market results in lower rates of bias. This indicates that competition between media outlets is among alternative solutions for reducing media bias (Stucke & Grunes, 2009). It is worthy to note that the marketplace of ideas is also important to democracy, in the sense that democracy flourishes when there is a free flow of information (Stucke, 2008; Stucke & Grunes, 2009).

Policymakers should initiate policies and interventions that encourage other unbiased media to compete with biased media. Although there are competitive civil media organizations countering biased media, these organizations need to focus more on updating media technologies to be able to fortify their virtual communications as well as to spread their messages to large audiences. They should also increase their funds and financial resources to be able to manage high quality and wider media outlets.

Countering biased media should focus on the extreme, conservative and radical ideology behind particular corrupt media outlets. Government agencies should promote policies that prohibit false information and Islamophobic propaganda, while warranting freedom of expression for media users, in accordance with international laws. Policymakers should plan to increase workshops and training sessions for relevant stakeholders, including government agencies, to better recognize and understand the underlying media biases that manufacture negative stereotypical images and beliefs about Muslim minorities. Additionally, policymakers should urge internet companies and social media platforms to establish guidelines and restrictions against any form of false or hateful activities, including Islamophobia (Table 11.3). Policy changes by social media companies can have an impact on extremist activity by denying extremist groups' presence on media platforms (Davey et al., 2020). For example, Facebook and Twitter have banned Trump and other Islamophobes (Isaac & Conger, 2021; Lerman, 2021) from using their platforms.

11.3   Conclusion

Guided by the quality-of-life approach, this research has focused on economic, political, religious, cultural and media drivers of the Islamophobia industry in order to provide long-term policies and recommendations aimed at eradicating Islamophobia and anti-Muslim racism in North America and worldwide.

As stated earlier in this book, Muslim communities in North America face extreme and arduous challenges embodied in social, economic, political, religious and cultural discrimination as well as in Islamophobic propaganda and media bias. Islamophobia has created a climate of fear that has impacted Muslims' well-being as well as their human, civil and political rights. Despite North American governments' commitment to human rights, religious freedom and freedom of expression, religious minorities, including Muslims, have been stigmatized, marginalized, excluded, and deprived of justice.

Social policy is a planned process where the well-being of individuals, communities, and organizations is achieved through the adoption of ideas and strategies that improve the quality of life of people. Although the anti-Muslim forces will surely lose (Fiedler, 2016), attitudes toward Muslims will not be easy to alter or change in a short period of time. But change is a necessity and might be possible when effective policies and interventions are designed and successfully implemented.

This monograph urges North American governments, institutions, and agencies to uphold laws and respect the civil rights of all minority groups, including Muslims. More public policies countering Islamophobia or any sort of discrimination, whether it is, economic, political, religious, cultural, racial, or gender should be researched, designed, and implemented.

This research has shown that it is essential to advance the quality of education of Muslim students at all levels in North America by eliminating discrimination and Islamophobia in schools. Effective education policies are viewed as an important means of enhancing the overall well-being of all people, Muslims and non-Muslims. When considering educational policies, it is worthy to mention that the fourth objective of the United Nations' Sustainable Development Goals is to "ensure inclusive and equitable quality education and promote life-long learning opportunities for all" (United Nations, 2018).

In addition to the author's recommendations, this research has addressed counter-Islamophobia policies and interventions provided by international, regional and national.

Institutions, such as the United Nations, the Human Rights Watch, the governments of Canada and the U.S., NGOs and advocacy (Muslim and non-Muslim) organizations. For example, the International Covenant on Civil and Political Rights (United Nations, 1966) proclaimed that any propaganda for war and any advocacy of national, racial or religious hatred that constitutes incitement to discrimination, hostility or violence shall be prohibited by law. Locally and regionally, in addition to public policies provided by North American governments, advocacy organizations and their leaders in the U.S and Canada are active agents confronting Islamophobia and supporting human rights. The following are the key recommendations for the governments, NGOs, and individuals of North America to address in countering Islamophobia (and summed up in Table 11.3):

- Support the United Nations' efforts to promote human rights and eliminate racial discrimination.
- Oppose discrimination and strive to attain equal political and civil rights for all citizens, including Muslims, within the standards acknowledged by the United Nations' Universal Declaration of Human Rights.

- Intensify recognition and resistance against far-right groups, white supremacist and other extremist groups that hurt not only Muslims, but all citizens (as was the case when extremists stormed the U.S. Capitol on January 6, 2021).
- Focus on the demand side of the Islamophobia industry/market, implicit or explicit in religious-political-ideological drivers that have encouraged Islamophobes to retail and distribute their Islamophobic products in North America.
- Combat religion-based hate violence and promote religious reflection, freedom and tolerance.
- Support Muslims' demand for equality and justice.
- Reduce inequalities in economic well-being within and across North American countries.
- Address far-right, conservative and radical religious-political ideologies behind media bias and corrupt media outlets that spread Islamophobic images and false information about Islam and Muslims.
- Develop savvy and far reaching networks of competitive media, web sites, online services and virtual platforms to confront the ideologies and actions of Islamophobes and their agents.
- Improve the quality of education at all levels by eliminating discrimination in schools, and updating curricula about Muslim culture.
- Promote more public policies countering Islamophobia, conspiracy theory and any sort of discrimination, whether it is, economic, political, religious, cultural, racial, or gender.
- Redefine patriotism to reflect inclusion rather than exclusion of minority groups.

Finally, this monograph has suggested that countering Islamophobia necessitates plans and action from religious, political, economic, educational and social institutions as well as communities and individuals to face, identify and reduce damaging impact of Islamophobia in North America. North American governments should use well-being research outcomes to facilitate and develop public policies that sustain comprehensive efforts within religious, cultural, economic, political, educational and media spheres, to reduce Islamophobia and improve the overall quality of life of American citizens.

Muslims' well-being in North America is intrinsically linked to global well-being. The United Nations' aforementioned strategies are directed toward denouncing any sort of prejudice or discrimination, promoting people's overall well-being, sustaining a culture of peace, and encouraging mutual respect for cultures, religions, and social values and beliefs. Such strategies might increase cultural understanding and rational dialogues between Muslims and non-Muslims, leading to the establishment of effective and peaceful policies (el-Aswad, el-S., 2012). While negative attitudes about Muslims as a cultural 'other' or outgroup may persist over time, discrimination against religious groups tends to diminish as citizens in the societal mainstream intercontact with members of these groups and become more familiar with them. This is to say that people who know Muslims do not view Islam as encouraging violence. And those who are most familiar with Islam and Muslims express favorable views of Muslims and to see similarities between Islam and their own religion.

It is also interesting to observe that while Muslims say they face a number of challenging problems and express a variety of concerns about life in North America, the picture they paint of their experiences implies promising messages. For instance, 55% of Muslim Americans say the American people, altogether, are friendly toward Muslims, and an additional 30% say the American people are neutral toward Muslims, though about 14% say Americans are unfriendly toward Muslim Americans (Pew Research Center, 2017). Cultural dialogue and engagement within and across local, regional and global communities can lead not only to the reduction or elimination of the adverse influence of Islamophobes, but also to the adoption of values, such as tolerance and peace, as well as the development of proactive security solutions, locally, regionally and globally.

References

Allport, G. W. (1979). *The nature of prejudice*. Addison-Wesley.

Babin, B. J., Boles, J. S., & Darden, W. R. (1995). Salesperson stereotypes, consumer emotions, and their impact on information processing. *Journal of the Academy of Marketing Science, 23*, 94–105. https://doi.org/10.1177/0092070395232002

Baldwin, J. (2017, January 25). Culture, prejudice, racism, and discrimination. In *Oxford research encyclopedia of communication* (pp. 1–26). Oxford University Press. https://doi.org/10.1093/acrefore/9780190228613.013.164

Benkler, Y., Faris, R., Roberts, H., & Zuckerman, E. (2017, March 13). Study: Breitbart-led right-wing media ecosystem altered broader media agenda. *Columbia Journalism Review*. Retrieved from https://www.cjr.org/analysis/breitbart-media-trump-harvard-study.php

Birkland, T. A. (2016). *An introduction to the policy process: Theories, concepts, and models of public policy making*. Routledge.

Boushey, H., & Park, S. (2021, April 16). *The coronavirus recession and economic inequality: A roadmap to recovery and long-term structural change*. Washington Center for Equitable Growth. Retrieved from https://equitablegrowth.org/the-coronavirus-recession-and-economic-inequality-a-roadmap-to-recovery-and-long-term-structural-change/

Braunstein, R. (2017). Muslims as outsiders, enemies, and others: The 2016 presidential election and the politics of religious exclusion. *American Journal of Cultural Sociology, 5*(3), 355–372. https://doi.org/10.1057/S41290-017-0042-X

Cader, F., & Kassamali, S. (2012, February 1). Islamophobia in Canada: A primer. *New Socialist: Ideas for Radical Change*. Retrieved from http://newsocialist.org/islamophobia-in-canada-a-primer/

Crane, R. D. (2010). Islamophobia, mimetic warfare and the bugaboo of Shari'a compliance: Counter-strategies for common ground. *Arches Quarterly, 4*(7), 54–61.

Cross, T. L., Bazron, B. J., Dennis, K. W., & Isaacs, M. R. (1989). *Towards a culturally competent system of care*. CAASP Technical Assistance Center.

Davey, J., Hart, M., & Guerin, C. (2020). *An online environmental scan of right-wing extremism in Canada: Interim report*. Institute for Strategic Dialogue. Retrieved from https://www.isdglobal.org/wp-content/uploads/2020/06/An-Online-Environmental-Scan-of-Right-wing-Extremism-in-Canada-ISD.pdf

Diab, K. (2007, July 14). A Christian jihad? *The Guardian*. Retrieved from https://www.theguardian.com/commentisfree/2007/jul/14/achristianjihad

Dixon, T. L., Weeks, K. R., & Smith, M. A. (2019, May 23). Media constructions of culture, race, and ethnicity. *Oxford Research Encyclopedia of Communication*. Oxford Press. Retrieved from https://doi.org/10.1093/acrefore/9780190228613.013.502.

el-Aswad, el-S. (2002). *Religion and folk cosmology: Scenarios of the visible and invisible in rural Egypt*. Praeger Press.

el-Aswad, el-S. (2006). The dynamics of identity reconstruction among Arab communities in the United States. *Anthropos: International Review of Anthropology and Linguistics, 101*, 111–121.

el-Aswad, el-S. (2007, December 15). Interfaith understanding: Not Islamo-fascism. *Insight on Islam and Middle East*. Retrieved from http://tabsir.net/?p=323

el-Aswad, el-S. (2011). Sindbad in America: Narrating the self among Arab Americans. *Journal of Human Sciences, 20*(2), 357–385. Retrieved from https://journal.uob.edu.bh/handle/123456789/1355

el-Aswad, el-S. (2012). *Muslim worldviews and everyday lives*. AltaMira Press.

el-Aswad, el-S. (2013a). Images of Muslims in Western scholarship and media after 9/11. *Digest of Middle East Studies, 22*(1), 39–56.

el-Aswad, el-S. (2013b). Muslim Americans. In C. E. Cortés (Ed.), *Multicultural America: A multimedia encyclopaedia* (pp. 1525–1530). Sage.

el-Aswad, el-S. (2013c). Arab Americans. In C. E. Cortés (Ed.), *Multicultural America: A multimedia encyclopedia* (pp. 265–270). Sage.

el-Aswad, el-S. (2016a). Political challenges confronting the Islamic world. In H. Tiliouine & R. J. Estes (Eds.), *The state of social progress of Islamic societies: Social, economic, political, and ideological challenges* (pp. 361–377). Springer International Publishing. https://doi.org/10.1007/978-3-319-24774-8_16

el-Aswad, el-S. (2016b). State, nation and Islamism in contemporary Egypt: An anthropological perspective. *Urban Anthropology, 45*(1–2), 63–92.

el-Aswad, el-S. (2019). *The quality of life and policy issues among the Middle East and North African countries*. Springer Nature.

el-Aswad, el-S., Sirgy, M., Estes, R., & Rahtz, D. (2020, December 17). Global jihad and international media use. *Oxford Research Encyclopedia of Communication* (pp. 1–29). Oxford University Press. https://doi.org/10.1093/acrefore/9780190228613.013.1151

Fiedler, M. (2016, February 4). *Islamophobia is just the latest culture war*. National Catholic Reporter. Retrieved from https://www.ncronline.org/blogs/ncr-today/islamophobia-just-latest-culture-war

Findley, P. (2001). *Silent no more: Confronting America's false images of Islam*. Amana publications.

Gallup. (2021, February 4). *U.S. satisfaction sinks with many aspects of public life*. Retrieved from https://news.gallup.com/poll/329279/satisfaction-sinks-aspects-public-life.aspx?utm_source=alert&utm_medium=email&utm_content=morelink&utm_campaign=syndication

Gorski, P. (2017). Why evangelicals voted for trump: A critical cultural sociology. *American Journal of Cultural Sociology, 5*(3), 338–354. https://doi.org/10.1057/s41290-017-0043-9

Hayoun, M. (2013, January 16). Islamophobia is bad for business: Anti-Arab and anti-Muslim sentiment has cost the United States and the West a number of business opportunities. *Boston Review: Political and Literary Forum*. Retrieved from http://bostonreview.net/world/islamophobia-bad-business

Huntington, S. P. (1993). The clash of civilizations? *Foreign Affairs, 72*, 22–49.

Iannaccone, L. (2006). The market for martyrs. *Interdisciplinary Journal of Research on Religion, 2*(4), 1–14.

Institute for Social Policy and Understanding. (2017). *American Muslim poll 2017: Muslims at the crossroads*. Retrieved from https://www.ispu.org/american-muslim-poll-2017/

Isaac, M., & Conger, K. (2021, May 5). Facebook bars Trump through end of his term. *New York Times*. Retrieved from https://www.nytimes.com/2021/01/07/technology/facebook-trump-ban.html

Johnston, D. M. (2016). Combating Islamophobia. *Journal of Ecumenical Studies, 51*(2), 165–173. https://doi.org/10.1353/ecu.2016.0022

Jones, R. P. (2020). *White too long: The legacy of white supremacy in American Christianity.* Simon & Schuste.

Jonson-Reid, M. (2015, July 2). Education policy. *Oxford Research Encyclopedia of Social Work.* Oxford University Press. https://doi.org/10.1093/acrefore/9780199975839.013.121

Kalkan, K. O., Layman, G. C., & Uslaner, E. M. (2009). 'Bands of others'? Attitudes toward Muslims in contemporary American Society. *Journal of Politics, 71*(3), 847–862.

Kazemipur, A. (2014). *The Muslim question in Canada: A story of segmented integration.* University of British Colombia (UBC) Press.

Krueger, A. B. (2003, May 29). Economic scene; cash rewards and poverty alone do not explain terrorism. *New York Times.* Retrieved from https://www.nytimes.com/2003/05/29/business/economic-scene-cash-rewards-and-poverty-alone-do-not-explain-terrorism.html (Business section).

Krueger, A. B. (2007). *What makes a terrorist: Economics and the roots of terrorism.* Princeton University Press.

Lean, N. (2017). *The islamophobia industry: How the right manufactures fear of Muslims.* Pluto Press.

Lerman, R. (2021, May 6). Trump remains banned from Twitter, Facebook. Here's how his messages could still get through. *Washington Post.* Retrieved from https://www.washingtonpost.com/technology/2021/05/06/twitter-facebook-trump-posts/

Levin, J. (1975). *The functions of prejudice.* Harper & Row.

Lewis, A. R. (2019, August 28). The inclusion-moderation thesis: The U.S. Republican Party and the Christian right. In *Oxford research encyclopedia of communication.* Oxford University Press. https://doi.org/10.1093/acrefore/9780190228637.013.665

Love, E. (2017). *Islamophobia and racism in America.* New York University Press.

O'Donnell, G., Deaton, A., Durand, M., Halpern, D., & Layard, R. (2014). *Wellbeing and policy.* [Technical report]. Legatum Institute. Retrieved from https://li.com/docs/default-source/commission-on-wellbeing-and-policy/commission-on-wellbeing-and-policy-report—march-2014-pdf.pdf

Perry, B., & Poynting, S. (2006). Inspiring islamophobia: Media and state targeting of Muslims in Canada since 9/11. *Paper presented at TASA conference*, University of Western Australia & Murdoch University, 4-7 December. Retrieved from https://web.archive.org/web/20180417175416/https://tasa.org.au/wp-content/uploads/2015/02/PerryPoynting.pdf

Pew Research Center. (2009, September 9). *Muslims widely seen as facing discrimination views of religious similarities and differences.* Retrieved from http://people-press.org/report/542/muslims-widely-seen-as-facing-discrimination

Pew Research Center. (2012, December 18). *The global religious landscape.* Retrieved from https://www.pewforum.org/2012/12/18/global-religious-landscape-exec/

Pew Research Center. (2017, July 26), *U.S. Muslims concerned about their place in society, but continue to believe in the American Dream.* Retrieved https://li.com/wp-content/uploads/2019/03/commission-on-wellbeing-and-policy-report-march-2014-pdf.pdf

Sirgy, M. J., R. Estes, el-Aswad, el-S., & Rahtz, D. (2019). *Combatting Jihadist terrorism through nation-building: A quality-of-life perspective.* Springer International Publishers.

Sheehi, S. (2011). *Islamophobia: The ideological campaign against Muslims.* Clarity Press.

Statistics Canada. (2019). *Insights on Canadian society: The role of social capital and ethnocultural characteristics in the employment income of immigrants over time.* Retrieved from https://www150.statcan.gc.ca/n1/pub/75-006-x/2019001/article/00009-eng.htm

Stewart, E., Edgell, P., & Delehanty, J. (2017). The politics of religious prejudice and tolerance for cultural others. *Sociological Quarterly.* https://doi.org/10.1080/00380253.2017.1383144

Stucke, M. E. (2008). Better competition advocacy. *St. John's Law Review, 82*(3), 951–1036. Retrieved from https://scholarship.law.stjohns.edu/cgi/viewcontent.cgi?article=1081&context=lawreview

Stucke, M. E., & Grunes, A. P. (2009). Toward a better competition policy for the media: The challenge of developing antitrust policies that support the media sector's unique role in our democracy. *Connecticut Law Review, 42*(1), 101. Retrieved from https://heinonline.org/HOL/LandingPage?handle=hein.journals/conlr42&div=6&id=&page

Sullivan, S. (2019). *White privilege*. Polity.

The White House. (2021, January 20). *Proclamation on ending discriminatory bans on entry to the United States*. Retrieved from https://www.whitehouse.gov/briefing-room/presidential-actions/2021/01/20/proclamation-ending-discriminatory-bans-on-entry-to-the-united-states/

Todd, D. (2011, October 30). The state of evangelicalism: Canada differs from U.S. *Vancouver Sun*. Retrieved from https://vancouversun.com/news/staff-blogs/the-state-of-evangelicalism-canada-different-from-u-s

Tutt, D. (2013, June 25). How should we combat islamophobia? *Huffpost*. Retrieved from https://www.huffingtonpost.com/daniel-tutt/how-should-we-combat-islamophobia_b_3149768.html

Tyrer, D. (2013). *The politics of islamophobia: Race, power and fantasy*. Pluto Press.

U.S. Commission on Civil Rights. (2014). *Federal civil rights engagement with Arab and Muslim American communities*. U.S. Commission on Civil Rights. Retrieved from https://www.usccr.gov/pubs/docs/ARAB_MUSLIM_9-30-14.pdf

United Nation. (2021). *Human rights*. Retrieved from https://www.un.org/en/sections/issues-depth/human-rights/

United Nations. (1966). International covenant on civil and political rights. *Office of the High Commissioner for human rights*. Retrieved from https://www.ohchr.org/en/professionalinterest/pages/ccpr.aspx

United Nations. (2018). *The sustainable development goals 2015–2030*. United Nations Association of Philadelphia. Retrieved from http://una-gp.org/the-sustainable-development-goals-2015-2030/

Valk, J. (2012). Christianity through a worldview lens. *Journal of Adult Theological Education, 9*(2):158–174. Retrieved from https://doi.org/10.1179/ate.9.2.hp430835g071v773

Walker, J. (2018, June 29). Hate speech and freedom of expression: Legal boundaries in Canada. Library of Parliament. Retrieved from https://perma.cc/8JPB-BMJ9

West, M. (2020). The fall of white supremacy in the USA: Reflections on the fight for racial equality and justice in the covid-19 era. *Insight, 2*(3), 5–14. Retrieved from http://thecordobafoundation.com/publications/the-fall-of-white-supremacy-in-the-usa/